Dietary Polyphenols and Neuroprotection

Dietary Polyphenols and Neuroprotection

Editors

Rui F. M. Silva
Lea Pogačnik

MDPI • Basel • Beijing • Wuhan • Barcelona • Belgrade • Manchester • Tokyo • Cluj • Tianjin

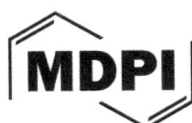

Editors
Rui F. M. Silva
Pharmaceutical Sciences and
Medicines
Universidade de Lisboa
Lisbon
Portugal

Lea Pogačnik
Department of Food Scence and
Technology
University of Ljubljana
Ljubljana
Slovenia

Editorial Office
MDPI
St. Alban-Anlage 66
4052 Basel, Switzerland

This is a reprint of articles from the Special Issue published online in the open access journal *Antioxidants* (ISSN 2076-3921) (available at: www.mdpi.com/journal/antioxidants/special_issues/ Dietary_Polyphenols_Neuroprotection).

For citation purposes, cite each article independently as indicated on the article page online and as indicated below:

LastName, A.A.; LastName, B.B.; LastName, C.C. Article Title. *Journal Name* **Year**, *Volume Number*, Page Range.

ISBN 978-3-0365-2883-0 (Hbk)
ISBN 978-3-0365-2882-3 (PDF)

© 2022 by the authors. Articles in this book are Open Access and distributed under the Creative Commons Attribution (CC BY) license, which allows users to download, copy and build upon published articles, as long as the author and publisher are properly credited, which ensures maximum dissemination and a wider impact of our publications.

The book as a whole is distributed by MDPI under the terms and conditions of the Creative Commons license CC BY-NC-ND.

Contents

About the Editors vii

Preface to "Dietary Polyphenols and Neuroprotection" ix

Rui F. M. Silva and Lea Pogačnik
Neuroprotective Properties of Food-Borne Polyphenols in Neurodegenerative Diseases
Reprinted from: *Antioxidants* **2021**, *10*, 1810, doi:10.3390/antiox10111810 1

Danilo Braga Ribeiro, Gabriela Santos Silva, Djanira Rubim dos Santos, Andressa Rose Castro Costa, Eliane Braga Ribeiro, Mihaela Badea and Gilvanda Silva Nunes
Determination of the Antioxidant Activity of Samples of Tea and Commercial Sources of Vitamin C, Using an Enzymatic Biosensor
Reprinted from: *Antioxidants* **2021**, *10*, 324, doi:10.3390/antiox10020324 5

Andrius Sakalauskas, Mantas Ziaunys, Ruta Snieckute and Vytautas Smirnovas
Autoxidation Enhances Anti-Amyloid Potential of Flavone Derivatives
Reprinted from: *Antioxidants* **2021**, *10*, 1428, doi:10.3390/antiox10091428 19

Urška Jug, Katerina Naumoska and Irena Vovk
()-Epicatechin—An Important Contributor to the Antioxidant Activity of Japanese Knotweed Rhizome Bark Extract as Determined by Antioxidant Activity-Guided Fractionation
Reprinted from: *Antioxidants* **2021**, *10*, 133, doi:10.3390/antiox10010133 33

Miriam Bobadilla, Josune García-Sanmartín and Alfredo Martínez
Natural Food Supplements Reduce Oxidative Stress in Primary Neurons and in the Mouse Brain, Suggesting Applications in the Prevention of Neurodegenerative Diseases
Reprinted from: *Antioxidants* **2021**, *10*, 46, doi:10.3390/antiox10010046 55

Monica Bucciantini, Manuela Leri, Pamela Nardiello, Fiorella Casamenti and Massimo Stefani
Olive Polyphenols: Antioxidant and Anti-Inflammatory Properties
Reprinted from: *Antioxidants* **2021**, *10*, 1044, doi:10.3390/antiox10071044 71

Valentina Novak, Boris Rogelj and Vera Župunski
Therapeutic Potential of Polyphenols in Amyotrophic Lateral Sclerosis and Frontotemporal Dementia
Reprinted from: *Antioxidants* **2021**, *10*, 1328, doi:10.3390/antiox10081328 95

Qiuchen Zheng, Micheal T. Kebede, Bethany Lee, Claire A. Krasinski, Saadman Islam, Liliana A. Wurfl, Merc M. Kemeh, Valerie A. Ivancic, Charles E. Jakobsche, Donald E. Spratt and Noel D. Lazo
Differential Effects of Polyphenols on Insulin Proteolysis by the Insulin-Degrading Enzyme
Reprinted from: *Antioxidants* **2021**, *10*, 1342, doi:10.3390/antiox10091342 111

Yuni Hong, Yun-Hyeok Choi, Young-Eun Han, Soo-Jin Oh, Ansoo Lee, Bonggi Lee, Rebecca Magnan, Shi Yong Ryu, Chun Whan Choi and Min Soo Kim
Central Administration of Ampelopsin A Isolated from *Vitis vinifera* Ameliorates Cognitive and Memory Function in a Scopolamine-Induced Dementia Model
Reprinted from: *Antioxidants* **2021**, *10*, 835, doi:10.3390/antiox10060835 123

Jennifer L. Robinson, Julio A. Yanes, Meredith A. Reid, Jerry E. Murphy, Jessica N. Busler, Petey W. Mumford, Kaelin C. Young, Zbigniew J. Pietrzkowski, Boris V. Nemzer, John M. Hunter and Darren T. Beck
Neurophysiological Effects of Whole Coffee Cherry Extract in Older Adults with Subjective Cognitive Impairment: A Randomized, Double-Blind, Placebo-Controlled, Cross-Over Pilot Study
Reprinted from: *Antioxidants* **2021**, *10*, 144, doi:10.3390/antiox10020144 . . . . **141**

About the Editors

Rui F. M. Silva

Prof. Dr. Rui Fernando Marques da Silva, Professor of Histology & Embriology and of Neurobiology at Universidade de Lisboa, Faculdade de Farmácia, Portugal (2001-present), is an expert on cell biology, namely nerve cell cultures, cell signaling, cell death mechanisms and neurotoxicology. His main research interests are on the neurosciences area, in the topics of neurobiology, neurotoxicology, neurodevelopment and glial function associated to neurologic conditions and neurodegeneration. Neuroprotection mechanisms is the most relevant area of intervention, embracing the neuroprotective properties of food natural products and food-borne molecules, either introduced in the regular diet or as additives or medicines, by several cell and molecular mechanisms, beyond the traditional antioxidant properties described for food polyphenols. He has published more than 90 research articles, mentored over 30 post-graduate students, and given more than 150 communications in scientific meetings in several countries. He is an Editorial Board Member of the scientific journal *Antioxidants*, guest editor of the Special Issue "Dietary Polyphenols and Neuroprotection" (*Antioxidants*) and Associate Editor of Frontiers in Cellular Neuroscience - Non-Neuronal Cells.

Lea Pogačnik

Prof. Dr. Lea Pogačnik, a professor of Chemistry, Food Analytical Chemistry and Biochemistry at University of Ljubljana, Biotechnical Faculty (2000-present), Slovenia, is an expert on preparation of extracts from different natural sources as well as their chemical and biological characterization. She has mentored over 60 graduate students and published more than 30 research articles. Her research focuses on the preparation and evaluation of bioactivities in extracts of different tissues of alien knotweed species, namely Japanese knotweed (*Fallopia japonica*), Giant knotweed (*F. sachalinensis*) and their interspecific hybrid –Bohemian knotweed (*F.* x *bohemica*), preparation and characterisation of cianobacteria species Arthrospira platensis extracts before and after the lactic acid fermentation and evaluation of brain accessibility, neuroprotection of different polyphenols, and simulation of digestion and evaluation of the stability of pomegranate juice anthocyanins. She has given almost 80 presentations on scientific meetings throughout the world. She is a scientific editor of *Sensors & Transducers* as well as guest editor of special issue of the journal *Antioxidants* (Dietary Polyphenols and Neuroprotection).

Preface to "Dietary Polyphenols and Neuroprotection"

As editors of this book, our aim was to collect new data from experienced authors in order to further advance the knowledge on the protective effects of polyphenols' intake, e.g., when included in the human diet, to modulate cellular functions and pathways associated with neurodegenerative diseases.

Most, if not all, edible vegetables included in human diet are rich sources of phenolic compounds. Such compounds are commonly used by the plants for several reasons, e.g., as metabolic intermediates, protective substances, reproductive attractants, etc. Many of those phytochemicals have been recognized as potent antioxidants, also sharing other important actions that can impact human health like their anti-inflammatory properties and their proposed capability to modulate several cell-signalling pathways and mediators.

Neurodegenerative diseases are among the main causes of death worldwide and, in most of them like Alzheimer's or Parkinson's, neurodegeneration occurs long before the onset of first symptoms, where a large population of brain neurons are already lost. Besides neurons, glial cells like astrocytes and microglia, are involved in oxidative and neuroinflammatory pathological pathways, making them interesting targets for neuroprotective strategies. Polyphenols are promising candidates for those strategies, either as prophylactic substances or as therapeutic molecules.

The proposed benefits of polyphenols, either as protective/prophylactic substances or as therapeutic molecules, may be achieved by the consumption of a natural polyphenol-enriched diet, by the use as food supplements or formulation as pharmaceutical drugs/nutraceuticals. It was also proved that the health effects of polyphenols depend on the amount consumed as well as on their bioavailability.

With this collection of original data and literature reviews, we hope to raise the interest of scientist, researchers, medical doctors and students in the promising field of polyphenols neuroprotection as a relevant approach to prevent or treat mental disorders, dementia and neurodegenerative diseases.

Rui F. M. Silva, Lea Pogačnik
Editors

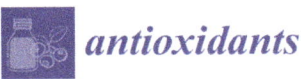

Editorial

Neuroprotective Properties of Food-Borne Polyphenols in Neurodegenerative Diseases

Rui F. M. Silva [1,*] and Lea Pogačnik [2]

1. Research Institute for Medicines (iMed.ULisboa) and Department of Biochemistry and Human Biology (DBBH), Faculty of Pharmacy, Universidade de Lisboa, 1649-003 Lisbon, Portugal
2. Department of Food Science and Technology, Biotechnical Faculty, University of Ljubljana, 1000 Ljubljana, Slovenia; lea.pogacnik@bf.uni-lj.si
* Correspondence: rfmsilva@ff.ulisboa.pt

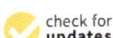

Citation: Silva, R.F.M.; Pogačnik, L. Neuroprotective Properties of Food-Borne Polyphenols in Neurodegenerative Diseases. *Antioxidants* 2021, *10*, 1810. https://doi.org/10.3390/antiox10111810

Received: 9 November 2021
Accepted: 11 November 2021
Published: 15 November 2021

Publisher's Note: MDPI stays neutral with regard to jurisdictional claims in published maps and institutional affiliations.

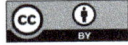

Copyright: © 2021 by the authors. Licensee MDPI, Basel, Switzerland. This article is an open access article distributed under the terms and conditions of the Creative Commons Attribution (CC BY) license (https://creativecommons.org/licenses/by/4.0/).

Fruits and vegetables are the richest source of polyphenols in the regular human diet. These substances belong to plants' secondary metabolites and can have several roles, such as being metabolic intermediates, reproductive attractants, and protective agents. Most of these molecules possess a high antioxidant capacity, as well as several other important activities that can affect human health, among which anti-inflammatory properties and the potential ability to modulate different cell signaling pathways seem to be the most important.

Taking into account these significant properties of polyphenols, together with their abundance in various food products that are a part of a healthy human diet, a wide range of different approaches, both in vitro and in vivo, address their potential role in the prevention and treatment of different pathological conditions associated with oxidative stress and/or inflammation.

The significance of food-borne polyphenols on human health has considerably increased the number of studies dedicated to their various proposed actions in many different pathologies such as cancer, and cardiovascular and neurodegenerative diseases, which has also resulted in a growing number of clinical trials on the acute or chronic use of dietary polyphenols. Studies in the field of cancer and neurodegenerative disorders are particularly important since an effective treatment is still not available. It was shown that food-borne polyphenols can be used either as protective/prophylactic molecules or as therapeutic substances. They can be consumed as part of a natural polyphenol-enriched diet, with the use of food supplements or as pharmaceutical drugs/nutraceuticals.

In this Special Issue of *Antioxidants*, several research papers and two reviews explore the chemical properties of naturally occurring polyphenols and some new possibilities for the therapeutic and/or prophylactic roles of these molecules in neurodegeneration and neurodegenerative diseases.

Ribeiro et al. [1] proposed the use of a new enzymatic biosensor to determine the antioxidant activity of commercially available teas, as well as the level of ascorbic acid in effervescent products, which can also be used to detect the real level of antioxidants in samples and depict the validity of "antioxidant" labeling in the product information. Using flavone derivatives, Sakalauskas et al. [2] further explored the potential of polyphenols to prevent amyloid aggregation, an important hallmark of Alzheimer's disease (AD) as well as other amyloid-related disorders. They demonstrated that after oxidation, flavones, particularly oxidized 6,2′,3′-trihydroxyflavone, not only keep but even increase their anti-amyloid properties, which might be a relevant addition to the discussion relating to whether, after physiologic metabolization, polyphenol derivatives still keep their beneficial properties.

Continuing with the study of the antioxidant properties of polyphenol-rich vegetables, Jug et al. [3] evaluated extracts of Japanese knotweed rhizomes produced by several extraction solvents. Knotweed is an invasive botanical species, and it is important to find novel economically viable applications for this destructive botanical species. Using size exclusion–high-performance liquid chromatography (SEC-HPLC)-UV and reversed-phase HPLC-UV coupled with multistage mass spectrometry to fractionate the extracts, they identified (−)-epicatechin as a potent and stable antioxidant.

The well-proven antioxidant properties of polyphenols can be explored in the prevention of or reduction in oxidative stress-induced injury. Accordingly, the results from Bobadilla et al. continue to reinforce the potential of natural food polyphenols to reduce neuronal demise by several mechanisms, as in the case of aluminum maltolate neurotoxicity, where several commercially available natural food supplements decreased neuronal cell death in vitro by reducing ROS levels and caspase-3 activity, and also increased the antioxidant enzyme activity in mice, preventing the formation of lipid peroxidation products in the brain [4].

The multiple targets for polyphenols and their beneficial effects on several human chronic diseases were reviewed by Bucciantini et al. [5]. These authors explore, in particular, the actions from polyphenols present in extra virgin olive oil, expanding from the antioxidant to the anti-inflammatory properties. They advance to the use of olive oil polyphenols in human chronic diseases that involve inflammation due to their inhibitory effects on oxidative stress-induced signaling pathways and minimal secondary effects.

The second review from this Special Issue reinforces polyphenols' multiple mechanisms of action, focusing on amyotrophic lateral sclerosis (ALS) and frontotemporal dementia (FTD), two of the neurodegenerative disorders still without effective treatments or cures. For that, Novak et al. [6] analyze the current therapeutical options for ALS and FTD in parallel with several of the more prominent polyphenols such as resveratrol, curcumin and green tea catechins, emphasizing the therapeutic potential of polyphenols.

In fact, according to the results from Zheng et al. [7], resveratrol might also influence the clearance of beta-amyloid peptide-42 (Aβ42), related to AD neurodegeneration, by modulating the insulin-degrading enzyme that also has a strong ability to degrade Aβ4.

Moving to in vivo studies, a crucial pre-clinical step, the findings from Hong et al. [8] show very important amelioration effects on cognitive and memory functions in models of neurodegeneration. Interestingly, ampelopsin A from Vitis vinifera was shown to have neuroprotective properties, increasing both cognitive and memory functions by, in part, elevating the BDNF/CREB-related signaling, in a mice model as well as in hippocampal brain slices (CA3-CA1 synapses), where neurodegeneration was induced by scopolamine.

Finally, in a pilot study performed in older human volunteers with memory complaints, but not AD, Robinson at al. [9] evaluated the effects of the administration of a whole coffee cherry extract nutraceutical, rich in polyphenols, using MRI and determination of BDNF blood levels. In summary, they found significant improvements in cognition that may be related to the increase in exosomal BDNF.

In conclusion, polyphenols seem to be effective molecules for preventive and therapeutic strategies in a wide range of pathological conditions. However, it will be important to take into account the possible issues raised by their dosage and toxicity and monitoring of their safe usage.

Funding: This work was supported by iMed.ULisboa, Fundação para a Ciência e Tecnologia (FCT), Portugal (UID/DTP/04138/2013), and the Slovene Research Agency (P4-0121).

Conflicts of Interest: The authors declare no conflict of interest.

References

1. Ribeiro, D.B.; Santos Silva, G.; Dos Santos, D.R.; Castro Costa, A.R.; Braga Ribeiro, E.; Badea, M.; Nunes, G.S. Determination of the Antioxidant Activity of Samples of Tea and Commercial Sources of Vitamin C, Using an Enzymatic Biosensor. *Antioxidants* **2021**, *10*, 324. [CrossRef] [PubMed]
2. Sakalauskas, A.; Ziaunys, M.; Snieckute, R.; Smirnovas, V. Autoxidation Enhances Anti-Amyloid Potential of Flavone Derivatives. *Antioxidants* **2021**, *10*, 1428. [CrossRef] [PubMed]

3. Jug, U.; Naumoska, K.; Vovk, I. (−)-Epicatechin-An Important Contributor to the Antioxidant Activity of Japanese Knotweed Rhizome Bark Extract as Determined by Antioxidant Activity-Guided Fractionation. *Antioxidants* **2021**, *10*, 133. [CrossRef] [PubMed]
4. Bobadilla, M.; Garcia-Sanmartin, J.; Martinez, A. Natural Food Supplements Reduce Oxidative Stress in Primary Neurons and in the Mouse Brain, Suggesting Applications in the Prevention of Neurodegenerative Diseases. *Antioxidants* **2021**, *10*, 46. [CrossRef] [PubMed]
5. Bucciantini, M.; Leri, M.; Nardiello, P.; Casamenti, F.; Stefani, M. Olive Polyphenols: Antioxidant and Anti-Inflammatory Properties. *Antioxidants* **2021**, *10*, 44. [CrossRef] [PubMed]
6. Novak, V.; Rogelj, B.; Zupunski, V. Therapeutic Potential of Polyphenols in Amyotrophic Lateral Sclerosis and Frontotemporal Dementia. *Antioxidants* **2021**, *10*, 1328. [CrossRef] [PubMed]
7. Zheng, Q.; Kebede, M.T.; Lee, B.; Krasinski, C.A.; Islam, S.; Wurfl, L.A.; Kemeh, M.M.; Ivancic, V.A.; Jakobsche, C.E.; Spratt, D.E.; et al. Differential Effects of Polyphenols on Insulin Proteolysis by the Insulin-Degrading Enzyme. *Antioxidants* **2021**, *10*, 1342. [CrossRef] [PubMed]
8. Hong, Y.; Choi, Y.H.; Han, Y.E.; Oh, S.J.; Lee, A.; Lee, B.; Magnan, R.; Ryu, S.Y.; Choi, C.W.; Kim, M.S. Central Administration of Ampelopsin A Isolated from Vitis vinifera Ameliorates Cognitive and Memory Function in a Scopolamine-Induced Dementia Model. *Antioxidants* **2021**, *10*, 835. [CrossRef] [PubMed]
9. Robinson, J.L.; Yanes, J.A.; Reid, M.A.; Murphy, J.E.; Busler, J.N.; Mumford, P.W.; Young, K.C.; Pietrzkowski, Z.J.; Nemzer, B.V.; Hunter, J.M.; et al. Neurophysiological Effects of Whole Coffee Cherry Extract in Older Adults with Subjective Cognitive Impairment: A Randomized, Double-Blind, Placebo-Controlled, Cross-Over Pilot Study. *Antioxidants* **2021**, *10*, 144. [CrossRef] [PubMed]

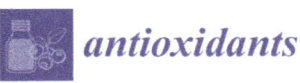

Article

Determination of the Antioxidant Activity of Samples of Tea and Commercial Sources of Vitamin C, Using an Enzymatic Biosensor

Danilo Braga Ribeiro [1], Gabriela Santos Silva [1], Djanira Rubim dos Santos [1], Andressa Rose Castro Costa [1], Eliane Braga Ribeiro [1], Mihaela Badea [2,*] and Gilvanda Silva Nunes [1,*]

1. Pesticide Residue Analysis Center, Federal University of Maranhão, UFMA. Av. Portugueses, CCET, Bacanga, CEP, São Luis, MA 65080-040, Brazil; danilobraga15@hotmail.com (D.B.R.); gabriela.santos@discente.ufma.br (G.S.S.); djanira.rubim@discente.ufma.br (D.R.d.S.); andressa.rcc@discente.ufma.br (A.R.C.C.); eliane.ribeiro@discente.ufma.br (E.B.R.)
2. Center for Fundamental Research and Prevention Strategies in Medicine, Department of Fundamental, Prophylactic and Clinical Specialties, Transilvania University of Brasov, 500039 Brasov, Romania
* Correspondence: mihaela.badea@unitbv.ro (M.B.); gilvanda.nunes@ufma.br (G.S.N.)

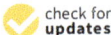

Abstract: Antioxidants are synthetic or natural compounds capable of preventing or delaying oxidative damage caused by chemical species that can oxidize cell biomolecules, such as proteins, membranes, and DNA, leading to the development of various pathologies, such as cancer, atherosclerosis, Parkinson, Alzheimer, and other diseases serious. In this study, an amperometric biosensor was used to determine the antioxidant activity of teas and effervescent products based on vitamin C, available on the market. A sensor composed of three electrodes was used. The performance of the following electrochemical mediators was evaluated: meldola blue combined with Reineck salt (MBRS), Prussian blue (PB), and cobalt phthalocyanine (CoPC), as well as the time of polymerization in the enzymatic immobilization process and the agitation process during chronoamperometric measurements. Prussian blue proved to be more efficient as a mediator for the desired purposes. After optimizing the construction stages of the biosensor, as well as the operational parameters, it presented stability for a period of 7 months. The results clearly indicate that the biosensor can be successfully used to detect fraud in products called "antioxidants" or even in drugs containing less ascorbic acid than indicated on the labels. The detection limit was set at 4.93 $\mu mol \cdot L^{-1}$.

Keywords: antioxidants; biosensors; xanthine oxidase; teas; drugs; vitamin C

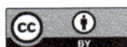

1. Introduction

Due to redox reactions that provide cells with the energy necessary for their functioning, external factors such as pollution, bad habits (smoking, alcohol consumption), and inadequate nutrition cause an increase in formation of free radicals in the human body [1].

Diabetes, cirrhosis, cardiovascular diseases, some types of cancer, and neurological disorders are examples of diseases often associated with irregular and uncontrolled processes in the production of these radicals. In excess, they can cause oxidative damage to cells, forming advanced glycation products, inactivating proteins (enzymes), and attacking membrane lipids, carbohydrates, and DNA [2–4].

The search for new methods of evaluating the antioxidant activity of several compounds potentially capable of inhibiting such damage in biological systems or even in food has increased in the last years, as shown by a search in the Web of Science database on 4 February 2021 (Supplementary Data)—1917 references since 1997 for antioxidant capacity detection, most of them from the last five years. From all the indicated references, 1801 (93.95%) were articles, 86 (4.46%) were proceedings papers, and 81 (4.23%) reviews. Considering the journals that published these papers, most of them are dealing with applications in food chemistry. Considering the entire group of proposed articles, an H-index—112 was generated, indicating in this way the importance of this topic for scientific media. We believe that also our study will be an important one due to the applications proposed in the sample of tea and commercial sources of vitamin C, using a novel methodology developed recently by our group and previously successfully applied for testing antioxidant capacity of fresh and frozen fruit. Of natural or synthetic origin, antioxidants are able to prevent or delay oxidative damage generated by oxidizing sources, even when in lower concentration compared to the oxidizable substrate [5]. The human body's antioxidant defense system consists of a range of bioactive compounds capable of neutralizing the action of free radicals, such as vitamins (A, C, E, K), glutathione, mineral salts, metalloproteins, enzymes (SOD—superoxide dismutase) and polyphenols [6,7]. Antioxidants of exogenous origin come from plant sources, such as fruits and teas, and are also found in commercially available supplements [8–10].

Over the years, the use of plants for medicinal purposes has grown considerably, either empirically or in complex compositions of the pharmaceutical industry and consumption in the form of teas has been quite expressive due mainly to the incentive to use natural products.

Different methodologies based on electrochemical, spectrophotometric, and chromatographic techniques have been described in the literature in order to assess the antioxidant capacity in different matrices. In general, they differ in terms of the mechanisms for obtaining oxidizing species and in the way the final products are measured. However, they have the drawback of being relatively time consuming and employing expensive bioreagents [11–13]. In addition, due to the presence of unsaturation in its chemical structure, antioxidants from natural products can present stability problems that make them sensitive to exposure to heat, light, and the presence of oxygen [14].

On the other hand, in recent years, electrochemical biosensors have been considered as a promising tool in determining the antioxidant potential, due to their characteristics as selectivity, low cost of obtaining, ease of storage, miniaturization capacity, easy automation, and portability, which combined make possible in situ analysis, reducing the risk of interference resulting from the destabilization of compounds [15,16].

Therefore, this work aims to improve and apply an analytical device in the determination of the antioxidant capacity in samples of teas and commercial sources of vitamin C, which offers the additional advantages of facilitated construction, high precision, and sensitivity of detection and that allows use both in the laboratory and in situ. In this paper, electrochemical evaluations will be performed using the cyclic voltammetry (CV) technique and chronoamperometric measurements, comparing with the previous paper [12] by our group where amperometry was used.

2. Materials and Methods

2.1. Reagents and Solutions

All reagents used were of analytical grade and the water used was deionized (Milli-Q Millipore 18.2 MΩ cm^{-1}). Prussian blue or ferric ferrocyanide (PB) was obtained from Gwent Group (Torfaen, United Kingdom). Water-soluble polyvinyl alcohol photopolymer (PVA-AWP) was purchased from Toyo Kogyo Corporation (Chiba, Japan). Monobasic potassium phosphate (KH_2PO_4), dibasic potassium phosphate (K_2HPO_4), potassium chloride (KCl), hypoxanthine (HX), bovine milk xanthine oxidase enzyme (XOD) were all purchased from Sigma Aldrich Corporation (Nasdaq-Sial, Darmstarm, Darmst, Germany). Ascorbic acid ($C_6H_8O_6$) was purchased from Merck (Seelze, Germany). The 50 mmol·L^{-1} K-PBS buffer solution (K_2HPO_4 33.33 mmol·L^{-1}, KH_2PO_4 16.67 mmol·L^{-1}) containing 10 mmol·L^{-1} KCl (pH 7.5) was used in the preparation of the enzymatic solutions (stock and work), solutions of the substrate hypoxanthine (HX) 5 mmol·L^{-1} and as the electrolyte in electrochemical measurements. It was also used as a solvent in tea infusions and dissolution of effervescent vitamins C.

2.2. Instrumentation

The electrochemical measurements using the biosensors were made in a a Ivium-n-stat potentiostat/galvanostat controlled by the IviumSoft software (Ivium Technologies, Eindhoven, Netherland). The working, reference, and auxiliary electrodes were printed on a thin transparent polyvinyl chloride (PVC) plate, which constituted the electrochemical sensor. The reference pseudo electrode was constituted by a straight line 5 × 1.5 mm in diameter, and is formed by a mixture (paste) of Ag/AgCl. The working electrode consisted of a 4 mm diameter disk, formed by a commercial graphite paste containing Prussian blue salt (PB) or Meldola blue with Reinecke salt (MBRS) or cobalt phthalocyanine (CoPC) as a modifier. The auxiliary electrode, formed by a 16 × 1.5 mm curved line, contained only the commercial graphite paste. Screen-printed electrodes (SPE) were produced in laboratory of University of Perpignan via Domitia, using a DEK 248 printing machine, and offered for these studies by Prof. Dr. Jean-Louis Marty.

2.3. Electrochemical Characterization

Electrochemical evaluations of sensors and biosensors were performed using the cyclic voltammetry (CV) technique. The biosensors were initially prepared according to the methodology developed in our research group [12]. An enzymatic charge of 8 mU XOD was immobilized under the surface of the modified working electrode, from the deposition of 3 μL of a homogeneous mixture of the enzymatic solution and PVA-AWP in the proportion 1:2 and later polymerization under neon light at 4 °C for 30 min. The effect of pH on the biosensor response was also evaluated.

2.4. Chronoamperometric Measurements and Parameter Optimization

All chronoamperometric measurements were performed at room temperature using a 10 mL dark electrochemical cell. The biosensor was previously subjected to 10 voltametric cycles and the current generated was then measured at a fixed working potential of −100 mV vs Ag/AgCl, where there is a reduction in H_2O_2. The intensity of the initial current was recorded after swelling of the PVA-AWP, followed by signal stabilization, in a total time of approximately 20 min. Then, an analytical curve was constructed by successively adding aliquots of the HX 5 mmol·L^{-1} solution under constant stirring. Then, the polymerization time (30 and 60 min) and the stirring conditions during measurements were optimized, as well as the current measurement time.

2.5. Determination of the Antioxidant Capacity of Real Samples

As a negative control, the production of reactive oxygen species (ROS) was used without neutralizing them by antioxidants. An analytical curve of current intensity (at the end of 75 s) as a function of the concentration of the hypoxanthine substrate (HX) was constructed, and the angular coefficient recorded (ma). Then, a new analytical curve was built, but in the presence of the antioxidant solution (standards or samples), and the antioxidant potential of the solution or sample was determined. The antioxidant capacity was expressed by the percentage of ROS inhibition by comparing the slope obtained in the curves constructed in the absence (ma) and the presence of antioxidants (mb), according to the Equation (1):

$$Antioxidant\ capacity\ \% = 100 * \left[1 - \left(\frac{mb}{ma}\right)\right]. \quad (1)$$

Sample Preparation and Analysis

Samples of teas (fennel, chamomile, mint, cimegripe tea) and effervescent vitamin C were obtained from pharmacies in the city of São Luís, Maranhão, Brazil.

In assessing the antioxidant capacity of the tea, a volume of 50 mL of an infusion in K-PBS buffer was prepared by heating for 10 min on a magnetic stirrer with heating. A 10 mL volume of the infusion was transferred to the electrochemical cell. Then, analytical curves were constructed in the presence of HX in different concentrations, and the slopes of the curves constructed in the presence and absence of the samples were compared.

The samples of effervescent vitamin C were prepared by dissolving the mass of the tablet corresponding to 500 mg of ascorbic acid in 20 mL of K-PBS buffer. An aliquot of 20 μL of this solution was then transferred to the electrochemical cell, and the volume was made up to 10 mL with K-PBS. The curves were constructed, according to the procedure described above, and the antioxidant capacity determined.

The experiments were carried out using an infrared spectrometer from Shimadzu, model IR-Prestige-21 with an extended KBr (potassium bromide) beam splitter. The data were collected in a range of 500 to 4000 cm^{-1}, at a resolution of 4 cm^{-1} using a spectral medium of 40 scans in potassium bromide.

The content of ascobic acid in the drugs was determined by the standard addition method. Then, 100 μl aliquots of the samples were transferred to a 50 mL volumetric flasks and volumes (500, 1000, 1500, 2000, and 2500 μL) of a 1 mg·L^{-1} solution of pure ascorbic acid was added to them, completing them with water. The absorbance was measured at a wavelength of 264 nm, using a UV-VIS spectrophotometer (Themoscientific, Orion AquaMate 8000), quartz cuvette 1 cm of optical path.

3. Results and Discussions

3.1. Electrochemical Characterization

The sensors used were built on a flexible and chemically inert base (PVC), where the three electrodes were printed, using a simple methodology based on semi-automatic screen printing. Such technology enables the manufacture of economic, portable, quick-response electrodes, with high sensitivity, low power required, disposable, and with the ability to operate at room temperature, thus enabling the performance of in situ analyses [17].

The O_2 and H_2O_2 molecules monitored in the system proposed here are electroactive species that undergo oxidation and/or reduction when subjected to high work potentials, generating an electrical signal. Uric acid, the product of the enzymatic reaction, as well as several antioxidant compounds (ascorbic acid, for example), are also oxidized when they occur at high potentials, which can generate interference in the measured current [18]. Thus, the use of electrochemical mediators aims to annul or reduce such interference since it allows working with lower potentials [19]. Mediators are chemical species capable of donating or receiving electrons, thus helping to regenerate the oxidation state of the enzyme and its active center in an enzymatic reaction. The modifying agent has the function of increasing the sensitivity of the electrodes and can be incorporated into the carbon paste by directly adding a certain mass of the modifier in a mixture of graphite powder and binder [20].

The generated H_2O_2 is reduced on the polarized (-100 mV vs. Ag/AgCl) WE surface, in presence of PB mediator, which has a specific catalytic effect for the H_2O_2 reduction due to its structure [21]. The $O_2\bullet-$ radicals and/or H_2O_2 are scavenged with a decrease of the cathodic current which permits the quantification of the antioxidant capacity of different samples. In the Figure 1, the principle of detection using XOD based biosensor, using PB as mediator, is shown.

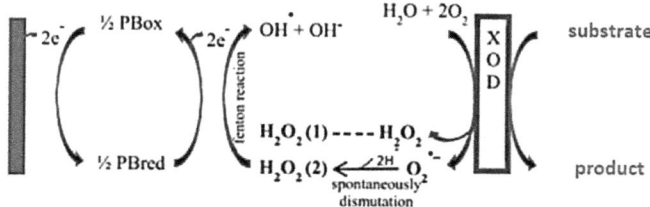

Figure 1. Principle of detection using XOD based biosensor, using Prussian Blue (PB), as mediator.

It is important to note that a range of working potential between 0 and −200 mV is quite desirable, when the focus of the electrochemical system is the determination of antioxidant capacity since at potentials below −200 mV there is a reduction in molecular oxygen, that at potentials above 0 mV oxidation of antioxidant compounds occurs [12,22].

Figure 2 shows the cyclic voltammetry of printed electrodes of carbon paste, bare and modified, as well as the electrochemical response after immobilization of the enzyme xanthine oxidase.

There is a limitation for the printed carbon paste electrode in the cathodic region at potentials below −0.5 V and anodic above 0.5 V vs. Ag/AgCl, regions in which the supporting electrolyte is discharged. However, such behavior did not produce interference, as it is outside the desired potential window.

The use of Prussian blue (PB) as a mediator proved to be feasible for application in determining the antioxidant capacity, as it has a cathodic peak at −133 mV, within the desired potential window (0 to −200 mV). An increase in cathodic and anodic current was also observed with the immobilization of the enzyme, indicating that the electronic transfer process was favored, demonstrating an electrochemical affinity between the enzyme and the mediator. In addition, the incorporation of the PB mediator into the working electrode has been described as a simple, cost-effective, and highly stable process in acid and neutral media.

The intensity of cathodic and anodic current obtained with the biosensors when MBRS was the mediator was greater, demonstrating that there is an electrochemical affinity between the enzyme and this mediator as well. In the case of CoPC, in addition to not having seen such an increase, there was also a negative shift in the cathodic peak potential. It is also noted that, in the region of interest, there is no electrocatalytic activity, making its use unfeasible in this study.

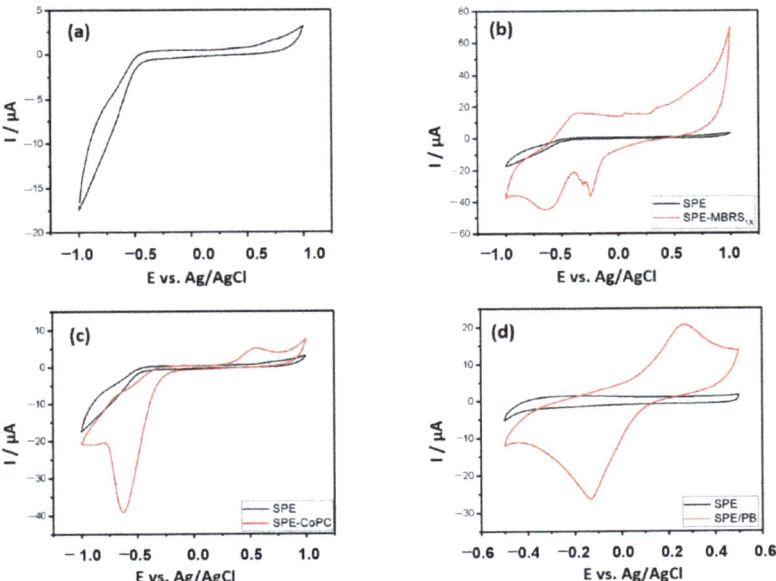

Figure 2. *Cont.*

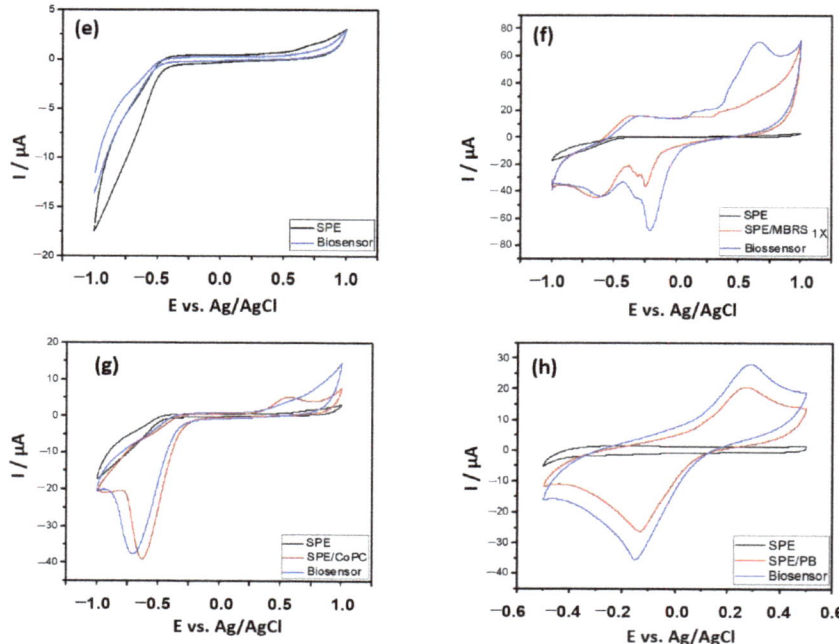

Figure 2. Cyclic voltamogram of (**a**) carbon paste electrode (SPE), (**b**) SPE modified with meldola blue with Reinecke salt (MBRS), (**c**) SPE modified with Cobalt phthalocyanine (CoPC), (**d**) SPE modified with PB and biosensors (**e**) without mediator and mediated with (**f**) MBRS, (**g**) CoPC, and (**h**) (PB) in K-PBS 50 mmol·L^{-1} pH 7.5. Scan rate 50 mV·s^{-1}.

In Figure 3, it can be seen that the electrochemical activity of PB is even more favored in an acidic environment. Due to the affinity of the enzyme with MBRS, its behavior at other pH was investigated, envisioning a possible application. However, considering the preservation of the enzyme activity, the medium with a pH close to neutrality was chosen as the working medium.

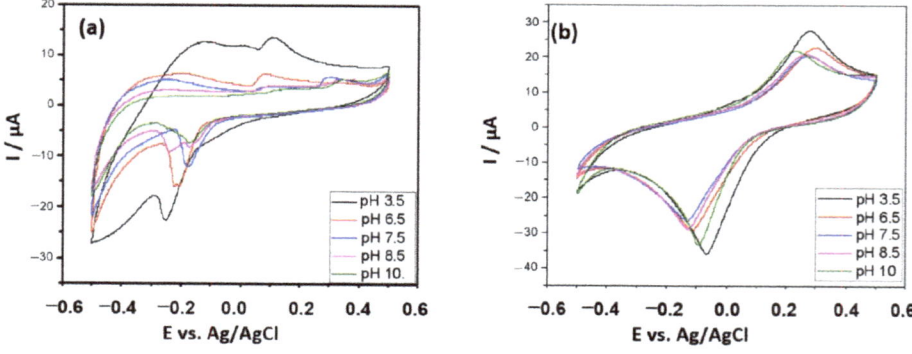

Figure 3. Evaluation of the effect of pH on the electrochemical behavior of the biosensor modified with (**a**) MBRS and (**b**) PB in K-PBS buffer as a function of the mediator's immediate behavior. Scan rate: 50 mV·s^{-1}.

Oxidation processes can be favored or compromised at specific pH levels, generating different oxidation and reduction potentials (greater or lesser), as well as greater sensitivity (higher peak currents). For the MBRS mediator, despite its high efficiency in the electronic transfer process, proven in the present study, the negative shift in the cathodic peak potential at pH 3.5 and pH 6.5 disadvantaged its use. In a more alkaline environment, there is a decrease in the cathodic current and the formation of ill-defined peaks, which may be possibly caused by problems in electronic kinetics.

It is also noteworthy that the catalytic properties of Prussian blue on the reduction of hydrogen peroxide are well known and have been discussed previously by several researchers [23–25].

3.2. Biochemical Principles and Electrochemical Characterization of the Biosensor

The detection principle explored in the present work was based on the measurement of the H_2O_2 reduction current generated as a final product of the hypoxanthine (HX) oxidation reaction to uric acid, catalyzed by the XOD enzyme. The current was proportional to its concentration. Antioxidants inhibit such ROS, causing a decrease in the cathodic current, thus evaluating the antioxidant capacity.

In accordance with the methodology described in the experimental part, analytical curves were constructed (Figure 4), evaluating the signal obtained when using different polymerization times in the enzymatic immobilization step, and a calibration curve was subsequently constructed.

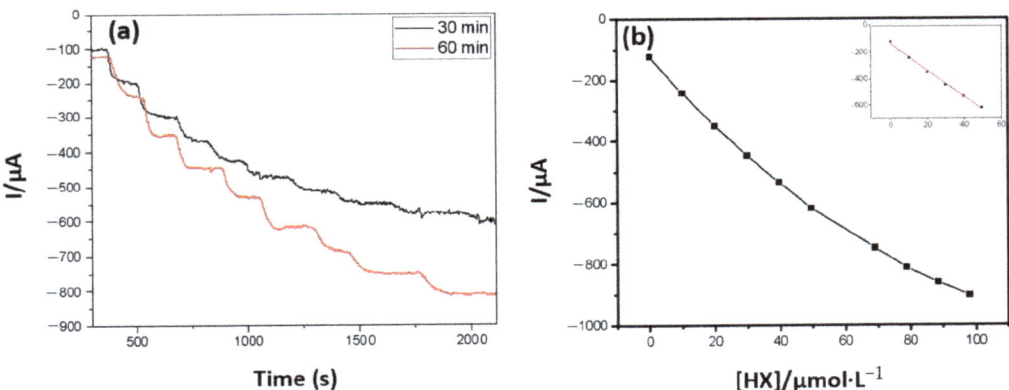

Figure 4. (a) Response of the amperometric biosensor with the successive addition of HX under constant agitation of 300 rpm, with the PB as a mediator and 8 mU of immobilized enzyme load, with polymerization times of 30 and 60 min. E = −100 mV. (b) Calibration curve of the amperometric biosensor modified with PB, when polymerization time of 60 min is used.

The reduction of hydrogen peroxide was more favored when a 60 min enzyme polymerization time was used in the graphite network, under neon radiation, becoming evident that the degree of polymerization depends on the time of exposure to neon light and interferes with enzyme retention in polymer and permeability of substrate and enzyme reaction products.

The agitation conditions also interfered with the biosensor response (Figure 5); therefore, the best conditions for carrying out the measurements were determined.

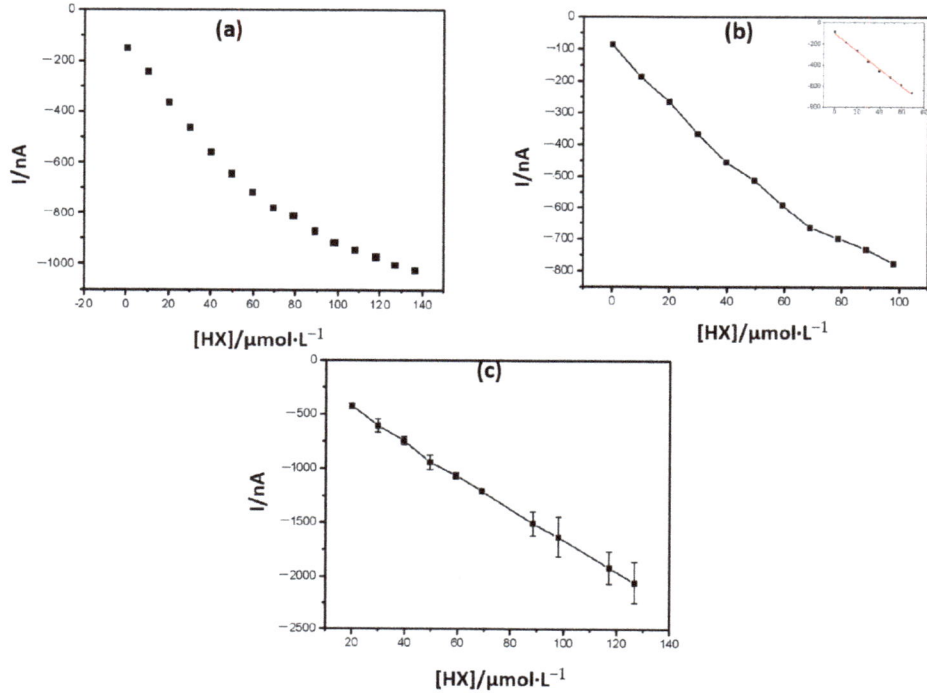

Figure 5. Curves obtained under different conditions: (**a**) 15 s of agitation, 15 s of rest, and 75 s measuring the current, fixed the time of 60 min of polymerization, (**b**) 30 s of agitation, 15 s of rest, and 60 s measuring the current, fixed the time of 60 min of polymerization, and (**c**) 15 s agitation, 15 s rest, 60 s current measurement, fixed the time of 60 min of polymerization.

From an analytical point of view, a greater linear range of work allows numerous alternatives for using the prototype, due to the variability of antioxidant capacities Table 1. Linear range and similar sensitivities, in amperometric biosensors, using printed electrodes modified with PB were achieved, fixing the work potential at −100 mV [25,26].

Table 1. Shows the analytical efficiency of the biosensor in terms of R^2, sensitivity, and linear range, under constant or controlled agitation.

Equation	R^2	Sensitivity	Linear Range ($\mu mol \cdot L^{-1}$)
$I^1 = -137.91 + (-9.98) \times [HX]$	0.994	−9.98	0–50
$I^2 = -165.43 + (-9.29) \times [HX]$	0.991	−9.29	0–69
$I^3 = -102.36 + (-8.33) \times [HX]$	0.995	−8.33	0–69
$I^4 = -0.12 + (-0.02) \times [HX]$	0.999	−0.02	20–136

[1] Constant agitation (300 rpm); [2] 15 s agitation, 15 s rest, 75 s current measurement; [3] 30 s agitation, 15 s rest, 60 s current measurement; [4] 15 s agitation, 15 s rest, 60 s current measurement. A new chronoamperometric run was performed at each substrate concentration.

The operating conditions were fixed at 15 s of agitation, 15 s of rest, and 60 s of current measurement and detection and quantification limits were set at 4.93 $\mu mol \cdot L^{-1}$ and 16.43 $\mu mol \cdot L^{-1}$, respectively. They were calculated by the ratio between the average of

10 blanks measurements and an inclination of the analytical curve, multiplied by a factor of 3 and 10, respectively [12].

3.3. Determination of the Antioxidant Capacity of Commercial Samples

3.3.1. Tea Samples

As shown in Figure 6a, the initial currents recorded for the samples of chamomile tea and cimegripre® tea, were discrepant in relation to that obtained in the absence of antioxidant and other samples. This may be the result of the different resistivity of the medium depending on the composition of the samples. However, it is noticeable in all cases the decrease in the cathodic current resulting from the reduction of H_2O_2 when compared to that obtained in the absence of the samples, resulting in smaller angular coefficients. Based on this difference, the total antioxidant capacity of the teas was calculated and the result shown in Figure 5b.

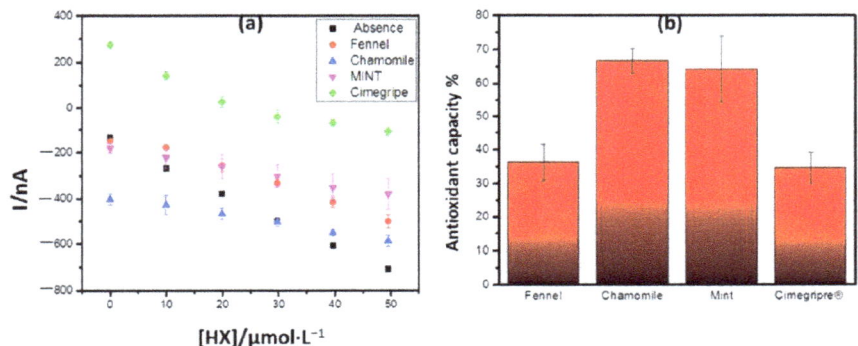

Figure 6. (a) Response of the biosensor in the presence of the antioxidant samples. (b) Antioxidant capacity.

The wide variety of antioxidants, which may respond differently to the different oxidizing sources, makes it difficult to develop a single, simple, and universal method to assess antioxidant capacity, which is why different methods are generally used to characterize a sample [27].

The antioxidant capacity in the analyzed ones followed the order: chamomile > mint > fennel > cimegripe. This result is in agreement with that obtained by Nakamura et al. [28] when investigating the total antioxidant capacity of the infusions of chamomile, mint, and fennel teas by the CUPRAC (Cupric Reducing Antioxidant Capacity) method, based on the reduction of Cu^{2+} to Cu^{1+} when certain reducing agents are present in the medium, forming a complex of Cu^{1+}/NC of intense color with maximum absorption at 454 nm, using the chromogenic reagent. This corroborates the applicability of the biosensor.

The importance of the study could be related also to the connection of these plants with their neuroprotective properties. In many countries, traditional herbal medicines are used to prevent or treat neurodegenerative disorders, and some have been developed as nutraceuticals or functional foods [29,30].

Fennel (*Foeniculum vulgare* Mill.) is a herbal that has antioxidant properties, with effects for prevention and treatment of stress-induced neurological disorders [31]. Fennel oil and trans-anethole, the main component of fennel oil, significantly inhibit SOCE-induced [Ca^{2+}] increase in vascular endothelial cells and that these reactions may be mediated by NSC, IP3-dependent Ca^{2+} mobilization, and PLC activation [32]. Several clinical studies indicated fennel for its therapeutic potential to minimize neuronal toxicity by normalizing the expression levels of APP isoforms and oxidative stress markers [33]. Efficacy of oral fennel oil in the management of dysmenorrhea, premenstrual syndrome, amenorrhea, menopause, lactation, and polycystic ovary syndrome were confirmed according to results of clinical studies [34].

Matricaria chamomilla L. (chamomile) extract may produce clinically meaningful antidepressant effects in addition to its anxiolytic activity in subjects with a generalized anxiety disorder (GAD) and comorbid depression [35]. Chamomile had moderate antioxidant and antimicrobial activities, and significant antiplatelet activity in vitro. Animal model studies indicate potent anti-inflammatory action, some antimutagenic and cholesterol-lowering activities, as well as anti-spasmotic and anxiolytic effects [36].

Mints are aromatic plants traditionally used as a remedy and as culinary herbs. Methanolic extracts of Mentha x piperita and Mentha aquatica produced significant ($p < 0.05$) protection of the PC12 cells against oxidative stress. There were observed antioxidant and MAO-A inhibitory properties, M. x piperita being the most active. M. aquatica showed the highest affinity to the GABA(A)-receptor assay [37]. Its beneficial effect on the central nervous system as a neuroprotective potential, for example, has been explored. In addition, it targets multiple Alzheimer's disease events [38].

Cimegripe® is a mixture of paracetamol, clorfeniramina, and fenilefrina, with oral adult usage, for the relief of nasal congestion, runny nose, fever, and body pain present in flu-like states [39]. In the form of tea, its main ingredient is paracetamol. This medicine induces drowsiness, so it should not be used by vehicle drivers, machine operators, or those whose attention depends on the safety of others.

3.3.2. Commercial Sources of Vitamin C

The enzymatic biosensor was used to determine the antioxidant capacity, not only of ascorbic acid (pure standard), but also of commercial effervescent vitamin C formulations.

Vitamin C provides protection against uncontrolled oxidation in the aqueous medium of the cell, due to its high reducing power, being a water-soluble and thermolabile vitamin. Humans and other primates, as well as the guinea pig, are the only mammals unable to synthesize it, requiring its administration through feeding or artificial supplementation [40].

Figure 7a shows the analytical curves constructed in the presence of different concentrations of ascorbic acid, in increasing concentrations of the HX substrate. By fixing the ascorbic acid concentration at 50 μmol·L^{-1}, greater sensitivity was obtained and, in higher concentrations, a considerable loss of it (Figure 7b). A similar behavior was observed when samples of effervescent vitamin C were used as antioxidants in the system. For comparative purposes, the concentration of 0.53 mmol·L^{-1} of vitamin C was fixed, according to manufacturers' specifications, and the antioxidant capacity of the effervescent vitamin C samples was determined (Figure 7c,d).

According to the manufacturers, each tablet of the effervescent contained 1 g of pure ascorbic acid. Thus, by weighing the equivalent quantity of each product, in order to make a final concentration of ascorbic acid equal to the three brands, it was expected that the results found for the antioxidant capacity were the same or very close. However, these were quite different from each other. The actual vitamin C content in the formulations may be the cause of the discrepancies found.

The composition of the samples was investigated by infrared spectroscopy and their spectra were similar, demonstrating that there are no significant differences between them. The content of ascorbic acid in the samples was determined by the standard addition method. Although samples 1 and 3 exhibited different antioxidant capacities, both contained the same content of ascorbic acid. This shows that the antioxidant capacity of the drugs is influenced by other compounds present in them. Some studies have shown a negative correlation between vitamin C content and antioxidant capacity [41,42]. Therefore, the individual and combined contribution of each component of the sample can be studied in the future.

The results of this study are in accordance with other published data using differential pulse voltammetry for vitamin C detection in pharmaceutical samples [43].

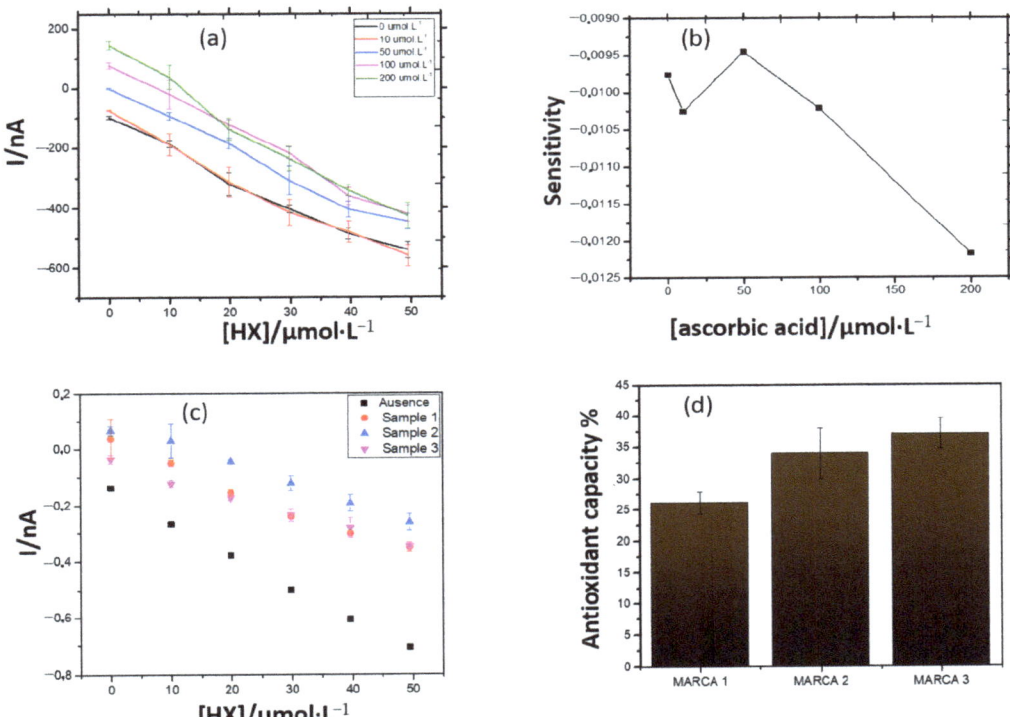

Figure 7. (a) Evaluation of the antioxidant capacity of ascorbic acid (standard) using the amperometric biosensor. (b) Sensitivity curve, in terms of the slopes of the curves showed in (a). (c) Response of the biosensor in the presence of the antioxidant samples. (d) Antioxidant capacity of drugs containing ascorbic acid against the biosensor.

3.4. Analytical Stability of the Amperometric Biosensor

Adequate quality control is necessary to obtain reliable results. The use of control charts can be an effective strategy to ensure that there has been no change in a particular process over time. It helps to detect variations outside a statistically acceptable standard, making it possible to correct them.

Figure 8 shows the statistical control chart, built from chronoamperometric measurements, obtained with the same biosensor, in a medium containing 9.9 $\mu mol \cdot L^{-1}$ HX, in the absence of antioxidants, over the course of 7 months. The biosensor proved to be statistically stable in this period, with the control lines not being exceeded once.

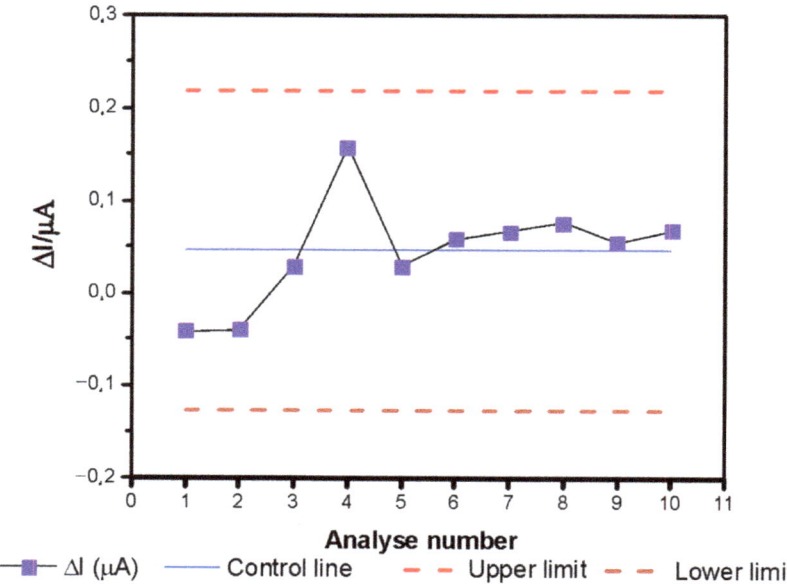

Figure 8. Statistical control chart for monitoring the biosensor stability.

4. Conclusions

The use of silk-screened sensors, whose working electrode contains graphite and the Prussian blue mediator (PB) proved to be efficient in determining the antioxidant capacity when the target molecule is hydrogen peroxide. This was possible due to the catalytic properties of this modifier, at the time of its reduction. The use of Meldola blue combined with Reinecke salt (MBRS) was not effective in the studied conditions. However, the possibility of future applications should not be ruled out, due to its high potential in electron transfer processes.

The method of immobilization by occlusion/entrapment of the enzyme xanthine oxidase (XOD) in polymeric PVA-AWE film on the surface of the carbon paste electrode modified with PB proved to be simple and efficient. However, the polymerization conditions must be properly controlled because a small variation in the polymerization time has considerably affected the analytical response of the biosensor

The elimination of the constant agitation process, during chronoamperometric measurements, for example, resulted in an increase in the linear range reached by the device. If higher levels of enzyme activity and substrate content are used, but always below the level of kinetic saturation, it is believed that the linear region can be further expanded.

The biosensor showed high stability and showed promise in determining the antioxidant capacity of teas and/or drugs that are sources of vitamin C and can also be used to detect fraud. Its use can be expanded to assess the antioxidant potential of fresh or processed foods and also to control different products used for their neuroprotective effects.

The developed biosensors could be used as possible tools to the monitoring of reactive oxygen species, the free radicals in different samples, as plants extracts, drugs, or other biological liquids, aiming to obtain a correlation between the index obtained from these indicators with the oxidative stress levels in the samples.

Supplementary Materials: The following are available online at https://www.mdpi.com/2076-3921/10/2/324/s1, Figure S1: Distribution of the references concerning antioxidant capacity detection, according with publication years—since 1997; Figure S2: Distribution of the references concerning antioxidant capacity detection, according with document type—since 1997; Figure S3: Distribution of the references concerning antioxidant capacity detection, according with source titles—since 1997; Figure S4: Distribution of the references concerning antioxidant capacity detection, according research area—since 1997; Figure S5: H-index related to the ISI WOS references dealing with antioxidant capacity detection—since 1997.

Author Contributions: Conceptualization, D.B.R. and G.S.N.; Data collection and experimentation, D.B.R., G.S.S. and A.R.C.C.; software and data curation, D.B.R., D.R.d.S. and E.B.R.; writing—original draft preparation, D.B.R.; writing—review and editing, M.B. and G.S.N. All authors have read and agreed to the published version of the manuscript.

Funding: This study was financed in part by the Coordenação de Aperfeiçoamento de Pessoal de Nível Superior—Brasil (CAPES)-Finance Code 001.

Institutional Review Board Statement: Not applicable.

Informed Consent Statement: Not applicable.

Data Availability Statement: Not applicable.

Conflicts of Interest: The authors declare no conflict of interest.

References

1. Nunez-Selles, A.J. Antioxidant therapy: Myth or reality? *J. Braz. Chem. Soc.* **2005**, *16*, 699–710. [CrossRef]
2. Barreiros, A.; David, J.M.; David, J.P. Oxidative stress: Relations between the formation of reactive species and the organism's defense. *Quim. Nova* **2006**, *29*, 113–123. [CrossRef]
3. Gliszczynska-Swiglo, A. Antioxidant activity of water soluble vitamins in the TEAC (trolox equivalent antioxidant capacity) and the FRAP (ferric reducing antioxidant power) assays. *Food Chem.* **2006**, *96*, 131–136. [CrossRef]
4. Vasconcelos, S.M.L.; Goulart, M.O.F.; Moura, J.; Manfredini, V.; Benfato, M.D.S.; Kubota, L.T. Reactive oxygen and nitrogen species, antioxidants and markers of oxidative damage in human blood: Main analytical methods for their determination. *Quim. Nova* **2007**, *30*, 1323–1338. [CrossRef]
5. Halliwell, B. Free radicals and antioxidants: Updating a personal view. *Nutr. Rev.* **2012**, *70*, 257–265. [CrossRef] [PubMed]
6. Carlsen, M.H.; Halvorsen, B.L.; Holte, K.; Bohn, S.K.; Dragland, S.; Sampson, L.; Willey, C.; Senoo, H.; Umezono, Y.; Sanada, C.; et al. The total antioxidant content of more than 3100 foods, beverages, spices, herbs and supplements used worldwide. *Nutr. J.* **2010**, *9*, 11. [CrossRef]
7. Li, S.; Li, S.K.; Gan, R.Y.; Song, F.L.; Kuang, L.; Li, H.B. Antioxidant capacities and total phenolic contents of infusions from 223 medicinal plants. *Ind. Crop. Prod.* **2013**, *51*, 289–298. [CrossRef]
8. Deng, G.F.; Lin, X.; Xu, X.R.; Gao, L.L.; Xie, J.F.; Li, H.B. Antioxidant capacities and total phenolic contents of 56 vegetables. *J. Funct. Foods* **2013**, *5*, 260–266. [CrossRef]
9. Li, A.N.; Li, S.; Li, H.B.; Xu, D.P.; Xu, X.R.; Chen, F. Total phenolic contents and antioxidant capacities of 51 edible and wild flowers. *J. Funct. Foods* **2014**, *6*, 319–330. [CrossRef]
10. Xu, D.P.; Li, Y.; Meng, X.; Zhou, T.; Zhou, Y.; Zheng, J.; Zhang, J.J.; Li, H.B. Natural Antioxidants in Foods and Medicinal Plants: Extraction, Assessment and Resources. *Int. J. Mol. Sci.* **2017**, *18*, 96. [CrossRef]
11. Becker, M.M.; Nunes, G.S.; Ribeiro, D.B.; Silva, F.; Catanante, G.; Marty, J.L. Determination of the Antioxidant Capacity of Red Fruits by Miniaturized Spectrophotometry Assays. *J. Braz. Chem. Soc.* **2019**, *30*, 1108–1114. [CrossRef]
12. Becker, M.M.; Ribeiro, E.B.; Marques, P.; Marty, J.L.; Nunes, G.S.; Catanante, G. Development of a highly sensitive xanthine oxidase-based biosensor for the determination of antioxidant capacity in Amazonian fruit samples. *Talanta* **2019**, *204*, 626–632. [CrossRef]
13. Pisoschi, A.M.; Negulescu, G.P. Methods for total antioxidant activity determination: A review. *Biochem. Anal. Biochem.* **2011**, *1*, 106. [CrossRef]
14. Rodriguez-Amaya, D.B. *A Guide to Carotenoid Analysis in Foods*; ILSI Press: Washington, DC, USA, 2011.
15. Lates, V.; Marty, J.L.; Popescu, I.C. Determination of Antioxidant Capacity by Using Xanthine Oxidase Bioreactor Coupled with Flow-through H2O2 Amperometric Biosensor. *Electroanalysis* **2011**, *23*, 728–736. [CrossRef]
16. Pereira, A.C.; de Santos, A.S.; Kubota, L.T. Tendências em modificação de eletrodos amperométricos para aplicações eletroanalíticas. *Quim. Nova* **2002**, *25*, 1012–1021. [CrossRef]
17. Hayat, A.; Marty, J.L. Disposable Screen Printed Electrochemical Sensors: Tools for Environmental Monitoring. *Sensors* **2014**, *14*, 10432–10453. [CrossRef] [PubMed]
18. Hoshi, T.; Saiki, H.; Anzai, J. Amperometric uric acid sensors based on polyelectrolyte multilayer films. *Talanta* **2003**, *61*, 363–368. [CrossRef]
19. Nunes, G.S.; Badea, M.; Medel, M.L.; Noguer, T.; Marty, J.L. Ultrasensitive biosensors for the detection of insecticide residues in fruit juices. *Bull. Transilv. Univ. Bras. Med. Sci. Ser.* **2008**, *1*, 29.
20. Saleem, M.; Yu, H.J.; Wang, L.; Zain ul, A.; Khalid, H.; Akram, M.; Abbasi, N.M.; Huang, J. Review on synthesis of ferrocene-based redox polymers and derivatives and their application in glucose sensing. *Anal. Chim. Acta* **2015**, *876*, 9–25. [CrossRef]

21. Ricci, F.; Palleschi, G. Sensor and biosensor preparation, optimisation and applications of Prussian Blue modified electrodes. *Biosens. Bioelectron.* **2005**, *21*, 389–407. [CrossRef] [PubMed]
22. Rosatto, S.S.; Freire, R.S.; Durán, N.; Kubota, L.T. Biossensores amperométricos para determinação de compostos fenólicos em amostras de interesse ambiental. *Quim. Nova* **2001**, *24*, 77–86. [CrossRef]
23. Pandey, P.C.; Pandey, A.K. Novel synthesis of Prussian blue nanoparticles and nanocomposite sol: Electro-analytical application in hydrogen peroxide sensing. *Electrochim. Acta* **2013**, *87*, 1–8. [CrossRef]
24. Varvari, L.; Popescu, I.C. New method for antioxidant activity evaluation using a H2O2 amperometric sensor. *Rev. Roum. Chim.* **2010**, *55*, 851.
25. Stoytcheva, M.; Zlatev, R.; Navarro, F.F.G.; Velkova, Z.; Gochev, V.; Montero, G.; Bautistaa, A.G.A.; Toscano-Palomar, L. PVA-AWP/tyrosinase functionalized screen-printed electrodes for dopamine determination. *Anal. Methods* **2016**, *8*, 5197–5203. [CrossRef]
26. Banerjee, S.; Sarkar, P.; Turner, A.P.F. Amperometric biosensor based on Prussian Blue nanoparticle-modified screen-printed electrode for estimation of glucose-6-phosphate. *Anal. Biochem.* **2013**, *439*, 194–200. [CrossRef] [PubMed]
27. Bhattacharyya, A.; Chattopadhyay, R.; Mitra, S.; Crowe, S.E. Oxidative stress: An essential factor in the pathogenesis of gastrointestinal mucosal diseases. *Physiol. Rev.* **2014**, *94*, 329–354. [CrossRef]
28. Nakamura, T.; Silva, F.S.; Silva DX da Souza MW de Moya, H.D. Determinação da atividade antioxidante e do teor total de polifenol em amostras de chá de ervas comercializadas em sachets. *Abcs Health Sci* **2013**, *38*, 56–74. [CrossRef]
29. Chung, V.; Liu, L.; Bian, Z.; Zhao, Z.; Fong, W.L.; Kum, W.F.; Gao, J.; Li, M. Efficacy and safety of herbal medicines for idiopathic Parkinson's disease: A systematic review. *Mov. Disord.* **2006**, *21*, 1709–1715. [CrossRef]
30. More, S.V.; Kumar, H.; Kang, S.M.; Song, S.Y.; Lee, K.; Choi, D.K. Advances in neuroprotective ingredients of medicinal herbs by using cellular and animal models of Parkinson's disease. *Evid.-Based Complement. Altern. Med.* **2013**, *2013*. [CrossRef]
31. Raman, S.; Asle-Rousta, M.; Rahnema, M. Protective effect of fennel, and its major component trans-anethole against social isolation induced behavioral deficits in rats. *Physiol. Int.* **2020**, *107*, 30–39. [CrossRef] [PubMed]
32. Han, A.Y.; Lee, H.S.; Seol, G.H. Foeniculum vulgare Mill. increases cytosolic Ca2+ concentration and inhibits store-operated Ca2+ entry in vascular endothelial cells. *Biomed. Pharm.* **2016**, *84*, 800–805. [CrossRef] [PubMed]
33. Bhatti, S.; Ali Shah, S.A.; Ahmed, T.; Zahid, S. Neuroprotective effects of Foeniculum vulgare seeds extract on lead-induced neurotoxicity in mice brain. *Drug Chem. Toxicol.* **2018**, *41*, 399–407. [CrossRef] [PubMed]
34. Mahboubi, M. Foeniculum vulgare as Valuable Plant in Management of Women's Health. *J. Menopausal Med.* **2019**, *25*, 1–14. [CrossRef] [PubMed]
35. Amsterdam, J.D.; Li, Q.S.; Xie, S.X.; Mao, J.J. Putative Antidepressant Effect of Chamomile (Matricaria chamomilla L.) Oral Extract in Subjects with Comorbid Generalized Anxiety Disorder and Depression. *J. Altern. Complement. Med.* **2020**, *26*, 813–819. [CrossRef]
36. McKay, D.; Blumberg, J. A Review of the bioactivity and potential health benefits of chamomile tea (*Matricaria recutita* L.). *Phyther. Res.* **2006**, *20*, 519–530. [CrossRef]
37. López, V.; Martín, S.; Gómez-Serranillos MPCarretero, M.; Jäger, A.; Calvo, M. Neuroprotective and neurochemical properties of mint extracts. *Phyther. Res.* **2010**, *24*, 869–874. [CrossRef] [PubMed]
38. Hanafy, D.M.; Burrows, G.E.; Prenzler, P.D.; Hill, R.A. Potential role of phenolic extracts of mentha in managing oxidative stress and Alzheimer's disease. *Antioxidants* **2020**, *9*, 631. [CrossRef]
39. De Bula, M. Cimegripe® 77 C. Available online: https://remediobarato.com/cimegripe-77c-bula-completa--cimed-industria-de-medicamentos-ltda--para-o-profissional.html#verpdf (accessed on 18 February 2021).
40. Penteado, M.D.V.C. *Vitaminas: Aspectos Nutricionais, Bioquímicos, Clínicos e Analíticos*; Manole: Sao Paulo, Brazil, 2021; 612p.
41. de Souza, A.V.; da Vieira, M.R.S.; Putti, F.F. Correlações entre compostos fenólicos e atividade antioxidante em casca e polpa de variedades de uva de mesa. *Braz. J. Food Technol.* **2018**, *21*. [CrossRef]
42. Guo, C.; Yang, J.; Wei, J.; Li, Y.; Xu, J.; Jiang, Y. Antioxidant activities of peel, pulp and seed fractions of common fruits as determined by FRAP assay. *Nutr. Res.* **2003**, *23*, 1719–1726. [CrossRef]
43. Badea, M.; Chiperea, S.; Bálan, M.; Floroian, L.; Restani, P.; Marty, J.L.; Iovan, C.; Țiț, D.M.; Bungău, S.; Taus, N. New approaches for electrochemical detection of ascorbic acid. *Farmacia* **2018**, *66*, 83–87.

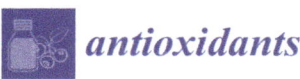

Article

Autoxidation Enhances Anti-Amyloid Potential of Flavone Derivatives

Andrius Sakalauskas, Mantas Ziaunys, Ruta Snieckute and Vytautas Smirnovas *

Life Sciences Center, Institute of Biotechnology, Vilnius University, LT-10257 Vilnius, Lithuania; andrius.sakalauskas@gmc.vu.lt (A.S.); mantas.ziaunys@gmail.com (M.Z.); r.snieckute@gmail.com (R.S.)
* Correspondence: vytautas.smirnovas@bti.vu.lt

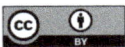

Citation: Sakalauskas, A.; Ziaunys, M.; Snieckute, R.; Smirnovas, V. Autoxidation Enhances Anti-Amyloid Potential of Flavone Derivatives. *Antioxidants* 2021, 10, 1428. https://doi.org/10.3390/antiox10091428

Academic Editors: Rui F. M. Silva and Lea Pogačnik

Received: 9 August 2021
Accepted: 1 September 2021
Published: 7 September 2021

Publisher's Note: MDPI stays neutral with regard to jurisdictional claims in published maps and institutional affiliations.

Copyright: © 2021 by the authors. Licensee MDPI, Basel, Switzerland. This article is an open access article distributed under the terms and conditions of the Creative Commons Attribution (CC BY) license (https://creativecommons.org/licenses/by/4.0/).

Abstract: The increasing prevalence of amyloid-related disorders, such as Alzheimer's or Parkinson's disease, raises the need for effective anti-amyloid drugs. It has been shown on numerous occasions that flavones, a group of naturally occurring anti-oxidants, can impact the aggregation process of several amyloidogenic proteins and peptides, including amyloid-beta. Due to flavone autoxidation at neutral pH, it is uncertain if the effective inhibitor is the initial molecule or a product of this reaction, as many anti-amyloid assays attempt to mimic physiological conditions. In this work, we examine the aggregation-inhibiting properties of flavones before and after they are oxidized. The oxidation of flavones was monitored by measuring the UV-vis absorbance spectrum change over time. The protein aggregation kinetics were followed by measuring the amyloidophilic dye thioflavin-T (ThT) fluorescence intensity change. Atomic force microscopy was employed to image the aggregates formed with the most prominent inhibitors. We demonstrate that flavones, which undergo autoxidation, have a far greater potency at inhibiting the aggregation of both the disease-related amyloid-beta, as well as a model amyloidogenic protein—insulin. Oxidized 6,2′,3′-trihydroxyflavone was the most potent inhibitor affecting both insulin (7-fold inhibition) and amyloid-beta (2-fold inhibition). We also show that this tendency to autoxidize is related to the positions of the flavone hydroxyl groups.

Keywords: aggregation; amyloid-beta; insulin; flavones; inhibition; autoxidation

1. Introduction

Protein aggregation into highly structured aggregates is associated with various amyloidoses, such as Alzheimer's disease (AD) and Parkinson's disease (PD) [1]. AD alone is recognized to be the most common cause of dementia (60–80%) [2] that affects more than 50 million people worldwide and, according to the World Alzheimer's Report, is set to increase up to 152 million by 2050. The cause of this forecast is that the onset of AD mostly occurs after 60 years of age, and the increasing life expectancy leads to more people suffering from dementia. The pathological hallmark of this disease is the increased concentration of the 42 amino acid peptide—amyloid-beta (Aβ_{42}) that prompts the formation of its oligomeric and fibrillar species [3].

The increasing focus on anti-amyloid-β compounds has led to many different in vitro studies showing positive effects against protein aggregation [4]. Despite this fact, many suggested disease-modifying compounds, ranging from small organic molecules to large monoclonal antibodies, have not led to an effective cure, leaving 99.5% of clinical trials unsuccessful [5,6]. Several potential problems with the very low clinical trial success rate are linked to targeting the wrong pathological substrates, concerns with drug development, and problems with methodologies [7,8]. Subsequently, it is of utmost importance to take into consideration the gap between the initial drug screening and human physiology [4,9].

The aggregation process of the Aβ_{42} peptide is exceptionally complicated; however, the mechanism is rather well described [10,11]. The process of several steps involves primary nucleation, elongation, fibril surface-catalyzed nucleation (often referred to as secondary nucleation), and fragmentation [12]. While primary nucleation causes the formation of nuclei that eventually grow into fibril aggregates, secondary nucleation is shown to be the main source of more cytotoxic oligomeric species that cause direct neurotoxicity [13–15]. For that reason, it is beneficial to find an anti-amyloidogenic compound that prevents primary and secondary nucleation as well as elongation processes [16].

Flavones are abundant in nature and found in a variety of herbs, fruits, vegetables, and spices [17]. This group of natural anti-oxidants has been reported to possess anti-amyloid characteristics, exhibit neuroprotective, anti-inflammatory, and anti-microbial properties [16,18]. In addition, flavone derivatives have shown positive effects when treating diabetes, cancer, malaria, asthma, and cardiovascular system diseases [19]. Studies have also shown that a variety of flavonoids function as acetylcholinesterase inhibitors (AChEI) [20,21]. AChEI is currently one of the most prominent options for symptomatic treatment of AD, mostly by increasing neurotransmitter acetylcholine concentrations in synaptic gaps of the nervous system [22,23]. If the same compound would also inhibit amyloid formation, it could be an ultimate anti-amyloid drug. Moreover, the small molecular weight and widely abundant flavonoids could be a better option for drug development. Compared to the large monoclonal antibody-based drugs, such molecules do pass Lipinski's rule of 5, have high availability and stability, and could potentially be used for less expensive prevention against the onset of neurodegenerative diseases [24].

Studies with flavones demonstrated properties against $A\beta_{42}$ aggregation in vitro [25,26]. In many cases, the anti-aggregation potential is evaluated via measurement of amyloidophilic dye thioflavin-T (ThT) fluorescence intensity [27,28], assuming that relatively lower fluorescence intensity correlates with fewer fibrils formed. While this hypothesis is quite prominent, various counterfactors exist. Typically, $A\beta_{42}$ aggregation is examined at neutral pH without evaluating the characteristics of the potential inhibitor in question. Numerous flavones have light absorbance properties in the same range as typically used fluorescent amyloid-dyes [29]. In addition, flavones could potentially bind to either the dye molecule itself or the formed aggregates, preventing its interaction with the fibril [30].

Many polyphenolic compounds, including flavones, are reported to undergo autoxidation at neutral or higher pH [31,32]. One particular study shows the oxidation mechanism of quercetin, suggesting that the process involves the breakdown of the flavone C ring, enabling different structure formations [32]. In another report, the $A\beta_{42}$ inhibitory effect is based on the autoxidation of (+)-taxifolin [28]. This leads to an assumption that molecule autoxidation could be the main cause of the inhibitory effect in vitro. Furthermore, several reports demonstrate low mono- and polyhydroxylated flavone oral bioavailability due to direct metabolism [33]. In addition, human cytochrome P450 enzymes oxidize the 5-hydroxyflavone to specific di- or trihydroxyflavones [34]. These aforementioned aspects raise questions about whether the tested molecule or its oxidized species inhibit amyloid formation in vitro.

In this work, we examined the oxidation potential of 64 mono- and polyhydroxylated flavones and tested their inhibitory effect on the aggregation of amyloid-beta and a commonly used model amyloid protein—insulin. We show that the positions of flavone hydroxy groups have a remarkably high impact on autoxidation which enables the inhibitory effect on both proteins under the tested conditions.

2. Materials and Methods

2.1. Flavone Solution Preparation

Each non-oxidized flavone stock solution was prepared by dissolving the flavones (Indofine Chemical Company, Inc., Hillsborough, NJ, USA) in dimethylsulfoxide (DMSO, Carl Roth, Karlsruhe, Germany) to a final concentration of 10 mM. The oxidation solution of each flavone was prepared by diluting 10 mM flavone stock solution with 10 mM sodium phosphate buffer (pH 8.0) and DMSO to yield a final flavone concentration of 0.2 mM in

9 mM sodium phosphate buffer solution containing 10% DMSO. The 10% DMSO buffer solution was used to increase the solubility of flavones.

2.2. Absorbance Measurements

The autoxidation of flavones was monitored by measuring UV-Vis absorbance spectrum changes over time using a ClarioStar Plus plate reader (BMG Labtech, Ortenberg, Germany). Each flavone oxidation solution was stored as 100 µL samples in a UV-clear 96-well plate (Thermo Fisher Scientific, Inc., Waltham, MA, USA, cat. No. 11670352) and incubated at 37 °C, while the measuring absorbance spectra were in the range from 240 nm to 800 nm. Data were collected each hour for a total of 100 h. Spectra was baseline corrected at 800 nm. The resulting samples, which are later referred to as "incubated" or "oxidized" flavones, were then used in aggregation kinetic experiments.

Samples for the measurement of ThT and flavone interaction were prepared by mixing 0.5 mM incubated flavone, 10 mM ThT stock solution, and 20 mM phosphate buffer solution (pH 7.0), yielding either separate 50 µM flavone and 20 µM ThT or combined 50 µM flavone and 20 µM ThT solutions in 20 mM phosphate buffer (pH 7.0). Samples were scanned using a Shimadzu UV-1800 spectrophotometer (1 nm steps). Separate 50 µM flavone and 20 µM ThT spectra were added together for comparison with their mixture. Each sample was scanned three times and averaged; the baseline was corrected at 800 nm.

2.3. Fluorescence Measurements

Samples for the fluorescence measurements were prepared by mixing 0.5 mM incubated flavone, 10 mM ThT stock solution, 2 µM of $A\beta_{42}$ aggregates, and 20 mM phosphate buffer solution (pH 7.0), yielding 1 µM of $A\beta_{42}$ fibril samples with either 20 µM ThT or 50 µM flavone samples with both ThT and flavone. The fluorescence intensity was scanned using a Varian Cary Eclipse fluorescence spectrophotometer, with excitation and emission wavelengths being 440 nm and 480 nm, respectively (5 nm excitation and 2.5 nm emission slit widths). The intrinsic fluorescence emission intensity, occurring from non-fibril-bound ThT or flavones, was subtracted from their respective fibril-compound sample intensities. This was done by acquiring fluorescence emission intensity values of ThT or flavone samples in the absence of $A\beta_{42}$ aggregates.

2.4. Purification of Recombinant $A\beta_{42}$

The expression vector of $A\beta_{42}$ was described previously [35]. The peptide was expressed in *E.coli* BL-21Star™ (DE3) (Invitrogen, Carlsbad, CA, USA) and purified as described previously [36]. In brief, the transformed cells were incubated on LB agar plates containing ampicillin (100 µg/mL) overnight at 37 °C. The next day, the overnight cultures were prepared from single colonies and grown in LB medium with ampicillin (100 µg/mL). The 1 mL of the culture was transferred to 400 mL of auto-inductive ZYM-5052 medium [37] containing ampicillin (100 µg/mL) and grown for 15 h. The collected cell pellet was washed 3 times to remove all soluble proteins. The procedure involves pellet homogenization, sonication, and centrifugation. After removing soluble proteins, the cell pellet was resuspended in 50 mL of 20 mM Tris/HCL pH 8.0 buffer solution containing 8 M urea and 1 mM EDTA, homogenized, and centrifuged as in the previous steps. The collected supernatant was diluted with 150 mL of 20 mM Tris/HCL (pH 8.0) buffer containing 1 mM EDTA, mixed with 60 mL DEAE-sepharose and agitated at 80 rpm for 30 min at 4 °C. The chromatography procedure was performed using a Buchner funnel with Fisherbrand glass microfiber paper on a vacuum glass bottle. The resin with bound proteins was washed with 20 mM Tris/HCL pH 8.0 buffer containing 1 mM EDTA in increasing NaCl concentrations in a step-gradient (0, 20, 150, 500 mM). The target protein fractions were collected by washing the resin with a 50 mL buffer solution (containing 150 mM NaCl) four times. Collected fractions were mixed together, lyophilized, and stored at -20 °C.

The $A\beta_{42}$ peptide powder was dissolved in a 20 mM sodium phosphate buffer solution (pH 8.0) containing 5 M guanidine thiocyanate (GuSCN, Carl Roth). The dissolved sample was loaded on a Tricorn 10/300 column (packed with Superdex 75) and eluted at 1 mL/min using a 20 mM sodium phosphate buffer solution (pH 8.0) containing 0.2 mM EDTA and 0.02% NaN$_3$. Collected fractions were mixed together, lyophilized, and stored at -20 °C. Before aggregation experiments, the purification procedure was repeated, but this time the collected fraction (0.75 mL) was purified Aβ_{42} was stored on ice for 5 min. The concentration was determined by calculating the integrated chromatographic UV absorbance peak (ε_{280} = 1 490 M^{-1} cm^{-1}). Afterward, it was diluted and immediately used for aggregation experiments.

2.5. Aggregation Kinetics of Aβ_{42} Peptide

The purified peptide fraction (1.5 mL, pH 8.0) was mixed with 3 mL of 20 mM sodium phosphate buffer solution (pH 6.33) to yield a 3-fold diluted peptide solution (pH 7.0). The peptide and each oxidized or incubated flavone solution was mixed together with 20 mM sodium phosphate buffer solution (pH 7.0), 10 mM ThT stock solution, and DMSO to a final reaction mixture, containing 1 µM Aβ_{42}, 20 µM ThT, 50 µM of selected flavone compound and 1% DMSO. The kinetic aggregation measurements were performed in non-binding 96-well plates (Fisher, Waltham, MA, USA, cat. No. 10438082) (sample volume was 80 µL) at 37 °C by measuring ThT fluorescence using 440 nm excitation and 480 emission wavelengths in a ClarioStar Plus (BMG Labtech, Ortenberg, Germany).

2.6. Aggregation Kinetics of Insulin

Human recombinant insulin powder (Sigma-Aldrich, St. Louis, MO, USA, cat. No. 91077C) was dissolved in a 20% acetic acid solution (prepared from 100% acetic acid; Carl-Roth) containing 100 mM NaCl (Fisher) to a protein concentration of 400 µM. This insulin stock solution was mixed with non-oxidized/incubated or oxidized/incubated flavone solutions and 10 mM ThT stock solution to a final insulin concentration of 200 µM, 100 µM ThT, and 20 µM of each flavone. The aggregation kinetic measurements were performed similarly as in the case of Aβ_{42}, but at 60 °C.

2.7. Kinetic Data Analysis

After reaching the plateau, kinetic aggregation curves were fit using Boltzmann's sigmoidal equation:

$$y = \frac{(A_1 - A_2)}{\left(1 + e^{\frac{x - x_0}{dx}}\right)} + A_2 \tag{1}$$

where, A_1 is the starting fluorescence intensity, A_2—final fluorescence intensity, x_0—aggregation halftime. The relative halftime and relative ThT fluorescence intensity values were calculated based on the control sample in their specific microplate. These values were calculated by dividing each sample's average value by the average control value. Data were processed using Origin software (OriginLab, Northampton, MA, USA).

2.8. Atomic Force Microscopy (AFM)

The samples for AFM images were collected after kinetic measurements and scanned similarly as previously described [31,38]. In short, 40 µL of 1% (v/v) APTES (Sigma-Aldrich, cat. No. 440140) in MilliQ water was deposited on freshly cleaved mica and incubated for 5 min. Then, mica was rinsed with 2 mL of MilliQ water and dried under gentle airflow. Each sample was deposited (40 µL) on the functionalized surface and incubated for another 5 min. Prepared samples were rinsed with 2 mL of MilliQ water and dried under gentle airflow. AFM imaging was performed using a Dimension Icon (Bruker, Billerica, MA, USA) atomic force microscope. Images were 1024 × 1024 pixel resolution and were analyzed using Gwyddion 2.5.5 software. Fibril heights were determined by tracing perpendicular to each fibril's axis.

2.9. FTIR

Aβ$_{42}$ fibrils were separated from the buffer solution by placing the mixture in the 0.5 mL 10 kDa concentrators (Fisher, cat. No. 88513) and spinning at 10,000 g for 10 min. Then 0.5 mL of D$_2$O was added, and the process of buffer exchange to D$_2$O was repeated 3 times. After the last spinning step, fibrils were resuspended in 0.1 mL of D$_2$O. FTIR spectra were recorded using an Invenio S IR spectrophotometer equipped with an MCT detector. The sample was placed in the CaF$_2$ transmission windows with 0.05 mm Teflon spacers, 256 interferograms of 2 cm^{-1} resolution were averaged per spectrum. All spectra were normalized in the 1705–1595 cm^{-1} region, and baseline corrected after subtracting the D$_2$O and water vapor spectrums. The data were processed using GRAMS software (Thermo Fisher Scientific, Inc., Waltham, MA, USA).

3. Results

We first incubated flavones at 37 °C in order to evaluate potential structural transitions that occur due to autoxidation. The time-dependent changes in the UV-vis spectra of flavones were recorded over a period of 100 h, comparing the absorbance in the 240–800 nm region. At the start of the experiment, each flavone spectrum (Figure 1) exhibited two characteristic maxima that are associated with the $\pi \rightarrow \pi^*$ transitions within rings A and C, referred to as benzoyl system, band II (~240–290 nm), and ring B that is conjugated with the carbonyl of ring C, referred to as cinnamoyl system, band I (~300–415 nm) [39] (Figure S1). A decrease in the magnitude of these bands was observed in all displayed spectra that led to no characteristic maxima (No. 11, 22, 31, 38, 44, 46, 48, 51–52, 57, 59, 64) or appearance of new maxima peaks in other cases. The absorbance spectra changes and reduced characteristics of the band I indicate structural changes, loss of conjugation in a chromophore, and development of different intra- and intermolecular interactions [40]. A few trihydroxyflavones (THF) (No. 38, 46), tetrahydroxyflavones (TeHF) (51–52), and most of penta- and hexahydroxyflavones (PHF and HHF) (No. 59, 61, 63, 64) had major spectrum changes within the first 5 h. Most of the other flavones, including dihydroxyflavones (DHF), THF, and TeHF (No.10, 11, 22, 31, 38, 42, 44, 46, 48, 53, 55, 57), had significant absorbance changes within a 5–40 h period, while only a few (No. 1, 32, 37, 58) exhibited most of their spectrum transitions only after > 40 h of incubation. The rest of the flavones had minor spectra changes during incubation that are reflected in slight transitions of the maxima positions (No. 30, 45, 54, 56, 60, 62) or a decrease in the magnitude of the maxima in the 380–420 nm region (No. 21, 43).

Examining the effect of non-oxidized flavones reveals that only the presence of luteolin (Figure 2A,B No. 56) slightly increased the aggregation halftime of insulin (Table S1) while not affecting the fluorescence intensity. Other flavone relative halftime and ThT fluorescence intensity did not change, except for a few cases, where they even decreased the aggregation halftime (Figure 2A No. 10, 21–22, 48, 53, 54, 59, 61–63). However, once flavones were oxidized, many of them displayed substantial inhibitory potential. Some flavones (Figure 2A,B No. 31, 59, 63) increased the aggregation halftime more than five-fold, which correlates with the ten-fold elevated fluorescence intensity (compared to the control sample). In most cases, oxidized flavones inhibited insulin aggregation, except for a few (Figure 2A,B No. 1, 30, 32, 37, 46, 54–55, 58) that did not possess such properties, as neither ThT fluorescence intensity nor halftime changed compared to the previously tested non-oxidized forms. A completely different effect was seen on Aβ$_{42}$ aggregation. Here, the fluorescence intensity (Figure 2D) was diminished in all cases, except for four flavones (Figure 2D No. 1, 30, 32, 37) which seem to have had no impact on either protein aggregation process, while several oxidized compounds (Figure 2D No. 22, 31, 52, 59) showed reduced intensity values ranging from 93% to 98%, which also reduced the aggregation rate. Despite the fact that most oxidized flavones inhibited insulin aggregation, only thirteen (Figure 2C No. 22, 31, 38, 43, 46, 48, 51, 52, 56–57, 59–60, 63) appeared to increase Aβ$_{42}$ relative halftime and only three (Figure 2C No. 22, 31, 52) slowed the aggregation by at least 50%.

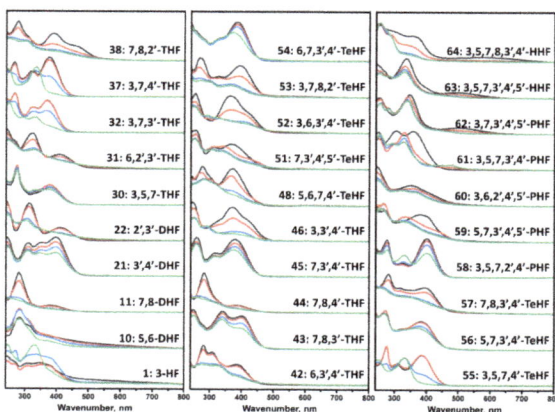

Figure 1. UV-visible absorbance spectra of flavones, recorded at 0 h (black), 5 h (red), 40 h (blue), and 100 h (green). Spectra were baseline corrected at 800 nm. Most of the flavone spectra experienced a significant change in the 250–450 nm region. In contrast, 21, 30, 43, 45, 54, 56, 60, and 62 experienced only a slight transition of maxima or decrease in the magnitude of the initial absorbance spectrum.

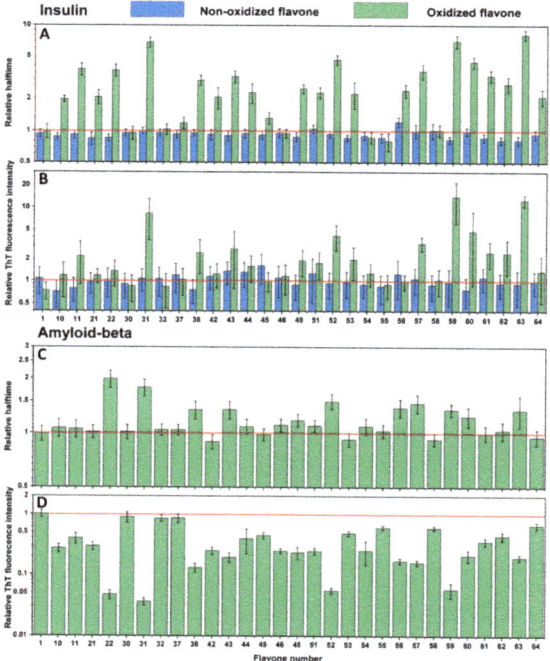

Figure 2. Effects of non-oxidized and oxidized flavones on insulin aggregation kinetics (**A**) and relative ThT fluorescence intensity (**B**). Effect of oxidized flavones on $A\beta_{42}$ aggregation kinetics (**C**) and relative ThT fluorescence intensity (**D**). Error bars are for one standard deviation ($n = 4$). None of the non-oxidized flavones, except 56, inhibited insulin aggregation; after the oxidation, more than half of the flavones showed an inhibitory effect, with 31, 59, and 63 having the most significant impact. Oxidized flavones 22, 31, 52, and 59 increased the relative halftime of $A\beta_{42}$ the most, while 1, 30, 32, 37 did not affect the relative halftime nor the relative ThT fluorescence intensity.

The flavone autoxidation experiment described above allowed us to evaluate the effect of oxidized flavones on protein aggregation. Nevertheless, not all compounds may undergo structural changes in the reaction mixture; thus, an additional number of flavones were incubated at the experimental conditions to evaluate whether UV-vis spectrum changes occur. Every tested flavone maintained the absorbance of Band I and Band II, with no major changes in the tested region (Figure 3). However, spectra of many compounds exhibited intensity changes with no shape or maximum transitions (No. 3, 6, 8, 9, 12, 13, 14, 19, 23, 26, 33, 47) that may be related to the solubility of each molecule, especially when the change occurred between the first two scans.

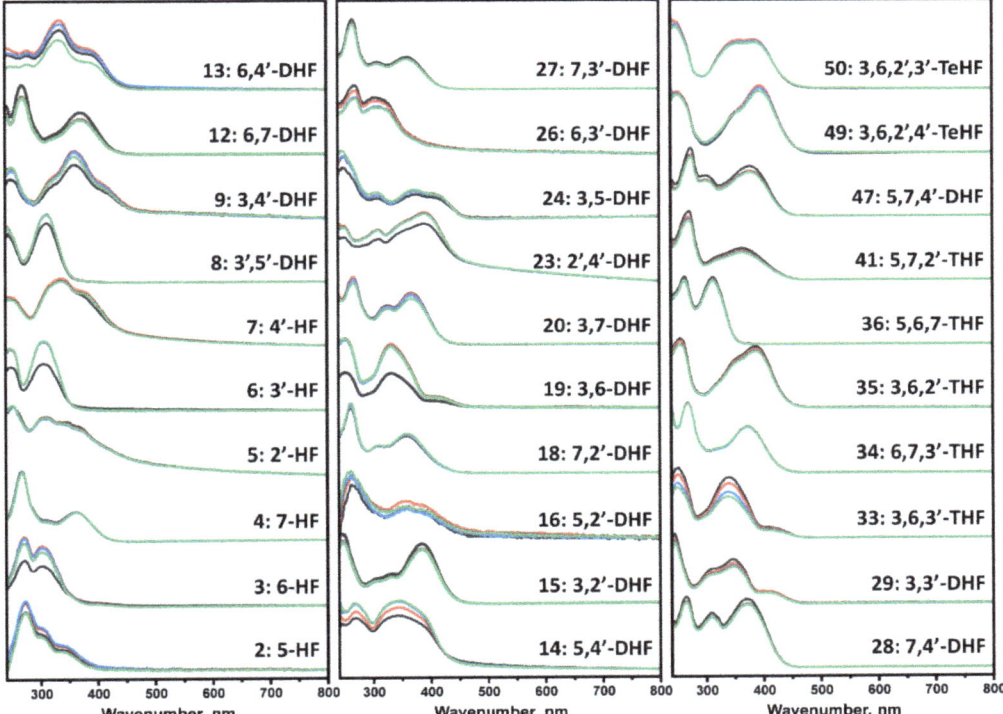

Figure 3. UV-visible absorbance spectra of flavones, recorded at 0 h (black), 5 h (red), 40 h (blue), and 100 h (green). Spectra were baseline corrected at 800 nm. Numbers 3, 6, 13, 14, 19, 23, 33 experienced the most significant decrease in the magnitude of the spectrum, while 4, 18, 27, 34, 36 had no notable change over the course of the experiment.

An identical experiment was conducted with the second set of flavones to evaluate their influence on insulin (Figure 4A,B) and $A\beta_{42}$ (Figure 4C,D) aggregation processes. Here, similar results were observed, where most of the non-incubated and incubated flavones did not inhibit insulin aggregation, yet some increased its rate (Figure 4A No. 2, 3, 7, 8, 9, 12, 13, 15, 16, 18, 19, 20, 49, 50). The majority of flavones did not affect $A\beta_{42}$ aggregation as well. However, a significant decrease in ThT fluorescence intensity was mostly evident for flavones with a higher number (Figure 4D No. 34–35, 41, 49–50), which represents THF and TeHF. In addition, dihydroxyflavones did not reduce the intensity value, except for no. 15. Three flavones (Figure 4C,D No. 5, 14, 16) that stand out appear to have altered the aggregation process by increasing the ThT fluorescence intensity and decreasing $A\beta_{42}$ aggregation halftime.

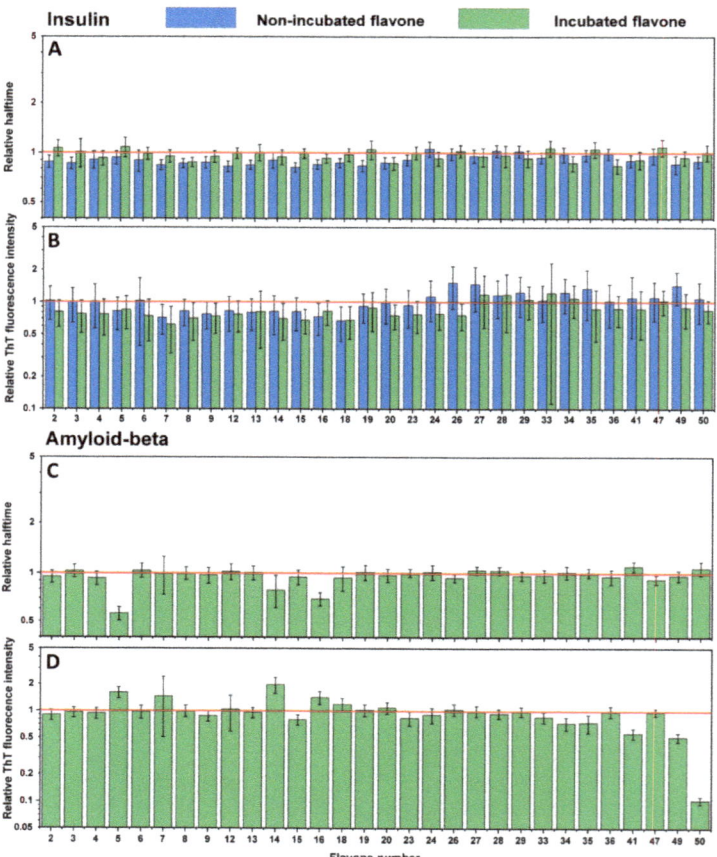

Figure 4. Effects of non-incubated and incubated flavones on insulin aggregation kinetics (**A**) and relative ThT fluorescence intensity (**B**). Effect of incubated flavones on $A\beta_{42}$ aggregation kinetics (**C**) and relative ThT fluorescence intensity (**D**). Error bars are for one standard deviation ($n = 4$). The non-incubated and incubated flavones did not impact insulin and $A\beta_{42}$ relative halftime, while incubated flavones 34, 35, 41, and 50 had the most significant impact on the relative ThT fluorescence intensity of $A\beta_{42}$.

Atomic force microscopy imaging was employed to observe whether fibrils were formed at the end of the $A\beta_{42}$ aggregation experiment (when plateau was reached). Five samples were tested that represented the control sample (Figure 5A,B) and $A\beta_{42}$ with incubated 2′,3′-DHF (Figure 5C,D), 6,2′,3′-THF (Figure 5E,F), 3,6,2′,3′-TeHF (Figure 5G,H), 3,6,3′,4′-TeHF (Figure 5I,J), 5,7,3′,4′,5′-PHF (Figure 5K,L). These particular compounds were selected due to their high impact on $A\beta_{42}$ aggregation rate and bound-ThT. All samples with flavones revealed $A\beta_{42}$ fibrillar aggregates on the mica, despite the fact that the surface was mostly covered by round-shaped oligomeric, very short fibrillar structures. Samples with 2′,3′-DHF, 6,2′,3′-THF, 3,6,2′,3′-TeHF, and 5,7,3′,4′,5′-PHF (Figure 5C,F,G,K) appeared to have clumps of fibrils with round-shaped oligomeric structures attached to them, leaving the area empty around this structure. This suggests that inhibition requires the binding of an active molecule to the protein or its oligomeric/fibrillar species. In order to further analyze AFM images, we measured the height of a hundred oligomeric structures or fibrils and compared their height distribution (Figure 5M). Structures formed with inhibitors had a dispersed height distribution, revealing that oligomeric structures may resemble clumped protofibrils. To understand this aspect more, the FTIR spectra of control Aβ$_{42}$ fibrils and the sample with 2′,3′-DHF (when both samples reached a plateau in the ThT intensity) were recorded (Figure 5N). Samples for this experiment were prepared by using 10 kDa concentrator tubes that aided in changing the reaction solution to D$_2$O. This method also eliminated monomeric species of amyloid-β. Notably, the FTIR spectrum of control fibrils exhibited the only major maximum at 1630 cm^{-1}, typical for β-sheet structures, commonly found in amyloid fibrils, while the spectrum of Aβ$_{42}$ + 2′,3′-DHF sample, had a less expressed β-sheet-related band at 1629 cm^{-1}, and another broad peak at 1675 cm^{-1}, which can mean the presence of substantial amounts of turns or different types of β-sheets. Unfortunately, the FTIR spectra could not be analyzed deeper; due to very low signal intensity, the signal-to-noise ratio was too high. It is necessary to note that, before spectra were normalized, the area of the amide I band of the sample with inhibitor was almost twice as small as the area of the amide I band of the control sample, leading to an assumption that less oligomeric and fibrillar species were present.

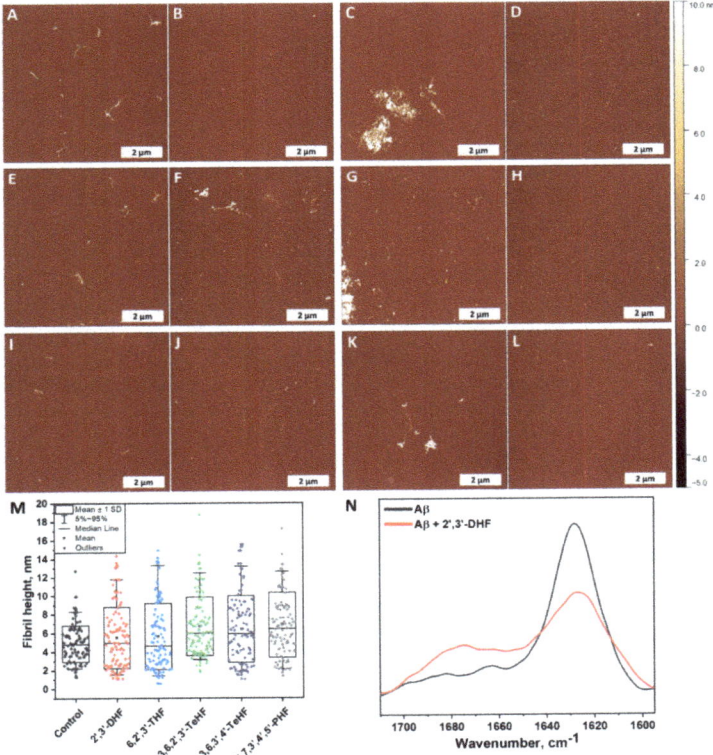

Figure 5. Atomic force microscopy images of Aβ$_{42}$ formed without (**A**,**B**) and with 50 µM of oxidized 2′,3′-DHF (**C**,**D**), 6,2′,3′-THF (**E**,**F**), 3,6,2′,3′-TeHF (**G**,**H**), 3,6,3′,4′-TeHF (**I**,**J**) and 5,7,3′,4′,5′-PHF (**K**,**L**) flavones. Fibril and oligomeric species height distribution (**M**), where box plots indicate mean ± SD and error bars are in the 5%–95% range (*n* = 100). FTIR spectra (**N**) of Aβ$_{42}$ fibrils formed alone and with 50 µM of 2′,3′-DHF. The AFM images of Aβ$_{42}$ aggregates formed with all inhibitors showed a similar distribution in height and revealed round shape structures that were not present in the image of the control sample. The FTIR spectrum of the sample with 2′,3′-DHF had less expressed β-sheet-related band at 1629 cm^{-1} than the control sample.

4. Discussion

The characteristics of insulin aggregation kinetic data show that 63 out of 64 tested non-oxidized flavones possess no anti-amyloid properties under the tested conditions (Table S1), while most flavones that undergo the autoxidation process slow down insulin fibril formation. This is expressed in altered relative aggregation halftime. However, compounds also change the ThT fluorescence intensity (Figure 2A,B), which can be explained based on our previous report, where we show that insulin is capable of forming distinct fibril conformations in 20% acetic acid solution, with one exhibiting ~10-fold higher bound-ThT intensity values [41]. Increased fluorescence intensity is also observed using oxidized gallic acid [38], leading to a hypothesis that oxidized flavones redirect insulin amyloid formation.

Contrary results are seen during the $A\beta_{42}$ aggregation process. Here, oxidized flavones led to a reduced ThT fluorescence intensity (Figures 2D and 4D), and only 14 oxidized flavones (Figures 2C and 4C) affected the aggregation rate. These diverse results introduce several potential explanations which may act simultaneously during the kinetic experiment. First, molecules that act as inhibiting agents should bind to monomers, intermediate oligomeric species, or aggregation nuclei to prevent the aggregation process [42]. Matos et al. revealed that quercetin, luteolin, and (+)-dihydroxyquercetin non-covalently bind to $A\beta_{42}$ lysine residues [27] and Sato et al. displayed the mechanism where catechol-type flavonoids, namely (+)-taxifolin, autoxidize forming an o-quinone on the B-ring that covalently binds to the amino group of lysine [28]. Second, the fluorescence quenching is unavoidable when using ThT as the excitation and emission wavelengths overlap with the majority of oxidized flavones absorbance region (Figures 1 and 3) and appear to form oxidized flavone-ThT interactions (as seen from differences in absorbance spectra, when the compounds are separate or together, Figure S2) that may lead to less bound-ThT on the fibril surface, reducing the fluorescence intensity even further (Figure S3). Therefore, most of the oxidized flavones (especially with more OH groups) suppress the fluorescence intensity in $A\beta_{42}$ aggregation experiments. This effect has been observed when two dye molecules interact alone or in the presence of fibrils [30].

Taking a deeper look into the AFM images, we see a tendency for the formation of major clumps when $A\beta_{42}$ aggregates with oxidized flavones, especially with 2',3'-DHF (Figure 5C) and 3,6,2',3'-TeHF (Figure 5G). This indicates that flavone derivatives bind to the surface of higher-level oligomeric particles as well as fibrils. While most of the mica is covered by oligomeric species, the AFM images may be analyzed, and it can be concluded that inhibitors redirect the aggregation pathway towards the arrangement of different structures. However, this explanation is just the tip of the iceberg, and a more revealing image is seen after a larger-scale analysis. The fibrillar clumps, which appear to be a combination of oligomeric structures and fibrils, consist mostly of aggregates present on the mica that is hardly found. Despite this, some oligomeric species that are found around these clusters led to the assumption that aggregation was partially stopped.

The main objective of this work was to understand the variety of flavones that may act as inhibiting molecules. There is a distinct correlation between the positions of hydroxyl groups, flavone oxidation, and inhibition of the insulin and the $A\beta_{42}$ aggregation process. Adjacent OH groups have a tendency to increase the solubility compared to other flavones and enable the autoxidation process, which was seen via UV-vis absorbance spectral data (Figures 1 and 3). Taking into consideration dihydroxyflavones, only four (5,6-DHF, 7,8-DHF, 2',3'-DHF and 3',4'-DHF) had an influence on the protein aggregation process. Surprisingly, 6,7-DHF does not autoxidize or affect protein aggregation. Despite this, the majority of hydroxyflavones that have neighboring hydroxy groups undergo oxidation leading to an enhanced inhibitory potential. This structural aspect is similar for 6,7,3'-THF and 5,6,7-THF, while 5,6,7,4'-TeHF and 6,7,3',4'-TeHF tend to oxidize, potentially due to the additional hydroxy groups on the flavone B ring. 2',3'-DHF appears to have the highest inhibition potential out of all tested flavones, which is then followed by 6,2',3'-THF. This may resemble a close connection between structures and the autoxidation end products.

Surprisingly, some of the flavonol derivates that do not have neighboring hydroxyl groups (3-hydroxyflavone, 3,5,7-THF, 3,7,3′-THF, 3,7,4′-THF, 3,5,7,4′-TeHF and 3,5,7,2′,4′-PHF) undergo autoxidation; however, these autoxidized molecules do not increase the Aβ_{42} aggregation time. This finding suggests a distinct autoxidation mechanism as well as different cinnamoyl system characteristics that are decisive for the developed anti-amyloid properties. Further, flavones with a higher number of hydroxyl groups that contain the aforementioned neighboring OH groups do autoxidize and inhibit insulin aggregation, but only some extend the Aβ_{42} aggregation time. These flavones can be categorized into two groups: 7,8-DHF derivatives (7,8,2′-THF, 7,8,3′-THF, and 7,8,3′,4′-TeHF) and flavones that have at least two hydroxyl groups on ring B (3,6,3′,4′-TeHF, 5,7,3′,4′-TeHF, 5,7,3′,4′,5′-PHF, 3,6,2′,4′,5′-PHF and 3,5,7,3′,4′,5′-PHF). Even though the number of effective inhibitors directly correlates with the number of OH groups on the molecule, the penta- and hexahydroxyflavone groups are far more complex. One probable scenario is that the flavone inhibitory effect is enabled by the appearance of particular molecular structures that form during the autoxidation process. These molecules should be structurally related, as the positions of OH groups on the molecule repeat, potentially leading to similar autoxidation mechanisms and products. While this study shows that the autoxidation of flavones leads to the formation of different structures, it is essential to note that due to this process, flavones may lose their initial characteristics, such as being inhibitors of AChE or anti-oxidants.

5. Conclusions

Taking everything into account, non-oxidized flavones do not inhibit the aggregation process of insulin or amyloid-beta, while their oxidized forms show potential against fibril formation. We also show that flavone autoxidation and inhibition are strictly related to the structure of the molecule and depend highly on the position of hydroxyl groups.

Supplementary Materials: The following are available online at https://www.mdpi.com/article/10.3390/antiox10091428/s1, Figure S1: Flavone structure; Figure S2: Absorbance spectra of incubated flavone mixed with ThT (red) and combined spectra of incubated flavone and ThT when they are scanned separately (black); Figure S3: Fluorescence intensity values of preformed Aβ_{42} aggregates mixed with incubated flavone (red), ThT (blue) and incubated flavone with ThT (green); Table S1: Relative halftime and ThT fluorescence intensity values of Insulin and Amyloid-β aggregation.

Author Contributions: A.S. and V.S. designed the experiments; A.S., M.Z., and R.S. performed the experiments; A.S., M.Z., and V.S. analyzed the data and prepared the manuscript. All authors have read and agreed to the published version of the manuscript.

Funding: This research was funded by grant no. S-SEN-20-3 from the Research Council of Lithuania.

Institutional Review Board Statement: Not applicable.

Informed Consent Statement: Not applicable.

Data Availability Statement: The data presented in this study are available in this manuscript.

Conflicts of Interest: The authors declare no conflict of interest.

References

1. Chiti, F.; Dobson, C.M. Protein Misfolding, Amyloid Formation, and Human Disease: A Summary of Progress Over the Last Decade. *Annu. Rev. Biochem.* **2017**, *86*, 27–68. [CrossRef]
2. Anand, A.; Patience, A.A.; Sharma, N.; Khurana, N. The present and future of pharmacotherapy of Alzheimer's disease: A comprehensive review. *Eur. J. Pharmacol.* **2017**, *815*, 364–375. [CrossRef] [PubMed]
3. Gouras, G.K.; Tampellini, D.; Takahashi, R.H.; Capetillo-Zarate, E. Intraneuronal β-amyloid accumulation and synapse pathology in Alzheimer's disease. *Acta Neuropathol.* **2010**, *119*, 523–541. [CrossRef]
4. Mallucci, G.R.; Klenerman, D.; Rubinsztein, D.C. Developing Therapies for Neurodegenerative Disorders: Insights from Protein Aggregation and Cellular Stress Responses. *Annu. Rev. Cell Dev. Biol.* **2020**, *36*, 165–189. [CrossRef] [PubMed]
5. Mehta, D.; Jackson, R.; Paul, G.; Shi, J.; Sabbagh, M. Why do trials for Alzheimer's disease drugs keep failing? A discontinued drug perspective for 2010-2015. *Expert Opin. Investig. Drugs* **2017**, *26*, 735–739. [CrossRef] [PubMed]

6. Mathur, S.; Dewitte, S.; Robledo, I.; Isaacs, T.; Stamford, J. Rising to the challenges of clinical trial improvement in Parkinson's disease. *J. Parkinson's Dis.* **2015**, *5*, 263–268. [CrossRef] [PubMed]
7. Huang, L.K.; Chao, S.P.; Hu, C.J. Clinical trials of new drugs for Alzheimer disease. *J. Biomed. Sci.* **2020**, *27*, 18. [CrossRef]
8. Cummings, J.; Ritter, A.; Zhong, K. Clinical Trials for Disease-Modifying Therapies in Alzheimer's Disease: A Primer, Lessons Learned, and a Blueprint for the Future. *J. Alzheimer's Dis.* **2018**, *64*, S3–S22. [CrossRef]
9. Rekatsina, M.; Paladini, A.; Piroli, A.; Zis, P.; Pergolizzi, J.V.; Varrassi, G. Pathophysiology and Therapeutic Perspectives of Oxidative Stress and Neurodegenerative Diseases: A Narrative Review. *Adv. Ther.* **2020**, *37*, 113–139. [CrossRef]
10. Frankel, R.; Törnquist, M.; Meisl, G.; Hansson, O.; Andreasson, U.; Zetterberg, H.; Blennow, K.; Frohm, B.; Cedervall, T.; Knowles, T.P.J.; et al. Autocatalytic amplification of Alzheimer-associated Aβ42 peptide aggregation in human cerebrospinal fluid. *Commun. Biol.* **2019**, *2*, 365. [CrossRef] [PubMed]
11. Chaturvedi, S.K.; Siddiqi, M.K.; Alam, P.; Khan, R.H. Protein misfolding and aggregation: Mechanism, factors and detection. *Process Biochem.* **2016**, *51*, 1183–1192. [CrossRef]
12. Morris, A.M.; Watzky, M.A.; Finke, R.G. Protein aggregation kinetics, mechanism, and curve-fitting: A review of the literature. *Biochim. Biophys. Acta—Proteins Proteom.* **2009**, *1794*, 375–397. [CrossRef]
13. Mucke, L.; Selkoe, D.J. Neurotoxicity of amyloid β-protein: Synaptic and network dysfunction. *Cold Spring Harb. Perspect. Med.* **2012**, *2*, a006338. [CrossRef] [PubMed]
14. Tanokashira, D.; Mamada, N.; Yamamoto, F.; Taniguchi, K.; Tamaoka, A.; Lakshmana, M.K.; Araki, W. The neurotoxicity of amyloid β-protein oligomers is reversible in a primary neuron model. *Mol. Brain* **2017**, *10*, 4. [CrossRef] [PubMed]
15. Lee, S.J.C.; Nam, E.; Lee, H.J.; Savelieff, M.G.; Lim, M.H. Towards an understanding of amyloid-β oligomers: Characterization, toxicity mechanisms, and inhibitors. *Chem. Soc. Rev.* **2017**, *46*, 310–323. [CrossRef]
16. Pagano, K.; Tomaselli, S.; Molinari, H.; Ragona, L. Natural Compounds as Inhibitors of Aβ Peptide Aggregation: Chemical Requirements and Molecular Mechanisms. *Front. Neurosci.* **2020**, *14*, 619667. [CrossRef] [PubMed]
17. Herrmann, K. Flavonols and flavones in food plants: A review. *Int. J. Food Sci. Technol.* **1976**, *11*, 433–448. [CrossRef]
18. Phan, H.T.T.; Samarat, K.; Takamur, Y.; Azo-Oussou, A.F.; Nakazono, Y.; Vestergaard, M.C. Polyphenols modulate alzheimer's amyloid beta aggregation in a structure-dependent manner. *Nutrients* **2019**, *11*, 756. [CrossRef] [PubMed]
19. Singh, M.; Kaur, M.; Silakari, O. Flavones: An important scaffold for medicinal chemistry. *Eur. J. Med. Chem.* **2014**, *84*, 206–239. [CrossRef]
20. Yiannopoulou, K.G.; Papageorgiou, S.G. Current and Future Treatments in Alzheimer Disease: An Update. *J. Cent. Nerv. Syst. Dis.* **2020**, *12*, 1–12. [CrossRef]
21. Khan, H.; Marya; Amin, S.; Kamal, M.A.; Patel, S. Flavonoids as acetylcholinesterase inhibitors: Current therapeutic standing and future prospects. *Biomed. Pharmacother.* **2018**, *101*, 860–870. [CrossRef]
22. Uriarte-Pueyo, I.; Calvo, M.I. Flavonoids as Acetylcholinesterase Inhibitors. *Curr. Med. Chem.* **2011**, *18*, 5289–5302. [CrossRef]
23. Abeysinghe, A.A.D.T.; Deshapriya, R.D.U.S.; Udawatte, C. Alzheimer's disease; a review of the pathophysiological basis and therapeutic interventions. *Life Sci.* **2020**, *256*, 117996. [CrossRef]
24. Youdim, K.A.; Shukitt-Hale, B.; Joseph, J.A. Flavonoids and the brain: Interactions at the blood–brain barrier and their physiological effects on the central nervous system. *Free Radic. Biol. Med.* **2004**, *37*, 1683–1693. [CrossRef] [PubMed]
25. Yu, K.H.; Lee, C.I. Quercetin disaggregates prion fibrils and decreases fibril-induced cytotoxicity and oxidative stress. *Pharmaceutics* **2020**, *12*, 1081. [CrossRef]
26. Sonawane, S.K.; Balmik, A.A.; Boral, D.; Ramasamy, S.; Chinnathambi, S. Baicalein suppresses Repeat Tau fibrillization by sequestering oligomers. *Arch. Biochem. Biophys.* **2019**, *675*, 108119. [CrossRef] [PubMed]
27. Matos, A.M.; Cristóvaõ, J.S.; Yashunsky, D.V.; Nifantiev, N.E.; Viana, A.S.; Gomes, C.M.; Rauter, A.P. Synthesis and effects of flavonoid structure variation on amyloid-β aggregation. *Pure Appl. Chem.* **2017**, *89*, 1305–1320. [CrossRef]
28. Sato, M.; Murakami, K.; Uno, M.; Nakagawa, Y.; Katayama, S.; Akagi, K.I.; Masuda, Y.; Takegoshi, K.; Irie, K. Site-specific inhibitory mechanism for amyloid β42 aggregation by catechol-type flavonoids targeting the lys residues. *J. Biol. Chem.* **2013**, *288*, 23212–23224. [CrossRef] [PubMed]
29. Hudson, S.A.; Ecroyd, H.; Kee, T.W.; Carver, J.A. The thioflavin T fluorescence assay for amyloid fibril detection can be biased by the presence of exogenous compounds. *FEBS J.* **2009**, *276*, 5960–5972. [CrossRef]
30. Ziaunys, M.; Mikalauskaite, K.; Smirnovas, V. Amyloidophilic Molecule Interactions on the Surface of Insulin Fibrils: Cooperative Binding and Fluorescence Quenching. *Sci. Rep.* **2019**, *9*, 20303. [CrossRef]
31. Sneideris, T.; Sakalauskas, A.; Sternke-Hoffmann, R.; Peduzzo, A.; Ziaunys, M.; Buell, A.K.; Smirnovas, V. The Environment Is a Key Factor in Determining the Anti-Amyloid Efficacy of EGCG. *Biomolecules* **2019**, *9*, 855. [CrossRef] [PubMed]
32. Sokolová, R.; Ramešová, Š.; Degano, I.; Hromadová, M.; Žabka, J. The oxidation of natural flavonoid quercetin. *Chem. Commun.* **2012**, *48*, 3433–3435. [CrossRef] [PubMed]
33. Walle, T. Methylation of Dietary Flavones Greatly Improves Their Hepatic Metabolic Stability and Intestinal Absorption. *Mol. Pharm.* **2007**, *4*, 826–832. [CrossRef]
34. Nagayoshi, H.; Murayama, N.; Kakimoto, K.; Tsujino, M.; Takenaka, S.; Katahira, J.; Lim, Y.R.; Kim, D.; Yamazaki, H.; Komori, M.; et al. Oxidation of Flavone, 5-Hydroxyflavone, and 5,7-Dihydroxyflavone to Mono-, Di-, and Tri-Hydroxyflavones by Human Cytochrome P450 Enzymes. *Chem. Res. Toxicol.* **2019**, *32*, 1268–1280. [CrossRef] [PubMed]

35. Walsh, D.M.; Thulin, E.; Minogue, A.M.; Gustavsson, N.; Pang, E.; Teplow, D.B.; Linse, S. A facile method for expression and purification of the Alzheimer's disease-associated amyloid β-peptide. *FEBS J.* **2009**, *276*, 1266–1281. [CrossRef]
36. Vignaud, H.; Bobo, C.; Lascu, I.; Sörgjerd, K.M.; Zako, T.; Maeda, M.; Salin, B.; Lecomte, S.; Cullin, C. A structure-toxicity study of Aß42 reveals a new anti-parallel aggregation pathway. *PLoS ONE* **2013**, *8*, e80262. [CrossRef]
37. Studier, F.W. Protein production by auto-induction in high-density shaking cultures. *Protein Expr. Purif.* **2005**, *41*, 207–234. [CrossRef]
38. Sakalauskas, A.; Ziaunys, M.; Smirnovas, V. Gallic acid oxidation products alter the formation pathway of insulin amyloid fibrils. *Sci. Rep.* **2020**, *10*, 14466. [CrossRef]
39. Jomová, K.; Hudecova, L.; Lauro, P.; Simunkova, M.; Alwasel, S.H.; Alhazza, I.M.; Valko, M. A Switch between Antioxidant and Prooxidant Properties of the Phenolic Compounds Myricetin, Morin, 3′,4′-Dihydroxyflavone, Taxifolin and 4-Hydroxy-Coumarin in the Presence of Copper(II) Ions: A Spectroscopic, Absorption Titration and DNA Damage Study. *Molecules* **2019**, *24*, 4335. [CrossRef]
40. Wormell, P.; Rodger, A. Absorption Spectroscopy: Relationship of Transition Type to Molecular Structure. In *Encyclopedia of Biophysics*; Roberts, G.C.K., Ed.; Springer: Berlin/Heidelberg, Germany, 2013; pp. 35–38. ISBN 978-3-642-16711-9.
41. Sakalauskas, A.; Ziaunys, M.; Smirnovas, V. Concentration-dependent polymorphism of insulin amyloid fibrils. *PeerJ* **2019**, *7*, e8208. [CrossRef]
42. Ma, L.; Yang, C.; Zheng, J.; Chen, Y.; Xiao, Y.; Huang, K. Non-polyphenolic natural inhibitors of amyloid aggregation. *Eur. J. Med. Chem.* **2020**, *192*, 112197. [CrossRef] [PubMed]

Article

(−)-Epicatechin—An Important Contributor to the Antioxidant Activity of Japanese Knotweed Rhizome Bark Extract as Determined by Antioxidant Activity-Guided Fractionation

Urška Jug [1,2], Katerina Naumoska [1,*] and Irena Vovk [1,*]

[1] Department of Food Chemistry, National Institute of Chemistry, Hajdrihova 19, SI-1001 Ljubljana, Slovenia; urska.jug@ki.si
[2] Faculty of Chemistry and Chemical Technology, University of Ljubljana, Večna pot 113, SI-1000 Ljubljana, Slovenia
* Correspondence: katerina.naumoska@ki.si (K.N.); irena.vovk@ki.si (I.V.); Tel.: +386-1476-0521 (K.N.); +386-1476-0341 (I.V.)

Abstract: The antioxidant activities of Japanese knotweed rhizome bark extracts, prepared with eight different solvents or solvent mixtures (water, methanol, 80% methanol$_{(aq)}$, acetone, 70% acetone$_{(aq)}$, ethanol, 70% ethanol$_{(aq)}$, and 90% ethyl acetate$_{(aq)}$), were determined using a 2,2-diphenyl-1-picrylhydrazyl (DPPH) free radical-scavenging assay. Low half maximal inhibitory concentration (IC$_{50}$) values (2.632–3.720 µg mL^{-1}) for all the extracts were in the range of the IC$_{50}$ value of the known antioxidant ascorbic acid at t$_0$ (3.115 µg mL^{-1}). Due to the highest extraction yield (~44%), 70% ethanol$_{(aq)}$ was selected for the preparation of the extract for further investigations. The IC$_{50}$ value calculated for its antioxidant activity remained stable for at least 14 days, while the IC$_{50}$ of ascorbic acid increased over time. The stability study showed that the container material was of great importance for the light-protected storage of the ascorbic acid$_{(aq)}$ solution in a refrigerator. Size exclusion–high-performance liquid chromatography (SEC-HPLC)–UV and reversed phase (RP)-HPLC-UV coupled with multistage mass spectrometry (MS^n) were developed for fractionation of the 70% ethanol$_{(aq)}$ extract and for further compound identification, respectively. In the most potent antioxidant SEC fraction, determined using an on-line post-column SEC-HPLC-DPPH assay, epicatechin, resveratrol malonyl hexoside, and its in-source fragments (resveratrol and resveratrol acetyl hexoside) were tentatively identified by RP-HPLC-MS^n. Moreover, epicatechin was additionally confirmed by two orthogonal methods, SEC-HPLC-UV and high-performance thin-layer chromatography (HPTLC) coupled with densitometry. Finally, the latter technique enabled the identification of (−)-epicatechin. (−)-Epicatechin demonstrated potent and stable time-dependent antioxidant activity (IC$_{50}$ value ~1.5 µg mL^{-1}) for at least 14 days.

Keywords: *Polygonum cuspidatum*; Reynoutria; invasive species; phenolic compounds; flavan-3-ols; stilbenes; vitamin C; size-exclusion chromatography; DPPH test; DPPH derivatization

1. Introduction

Japanese knotweed (*Fallopia japonica* Houtt.; synonyms: *Polygonum cuspidatum* Siebold & Zucc., *Reynoutria japonica* Houtt., *Polygonum reynoutria* Houtt., *Pleuropterus cuspidatus* (Siebold and Zucc.) H. Gross, *Tiniaria japonica* (Houtt.) Hedberg), which is native to East Asia, is an invasive plant species in Europe and North America [1]. The Japanese knotweed rhizome has already been tested in various biological studies [2], and its extract or existing compounds showed antioxidant [3–11], estrogenic [12], antiproliferative [3], antibacterial [13], antiviral (anti-human immunodeficiency virus) [14], anti-inflammatory [15], antiatherosclerotic [16] activities, etc. A lot of health benefits of Japanese knotweed rhizome extract were correlated with the content of some antioxidant compounds [4].

Mechanisms of antioxidant activity, such as free radical scavenging, singlet oxygen quenching, transition metal chelation, enzyme mimetic activity, and enzyme inhibition, have been described [17]. There are several methods for evaluating antioxidant activity [18,19] that are based on different mechanisms and can give results that are not comparable. A universal test does not exist; therefore, the use of at least two different methods is strongly recommended [18]. The methods can be classified according to their performance ("in vitro" and "in vivo") [19], the type of the measurement (e.g., spectrophotometric [3,5–11], electrochemical [20,21], chromatographic (gas chromatography [22], HPLC [20,21], HPTLC [23–26])), and the type of the reaction used for the assay (hydrogen atom transfer (HAT)-based assays and electron transfer (ET)-based assays) [18,21].

Among the free radical-scavenging methods, the DPPH assay is the fastest, the most straightforward, relatively inexpensive, efficient, and, therefore, the most frequently employed. Many studies on DPPH assay-guided fractionation of various plant materials have already been performed [27–40], including *on-line* methods with pre-column [27] or post-column [28–33,41] DPPH reactions. *On-line* methods for measurement of the free radical-scavenging activity indicate the antioxidant fractions/compounds in a fast and inexpensive way, without the need to isolate and test them *off-line*, which is time consuming, as described in [28].

The antioxidant activity of the Japanese knotweed rhizome has been tested and confirmed using various assays: DPPH radical-scavenging capacity [3–5,7–11]; superoxide-scavenging (nitroblue tetrazolium (NBT) reduction) capacity [4]; 2′-azinobis-[3-ethylbenzthiazolin-6-sulfonic acid] (ABTS) radical-scavenging capacity [5,6]; electron spin resonance spectrometry (ESR) [3]; oxygen radical absorption capacity (ORAC) [6]; ferric-reducing antioxidant power (FRAP) [9]; chemiluminescence [5]; phosphomolybdenum reduction [10]; lipid peroxidation inhibition performed on linoleic acid [10] and on mouse brain tissue [4]; DNA strand scission assay [3,4]; and superoxide dismutase (SOD) inhibition assay–water-soluble tetrazolium salt-1 (WST-1) [8].

Tests for determining the total polyphenol content, such as the Folin–Ciocalteu assay [4,5,9,10] have also been frequently used to estimate the antioxidant capacity of Japanese knotweed rhizomes, as the polyphenol content is generally significantly correlated to the sample's total antioxidant activity [9,18,42,43]. Phenolic compounds act as reducing agents, hydrogen donors, singlet oxygen quenchers, and metal chelators [44].

The antioxidant activities of the extracts obtained from the rhizome of Japanese knotweed and from two other knotweed species, giant knotweed (*Fallopia sachalinensis* Schm.) and their hybrid Bohemian knotweed (*Fallopia* × *bohemica* Chrtek & Chrtková), using different solvents, have already been compared [10]. The choice of solvent was shown to be of great importance for the extraction of antioxidants [10]. The relationship between the antioxidant activity and the chemical content was determined using principal component analysis (PCA) [10], showing that proanthocyanidins are the most important contributors to the total antioxidant capacity [10].

Japanese knotweed rhizome extract is already commercially available as food supplements, marketed as a source of resveratrol as an antioxidant from the stilbenes. Analyses of the bioactive compounds of Japanese knotweed rhizome extract were predominantly performed by (ultra)high-performance liquid chromatography coupled with a UV detector and (multistage) mass spectrometry ((U)HPLC-UV-MS$^{(n)}$) [6,8,10,45–51] using RP stationary phase, although HPLC-UV [11,12], HPTLC [52–55], HPTLC-MS^n [52,53], and capillary electrophoresis [56,57] were also used.

The objectives of our work were: (1) to select the most suitable solvent or solvent mixture for the extraction of antioxidants from Japanese knotweed rhizome bark; (2) to determine the antioxidant activity of Japanese knotweed rhizome bark extract; (3) to determine the stability of the antioxidant activity of the selected extract over time; (4) to fractionate the extract by a new SEC-HPLC method and to determine its most potent antioxidant fraction by an *on-line* post-column reaction with DPPH; and (5) to further identify the compounds present in the isolated antioxidant SEC fraction(s) by RP-HPLC-MS and HPTLC.

2. Materials and Methods

2.1. Chemicals and Materials

All solvents were at least of analytical grade. Methanol (HPLC and LC-MS grade), acetone, and acetonitrile (LC-MS grade) were obtained from Honeywell Reagents (Seelze, Germany). Ethanol (absolute anhydrous) was purchased from Carlo Erba Reagents (Val de Reuil, France). Ethyl acetate, acetic acid (glacial (100%) and glacial (100%) LC-MS grade), concentrated hydrochloric acid (37%), and 4-(dimethylamino)cinnamaldehyde (DMACA) were acquired from Merck (Darmstadt, Germany). Ammonium acetate, 2,2-diphenyl-1-picrylhydrazyl (DPPH), (−)-epicatechin (90%), and (−)-catechin (98%) were acquired from Sigma-Aldrich (Steinheim, Germany). Ascorbic acid was obtained from Fluka, Sigma-Aldrich (Steinheim, Germany). (−)-Epicatechin (of high purity) was purchased from Fluka Chemie (Buchs, Switzerland), while (+)-catechin (98%) was obtained from Carl Roth (Karlsruhe, Germany). A Milli-Q water purification system (18 MΩ cm^{-1}; Millipore, Bedford, MA, USA) was used to obtain ultrapure water. Disposable plastic cuvettes were purchased from Brand (Wertheim, Germany).

2.2. The Preparation, Extraction Yield, and Antioxidant Activity of Various Extracts

Japanese knotweed (*Fallopia japonica* Houtt.) rhizomes were harvested in Ljubljana, Slovenia (Vrhovci, by a bridge over the Mali Graben, N 46°02′33.9″; E 14°27′00.9″). A voucher specimen was deposited in the Herbarium LJU (LJU10143477). After the rhizomes were cleaned with tap water, the bark was peeled and lyophilized at −50 °C for 24 h (Micro Modulyo, IMAEdwards, Bologna, Italy). The obtained dry material was frozen using liquid N_2 and pulverized by a Mikro-Dismembrator S (Sartorius, Göttingen, Germany) for 1 min at a frequency of 1700 min^{-1}. The lyophilized and pulverized rhizome bark (200 mg; eight replicates) was extracted with 2 mL of the following solvents or solvent mixtures: water, methanol, 80% methanol$_{(aq)}$, acetone, 70% acetone$_{(aq)}$, ethanol, 70% ethanol$_{(aq)}$, and 90% ethyl acetate$_{(aq)}$, followed by 5 min vortexing, 15 min ultrasonication, and 5 min centrifugation at 6700× g.

The supernatants were transferred into pre-weighted glass storage vials, where the solvents were evaporated under N_2 flow. The vials with obtained dry extracts of Japanese knotweed rhizome bark (JKRB) were weighed to calculate the extraction yield. The dry extracts were further dissolved in methanol (stock solutions, which also served as first working solutions: 400 µg mL^{-1}) and diluted with the same solvent to obtain additional working solutions with the following concentrations (µg mL^{-1}): 200, 100, 50, 25, 12.5, 6.25, 3.125, 1.563, 0.781, 0.391, and 0.195. Immediately after dilution, they were tested using the DPPH assay described in [58]. The DPPH reagent (1 mL of 200 µM methanolic solution of DPPH) was added to 3 mL of each working solution in triplicate (solution A) [59].

To prepare the sample blanks, 1 mL of methanol was added to 3 mL of separate working solutions (solution B) [59]. A control sample (for DPPH) was prepared by the addition of 1 mL of DPPH reagent to 3 mL of methanol in triplicate (solution C) [59]. All prepared solutions were vortexed for 5 s and stored in amber glass storage vials for 30 min in the dark at room temperature. Spectrophotometric measurements of the absorbances of solutions A, B, and C (named A_A, A_B, and A_C, respectively; Equation (1)) were performed at 517 nm using a Lambda 45 UV/Vis spectrometer (Perkin Elmer, Waltham, MA, USA) with methanol as a blank solvent for the instrument. The IC$_{50}$ values were calculated and the curves were plotted in GraphPad Prism 7 [60].

Calculation of the DPPH scavenging effect [59]:

$$\text{DPPH scavenging effect (\%)} = 100 - ((A_A - A_B) \times 100/A_C) \quad (1)$$

in which A_B is included in the case of yellow-colored working solutions to exclude their absorbance contributions [59].

2.3. Comparison between the Antioxidant Activities of the 70% Ethanol$_{(aq)}$ Extract of Japanese Knotweed Rhizome Bark and Ascorbic Acid over Time

A DPPH assay of the selected dry 70% ethanol$_{(aq)}$ extract, re-dissolved in methanol (400 µg mL^{-1}) and diluted to the concentrations (µg mL^{-1}): 200, 100, 50, 25, 12.5, 6.25, 3.125, 1.563, 0.781, 0.391, and 0.195, and a DPPH assay of ascorbic acid dissolved in methanol (1000 µM) and diluted to the concentrations (µM): 500, 250, 100, 50, 40, 30, 20, 10, and 1, were performed at t = 0, 2, 4, 6, 8, 10, 24, and 50 h, 7 and 14 days (at T = 25 °C) after the preparation of solutions.

The influence of glass vs. plastic storage containers on the stability of ascorbic acid was studied by a 24 h aging of 50 µM aqueous ascorbic acid solutions stored in the refrigerator (T = 4 °C) or at room temperature (T = 25 °C) and: (i) protected from light in plastic centrifuge tubes (T = 4 °C), (ii) protected from light in glass storage vials (T = 4 °C), (iii) exposed to daylight in plastic centrifuge tubes (T = 25 °C), and (iv) exposed to daylight in glass flasks (T = 25 °C). HPLC-UV analyses of ascorbic acid solutions were performed at t = 0 h and at t = 24 h after solution preparation using an in-house HPLC method (confidential) at 254 nm. As ascorbic acid degrades very quickly, three fresh ascorbic acid solutions were prepared at t = 24 h to confirm the intermediate precision of the method ($n = 6$; $t_R = 3.1$ min).

2.4. SEC-HPLC-UV Fractionation of the 70% Ethanol$_{(aq)}$ JKRB Extract Guided by an On-Line Post-Column Reaction with DPPH

The SEC-HPLC-UV method was developed for the fractionation of the 70% ethanol$_{(aq)}$ extract of JKRB using an Agilent Bio SEC-3 column (150 mm × 4.6; 3 µm, 100 Å) on an HPLC-PDA Agilent Technologies 1260 Infinity system (Santa Clara, California, USA), equipped with a fraction collector (Agilent 1260 Infinity II). OpenLAB CDS ChemStation software (Agilent) was used for data collection and analysis. A pre-mixed mobile phase was prepared with 150 mM ammonium acetate buffer and ethanol in the ratio 75:25 (*v/v*).

The ammonium acetate buffer was prepared by dissolving 5.778 g of ammonium acetate in 500 mL ultrapure water, and acetic acid was used to adjust the pH value to 4.8. An isocratic elution was performed with a flow rate of 0.325 mL min^{-1} and a run time of 40 min. The temperatures of the column and autosampler were set to 40 °C and 25 °C, respectively. The dry 70% ethanol$_{(aq)}$ extract of JKRB was re-dissolved in the mobile phase to achieve a concentration of 0.5 mg mL^{-1} and was filtered through a 0.45 µm polyvinylidene fluoride (PVDF) membrane filter before injection (5 µL). Chromatograms were recorded at different wavelengths (280, 300, and 360 nm), and absorption spectra were acquired as well.

To determine the antioxidant fractions, an *on-line* post-column reaction was performed using DPPH solution (400 µM in 80% methanol$_{(aq)}$) delivered at a flow rate of 5 µL min^{-1} through a syringe pump, leading to one inlet of a T-unit. The second inlet of the T-unit was connected to the column effluent capillary, while the outlet led to a 3.5 m long reaction coil (0.13 mm internal diameter (I.D.)) and later to the photodiode array (PDA) detector. The chromatographic conditions were as explained above. The reaction coil allowed a longer contact time between the eluting fractions' compounds and the DPPH reagent, thus enabling radical scavenging reactions before reaching the PDA detector. UV/Vis spectra were acquired, and the chromatograms were recorded at 280 and 517 nm.

The decrease in absorbance at 517 nm indicated the antioxidant activity of the fractions, visible as negative peaks on the chromatogram. The *on-line* post-column reaction of the SEC fractions was performed in triplicate. Blank and control analyses were executed as follows: (i) injection of the sample extract and post-column introduction of 80% methanol$_{(aq)}$; (ii) injection of the procedural blank (the mobile phase filtered through a 0.45 µm PVDF membrane filter) and post-column reaction with DPPH; and (iii) injection of the procedural blank and post-column introduction of 80% methanol$_{(aq)}$.

As expected, the reaction coil led to a shift of the retention times (t_Rs) to higher values. Therefore, it was used for all analyses, including fraction collection, although the reaction with DPPH was not applied during this step.

Fourteen fractions, detected at 280 nm, were selected for retention time-based collection (Section 3.4). The temperature of the fraction collector was maintained at 4 °C. The collected fractions were pooled, the solvent was evaporated under N_2 flow, and the solid residues were stored in a freezer at −20 °C.

2.5. Analyses of SEC Fractions and Determination of the Strongest Antioxidant by RP-HPLC-MS

The compounds of the isolated SEC fractions were analyzed using a UHPLC-UV-MS system (Accela 1250, coupled to an LTQ Velos MS, Thermo Fisher Scientific, Waltham, MA, USA). A new HPLC-UV-MS method was developed for the separation and characterization of the compounds from the 70% ethanol$_{(aq)}$ extract of JKRB using a Hypersil ODS column (150 × 4.6 mm; 5 μm I.D., Thermo A). SEC fractions (FRs) obtained from 122 (FRs 1–7, 9, and 14), 96 (FRs 10–13), and 77 (FR 8) runs were dried under a N_2 flow, dissolved in 150 (FRs 2, 5, and 7), 200 (FRs 1, 3, and 4), 250 (FRs 6 and 9), 300 (FR 8), 500 (FR 14), and 1000 μL (FRs 10–13) of solvent (water:ethanol, 3:1, *v/v*) and injected in different volumes (5 μL: FRs 10–13; 10 μL: FRs 1, 6, 9, and 14; 15 μL: FRs 2–5, 7, and 8).

These values were adapted to the peak heights and widths of the SEC fractions. The mobile phase, consisting of 0.1% acetic acid$_{(aq)}$ (A) and acetonitrile (B), and a linear gradient elution with a flow rate of 0.7 mL min^{-1} of 10–100% B (0–30 min), were used. The column and autosampler temperatures were maintained at 25 °C and 10 °C, respectively. Chromatograms were recorded at 280, 300, and 360 nm, and absorption spectra were acquired as well. For the ionization of compounds, heated electrospray ionization (HESI) in negative ion mode was used, and the MS parameters were as follows: heater and capillary temperatures of 400 and 350 °C, respectively, sheath gas 30 arbitrary units (a.u.), auxiliary gas 5 a.u., sweep gas 0 a.u., spray voltage 4 kV, and S-Lens RF level 69.0%.

To optimize the MS parameters, a methanolic standard solution of (−)-epicatechin (0.1 mg mL^{-1}, 10 μL min^{-1}) was combined with the column effluent (55% B, 0.7 mL min^{-1}) using a T-unit, thus directing the combined flow into the MS source. The MS spectra were recorded in the *m/z* range of 50–2000, while the precursor ions of interest were fragmented in MS^n using a collision energy of 35%. Xcalibur software (version 2.1.0, Thermo Fisher Scientific) was used to evaluate the collected chromatograms and spectra.

2.6. Identification of the Compounds in the Antioxidant Fraction by Orthogonal Methods and Confirmation of Their Antioxidant Activity by DPPH Assay

To confirm the presence of (−)-epicatechin in the isolated antioxidant fraction, commercially available standards of flavan-3-ols were used. Standards of (+)-catechin and (−)-epicatechin were used for the SEC-HPLC-UV and RP-HPLC-UV-MS analyses, while for the HPTLC analysis performed on an HPTLC cellulose stationary phase, which enables separation of enantiomers, a (−)-catechin standard was also applied. Standards were prepared in concentrations of 0.01 mg mL^{-1} (in water:ethanol (3:1, *v/v*) for SEC-HPLC-UV) and 0.1 mg mL^{-1} (in methanol for RP-HPLC-UV-MS and HPTLC). The injection volume was 5 μL for both HPLC methods.

The antioxidant fraction FR 8, collected from 77 runs (by SEC-HPLC method; Section 2.4), was dissolved in 200 μL of methanol. All standards (4 μL, 0.4 μg) and the antioxidant fraction (40 μL) were applied on an HPTLC cellulose plate (Merck, Art. No. 1.05786.0001, cut to 10 cm × 10 cm) as 8 mm bands, 8 mm from the bottom of the plate using a Linomat 5 (Camag, Muttenz, Switzerland). The plate was developed up to 90 mm (45 min) in a normal developing chamber (for 10 cm × 10 cm plates, Camag) using water as a developing solvent [23,61,62] and dried with a stream of warm air for 3 min after development.

Post-chromatographic derivatization was performed by immersing the plate for 1 s into DMACA detection reagent, prepared by dissolving 60 mg of DMACA in 13 mL of concentrated hydrochloric acid (37%) and diluted with ethanol to make up a total volume of 200 mL [61]. The plate was then dried with warm air for 2 min. The DigiStore 2 documentation system in conjunction with Reprostar 3 (Camag) was used for the documentation of the chromatograms at 254 nm, 366 nm, and white light illumination after development and 10 min after post-chromatographic derivatization with DMACA reagent.

After derivatization, the plate was also scanned with a slit-scanning densitometer (TLC Scanner 3, Camag) set in absorption/reflectance mode at 655 nm. The selected wavelength was derived from our previously published studies [61,63]. The other settings were as follows: slit length 6 mm, slit width 0.30 mm, and scanning speed 20 mm s^{-1}. Both instruments were controlled using winCATS software (version 1.4.9.2001).

As in Sections 2.2 and 2.3, the spectrophotometric DPPH assay of methanolic solutions of the (−)-epicatechin standard (Sigma-Aldrich; 1000, 500, 250, 100, 50, 40, 30, 20, 10, 1, and 0.1 µM) was performed at t = 0, 2, 4, 6, 8, 10, 24, and 50 h, 7 and 14 days (storage at T = 25 °C) after solution preparation to determine its IC_{50} value for the radical scavenging activity, as well as the stability of its antioxidant activity.

3. Results and Discussion

3.1. Extraction Yields and Antioxidant Activity of Various Extracts

The extraction of JKRB was performed with water, polar organic solvents (methanol, acetone, and ethanol), and aqueous solutions thereof (80% methanol$_{(aq)}$, 70% acetone$_{(aq)}$, 70% ethanol$_{(aq)}$, and 90% ethyl acetate$_{(aq)}$). The highest extraction yield was achieved by 70% ethanol$_{(aq)}$, and a slightly lower yield was achieved by 70% acetone$_{(aq)}$ (Table 1). Significantly lower extraction yields were obtained with pure ethanol and acetone. The difference between the extraction yields obtained with methanol and 80% methanol$_{(aq)}$ was not significant. Water gave a higher extraction yield than did pure acetone. The lowest extraction yield was obtained using 90% ethyl acetate$_{(aq)}$ (Table 1).

Table 1. The extraction yields and the calculated values of the half maximal inhibitory concentrations (IC_{50}) of antioxidant activity (GraphPad Prism 7 [60]) of extracts prepared with different solvents or solvent mixtures tested in the concentration range of 0.195–400 µg mL^{-1}.

	Extraction Solvents							
	Water	Methanol		Acetone		Ethanol		Ethyl Acetate
		100%	80% $_{(aq)}$	100%	70% $_{(aq)}$	100%	70% $_{(aq)}$	90% $_{(aq)}$
Extraction yield (w/w %)	25.8	38.1	37.2	21.1	42.6	29.3	44.3	14.9
IC_{50} (µg mL^{-1})	3.561	3.715	3.469	2.632	3.350	2.893	3.503	2.786
$LogIC_{50}$	0.552	0.570	0.540	0.420	0.525	0.461	0.544	0.445
$LogIC_{50}$ std. error	0.016	0.014	0.022	0.018	0.017	0.016	0.014	0.020
Hillslope	1.607	1.884	1.669	1.911	1.665	1.924	1.789	1.756
Hillslope std. error	0.083	0.105	0.125	0.136	0.097	0.123	0.093	0.124

The antioxidant activities of all dry extracts, re-dissolved in methanol, were tested using a DPPH assay. Re-dissolving all dry extracts in the same solvent (methanol) was preferred (providing equal polarity and pH of the reaction medium for all extracts) to enable comparison of the obtained DPPH assay results, as discussed in [58]. As all dry extracts and DPPH were soluble in methanol, this was selected as a reaction medium.

The obtained results of the DPPH radical scavenging assay are expressed as IC_{50} values, which represent the concentration of the antioxidant required to scavenge 50% of the DPPH free radicals and consequently lead to a 50% decrease in the DPPH absorption [64–66].

As different protocols of the same antioxidant assay may lead to incomparable results, a known antioxidant, ascorbic acid, was used as a reference. The IC_{50} values of all JKRB extracts (Figure 1) prepared by different extraction solvents and solvent mixtures were very low (2.632–3.715 µg mL^{-1}; Table 1) and in the range of the IC_{50} value of ascorbic acid at t_0 (3.115 µg mL^{-1}; Table 2). This indicates the high antioxidant potential of JKRB extracts, which may be attributed to the activity of the various phenolic compounds present in JKRB [67]. A JKRB extract prepared with 70% ethanol$_{(aq)}$ was used for further analyses due to the highest extraction yield (only 70% acetone$_{(aq)}$ resulted in a comparable yield) (Table 1). Additional reasons for the selection of this green extraction solvent include that ethanol is considered less harmful than other solvents when present as a residual solvent in pharmaceutical formulations [68], 70% ethanol$_{(aq)}$ is suitable for the preparation of tinctures, and ethanol is commercially available as a "food grade" solvent.

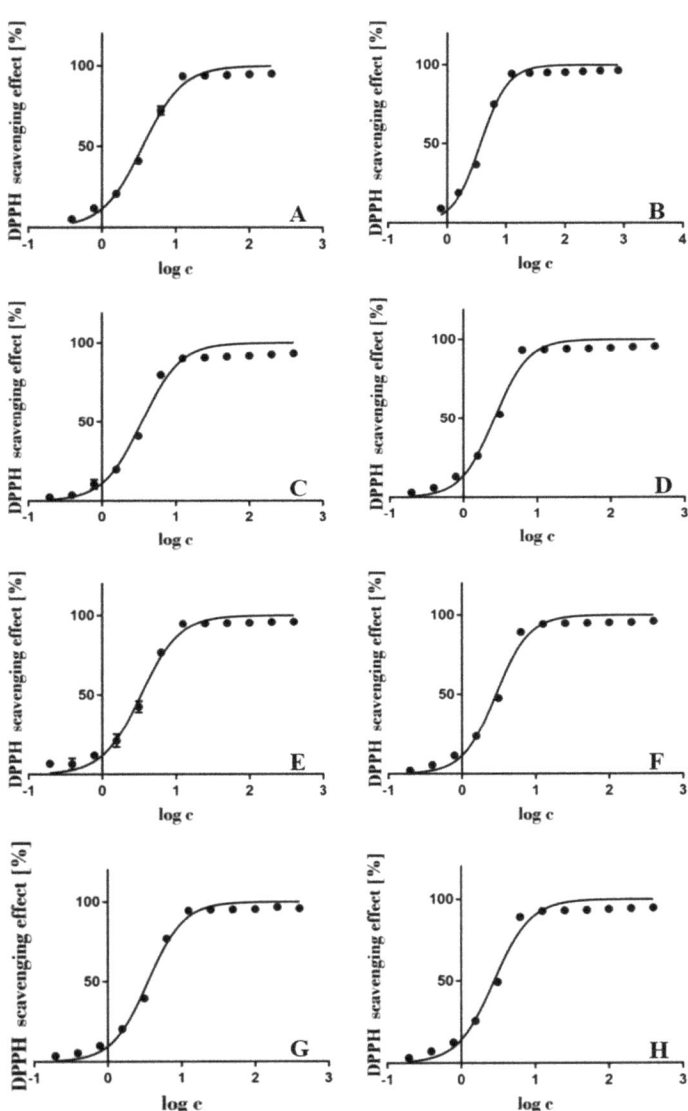

Figure 1. Logarithmic curves of the antioxidant activities of extracts of Japanese knotweed rhizome bark (JKRB) (n = 3) prepared with the following solvents and solvent mixtures: water (**A**), methanol (**B**), 80% methanol$_{(aq)}$ (**C**), acetone (**D**), 70% acetone$_{(aq)}$ (**E**), ethanol (**F**), 70% ethanol$_{(aq)}$ (**G**), and 90% ethyl acetate$_{(aq)}$ (**H**). The calculated values of IC$_{50}$ are 3.561 (**A**), 3.715 (**B**), 3.469 (**C**), 2.632 (**D**), 3.350 (**E**), 2.893 (**F**), 3.503 (**G**), and 2.786 (**H**) µg mL^{-1} (obtained by GraphPad Prism 7 [60]).

Table 2. The calculated IC_{50} values of the antioxidant activity of ascorbic acid (AA, in the range 1–1000 μM or 0.176–176.12 μg mL^{-1}) and JKRB 70% ethanol$_{(aq)}$ extract (in the range 0.195–400 μg mL^{-1}) over time.

	0 h	2 h	4 h	6 h	8 h	24 h	50 h	7 d	14 d
IC_{50} AA (μM)	17.6853.1	30.524	37.662	45.846	56.612	~96.886	164.933	~219.382	356.495
IC_{50} AA (μg mL^{-1})	15	5.376	6.633	8.075	9.971	~17.064	29.049	~38.637	62.787
$LogIC_{50}$ (μM)	1.248	1.485	1.576	1.661	1.753	~1.986	2.217	~2.341	2.552
$LogIC_{50}$ std. error	0.011	0.005	0.003	0.006	0.006	~1.293	0.020	~33.874	0.015
Hillslope	2.606	5.344	6.492	6.060	5.673	~17.640	7.444	~16.268	9.400
Hillslope std. error	0.149	0.304	0.254	0.566	0.383	~1659.493	0.771	~9712.611	0.938
IC_{50} JKRB (μg mL^{-1})	3.503	3.684	3.662	3.876	3.947	3.530	3.759	3.731	3.325
$LogIC_{50}$	0.544	0.566	0.564	0.588	0.596	0.548	0.575	0.572	0.522
$LogIC_{50}$ std. error	0.014	0.013	0.015	0.017	0.021	0.016	0.011	0.014	0.024
Hillslope	1.789	1.815	1.858	1.796	1.736	2.044	1.933	1.737	1.531
Hillslope std. error	0.093	0.086	0.106	0.117	0.128	0.140	0.085	0.088	0.118

The logarithmic curves representing the radical scavenging activity of the extracts of JKRB with different concentrations are shown in Figure 1.

A time-dependent decrease in the antioxidant activity (increase in the IC_{50} value) of the ascorbic acid solutions was observed, which is most likely a consequence of its oxidation, which can particularly be promoted by light, heat, and heavy metal cations [69]. Therefore, the preparation of the ascorbic acid solutions was carried out very quickly, and the time from their preparation to exposure to DPPH was kept as short as possible (10 min in the worst-case scenario). The addition of the chelating agent ethylenediaminetetraacetic acid (EDTA) to ascorbic acid solution was previously found to have an indirect stabilizing effect on the ascorbic acid molecule through the chelation of traces of heavy metals residing on the surface of glass containers [70]. To examine the influence of glass vs. plastic storage containers on the stability of ascorbic acid in solution, its content after storage in different containers was determined by the use of the HPLC-UV method (Section 3.2).

3.2. Antioxidant Activity over Time—Ascorbic Acid Compared to the JKRB 70% Ethanol$_{(aq)}$ Extract

The antioxidant activity of ascorbic acid continuously decreased over time (IC_{50} value increased from 3.115 up to 62.787 μg mL^{-1}, Table 2, Figure 2A), while the antioxidant activity of the JKRB 70% ethanol$_{(aq)}$ extract remained constant during the same time interval (0 h to 14 days) (Table 2, Figure 2B). These results suggest a potential use of the JKRB 70% ethanol$_{(aq)}$ extract as a strong antioxidant material. The potential applications might include the formulation of food supplements (e.g., tincture, powder, and solid dosage forms) or its utilization as a food antioxidant. On the other hand, the stability of ascorbic acid (and its antioxidant effect) in various beverages (bottled and left standing) rich in or enriched with ascorbic acid remains questionable.

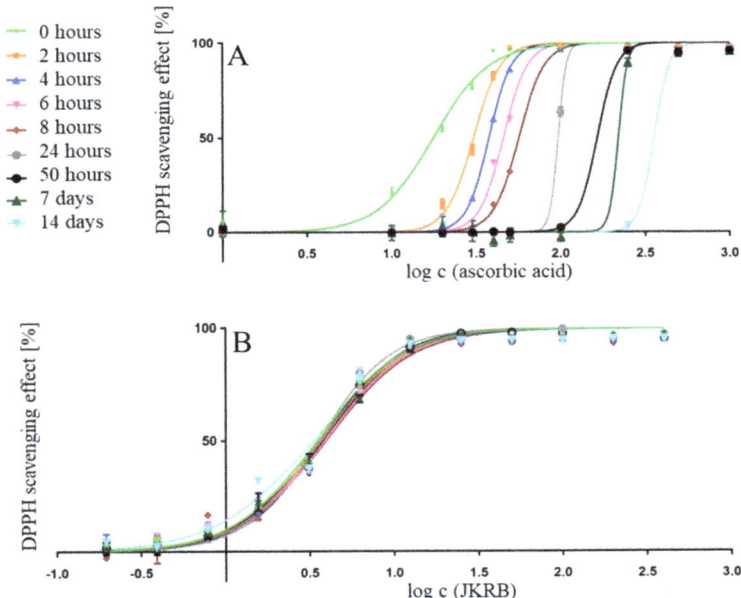

Figure 2. Logarithmic curves plotting the 2,2-diphenyl-1-picrylhydrazyl (DPPH) scavenging effect (%) of ascorbic acid (**A**) and JKRB 70% ethanol$_{(aq)}$ extract (**B**) against the concentration, measured over time.

As the mobile phase used for the HPLC quantification of ascorbic acid was aqueous based, ascorbic acid for the HPLC analyses was dissolved in water. After 24 h of aging in daylight and at room temperature, practically all ascorbic acid was lost (ascorbic acid <1%), regardless of the container material used for storage. On the other hand, the container material was of great importance for the light-protected storage of the ascorbic acid$_{(aq)}$ solution in the refrigerator. After 24 h of aging (dark, refrigerator) in a plastic container, the content of ascorbic acid$_{(aq)}$ was 65.19% of the initial concentration, while storage in a glass container resulted in a loss (<1% of the initial concentration) comparable to that reported for the room conditions (room temperature and daylight).

Based on these results, the combination of light and temperature, as well as trace metals on the glass surface, influence the stability of ascorbic acid in aqueous solution (Figure 3). On the other hand, the JKRB extract showed stable antioxidant activity for at least 14 days in the worst-case scenario conditions for ascorbic acid (light, room temperature, glass container). The flavan-3-ols, proanthocyanidins, and anthraquinones, which represent major groups of compounds in the JKRB extract [67], are proven chelating agents of glass surface ions [71,72], acting through their hydroxyl or both carbonyl and hydroxyl groups, located on the vicinal or *peri* positions [71]. This supports our findings regarding the stability of the measured antioxidant activity of the JKRB extract.

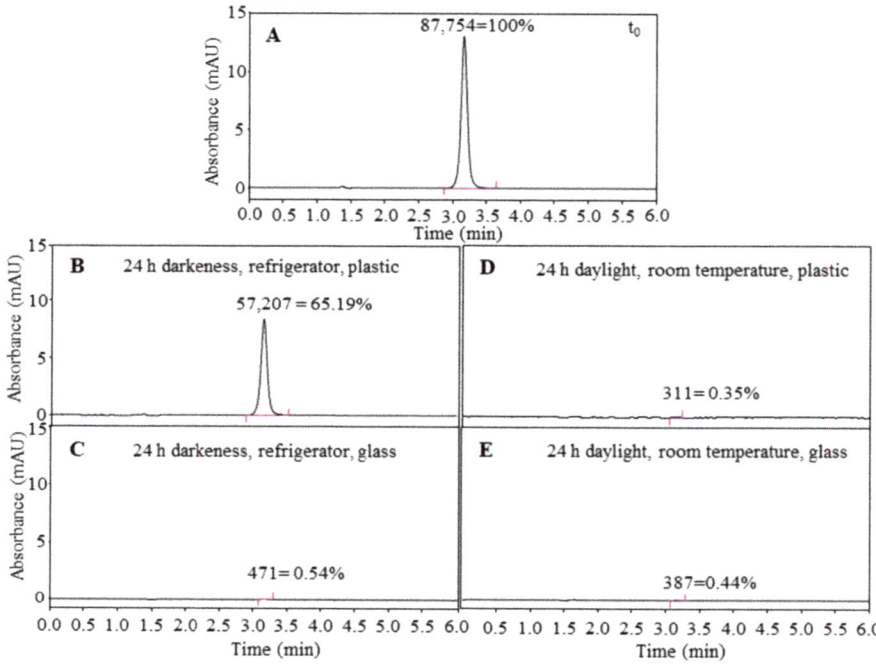

Figure 3. Ascorbic acid$_{(aq)}$ (50 µM) analyzed immediately after preparation (**A**) was subjected to 24 h of aging (**B–E**), stored in the refrigerator and protected from light (**B,C**) in plastic (**B**) and glass containers (**C**) or stored in daylight at room temperature (**D,E**) in plastic (**D**) and glass containers (**E**). The peak areas corresponding to ascorbic acid (t_R 3.1 min, 254 nm) in aged solutions were compared to the peak area of ascorbic acid in the fresh solution. The intermediate precision of the method was 3% (n = 6).

3.3. SEC-HPLC Fractionation of the JKRB 70% Ethanol$_{(aq)}$ Extract, On-Line Post-Column Reaction of the SEC Fractions with DPPH and Determination of the Antioxidant Fractions

A SEC-HPLC-UV method was developed for the first time to separate the compounds from the Japanese knotweed rhizome extract. A SEC column with a pore size of 100 Å was used to enable better separation of the smaller molecules from the extract. A high concentration of the buffer (150 mM) was used to reduce the secondary interactions on the column. Ethanol as a co-solvent, mixed with the buffer in a ratio of 25:75 (v/v), improved the solubility of JKRB compounds in the mobile phase. A higher percentage of ethanol in the mobile phase causes precipitation of the ammonium acetate buffer. The chromatograms were recorded at 280 nm, where the highest sensitivity for most of the compounds was achieved. Fourteen of the most abundant fractions (FR 1–FR 14) were selected for isolation.

The antioxidant potential of the Japanese knotweed rhizome bark was tested for the first time using the SEC-HPLC-UV/Vis method with an *on-line* post-column DPPH assay. Finding the right concentration, flow rate, and solvent for the DPPH reagent (insoluble in water and soluble in methanol) to be introduced into the mobile phase (buffer insoluble in methanol) was challenging. However, a 400 µM DPPH solution in 80% methanol$_{(aq)}$, delivered at a flow rate of 5 µL min^{-1}, proved to be a good choice as it did not cause precipitations in the system upon contact with the mobile phase. The isocratic elution of the SEC method enabled the constant solubility of the DPPH reagent in the mobile phase and equal chemical reaction conditions throughout the whole run, thus ensuring more relevant results related to the antioxidant activity in comparison to gradient mode chromatography (e.g., RP in the gradient mode).

The noisy baseline of the chromatogram at 517 nm (Figure 4) was most probably due to the imperfections of the in-house built equipment for *on-line* post-column derivatization. Therefore, some antioxidant fractions might have been overlooked, due to a potentially too low decrease in the baseline at 517 nm. However, FR 8, eluting at t_R 16.8–18 min (Figure 4), was undoubtedly determined as the most potent antioxidant (a clear baseline drop at 517 nm). Although only FR 8 showed antioxidant activity, all fractions (FR 1–FR 14, Figure 4) were collected and screened using RP-HPLC.

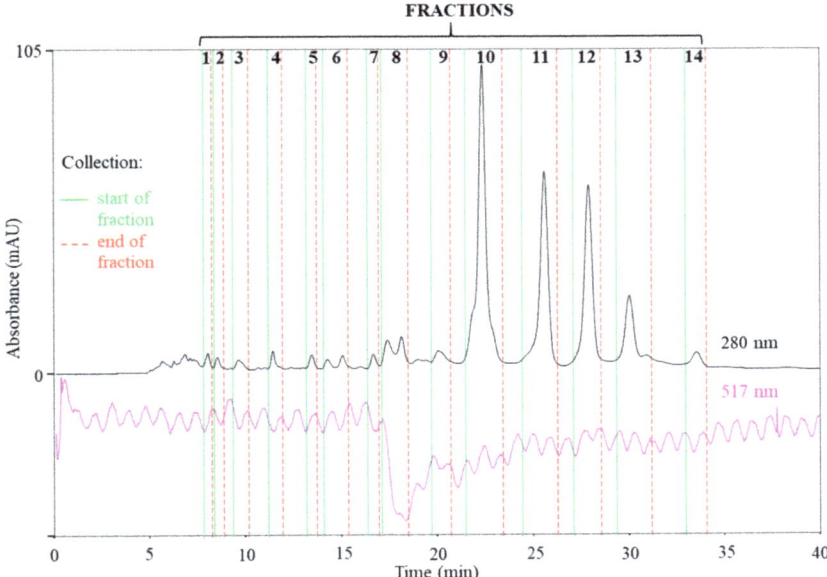

Figure 4. SEC-HPLC-UV/Vis chromatogram at 280 nm (without post-column reaction) and at 517 nm (after post-column reaction with DPPH). The fractions and time intervals selected for fraction collection are marked. Fraction 8 was determined to be the strongest antioxidant due to the decrease in the absorbance at 517 nm.

3.4. Characterization of the Compounds in the Isolated SEC Fractions, Identification of the Antioxidant Fraction Compounds by Orthogonal Methods, and their Antioxidant Activity over Time

An RP-HPLC-MS^n method was developed to analyze the compounds in the isolated SEC fractions. The compounds were tentatively identified by comparing the obtained and literature MS and MS^2 data (Table 3). For the antioxidant fraction FR 8, MS^3 was also performed. Although expected, the size distribution of the SEC eluting compounds (from larger to smaller molecular masses) was not obvious (Table 3). One of the possible explanations relates to the content of the organic solvent (25%) in the mobile phase, which might promote secondary interactions and might subsequently impact the distribution of the compounds.

The presence of flavan-3-ol monomer, as the main representative in the antioxidant fraction FR 8, was suspected based on the mass spectra and fragmentation patterns, which were compared to those of the (−)-epicatechin standard (Figure 5) and to the literature data [52,53,67]. MS signals of resveratrol malonyl hexoside, resveratrol, and resveratrol acetyl hexoside were also observed in FR 8, where the last two most likely corresponded to in-source fragments of resveratrol malonyl hexoside [67]. Additional MS signals (Table 3) were not identified due to their low abundance.

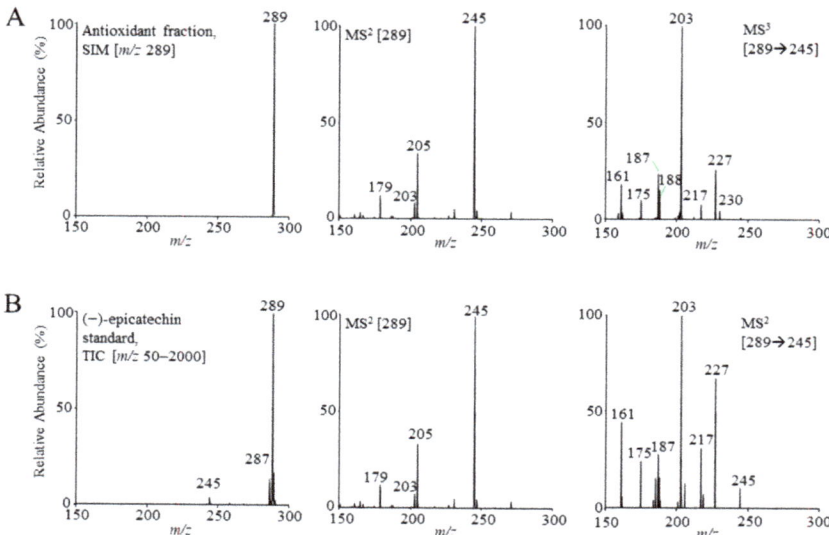

Figure 5. The flavan-3-ol monomer identified by (−)ESI-MS based on the mass spectra and fragmentation patterns obtained for the signal at t_R 6.4 min in the antioxidant fraction (FR 8) (**A**) and confirmed by (−)-epicatechin standard (**B**). Figure abbreviations: selected ion monitoring (SIM), and total ion current (TIC).

In our previous study [67], (+)-catechin and (−)-epicatechin were identified as the two main flavan-3-ol monomers in JKRB. Therefore, both standards were analyzed using the developed RP-HPLC-MS method, which resulted in the separation of (−)-epicatechin (t_R 6.4 min) and (+)-catechin (t_R 5.6 min) (Figure 6). The presence of epicatechin (Figure 6) was thus confirmed in FR 8 (Figures 5 and 6).

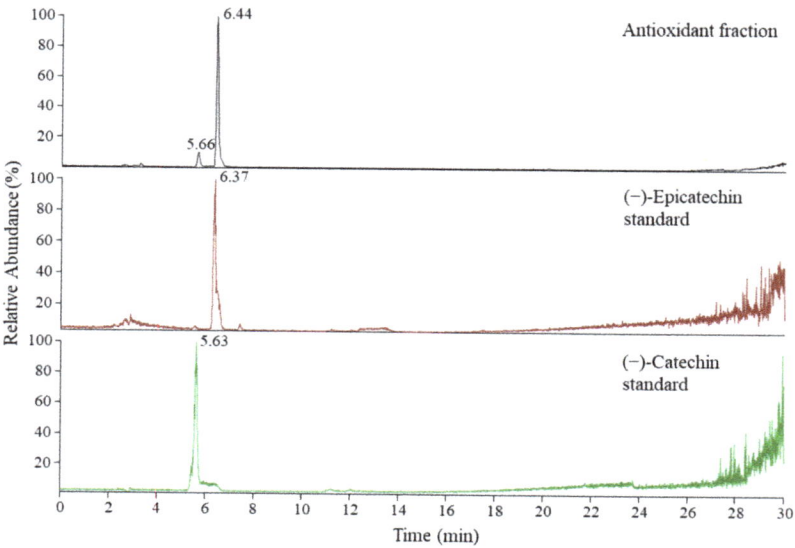

Figure 6. RP-HPLC-MS chromatograms of the antioxidant fraction (FR 8) in SIM mode (m/z 289), (−)-epicatechin and (+)-catechin standards (both in TIC mode; m/z 50–2000).

The (−)-epicatechin and (+)-catechin standards were also analyzed using the SEC-HPLC method and the t_R of (−)-epicatechin (17.2 min) matched the t_R range of the antioxidant fraction FR 8 (16.8–18.0 min) (Figure 7), while (+)-catechin (t_R 19.8 min) eluted at the t_R range of FR 9 (19.4–19.8 min). MS signals of flavan-3-ols at m/z 289 were observed by RP-HPLC-MS in both fractions (Table 3). Unexpectedly, catechin and epicatechin diastereoisomers were separated by SEC-HPLC (Figure 7), likely due to their conformational differences or as a consequence of secondary interactions in the column. However, C18-RP-HPLC and SEC-HPLC methods do not enable distinguishing between the enantiomers ((+)-catechin and (−)-catechin; (+)-epicatechin and (−)-epicatechin). According to our previous study [67], the presence of diastereoisomer (−)-epicatechin in FR 8 and (+)-catechin in FR 9, was suspected.

Matching UV spectra of the isolated epicatechin in FR 8 and (−)-epicatechin standard obtained by RP-HPLC and SEC-HPLC methods (λ_{max} at 230 and 280 nm—data not shown) showed that epicatechin is the main compound of the most potent antioxidant fraction, FR 8.

To confirm the presence of (−)-epicatechin, HPTLC analysis of FR 8 and three standards, (−)-epicatechin, (+)-catechin, and (−)-catechin, was performed on the cellulose stationary phase, which acts as a chiral selector. (+)-Epicatechin was not applied on the plate as it is not commercially available. Derivatization of the chromatograms with the DMACA detection reagent (flavan-3-ol-specific reagent) confirmed the presence of (−)-epicatechin in FR 8 (matching R_F values of the bands of FR 8 and the (−)-epicatechin standard; Figure 8). In addition to the band for (−)-epicatechin, another poorly resolved band appeared in FR 8 (Figure 8, track 1), which also showed a positive reaction with DMACA. The presence of the two peaks was also confirmed densitometrically (Figure 9).

Resveratrol malonyl hexoside, which was also detected in the antioxidant fraction, was reported for the first time in the Japanese knotweed rhizome in our previous study [67]. Unfortunately, the standard of this compound is not commercially available, thus, an additional confirmation of its presence in the antioxidant fraction was not possible (too low an amount for nuclear magnetic resonance (NMR) spectroscopy).

The antioxidant potential of resveratrol, an aglycone moiety of resveratrol malonyl hexoside, is already well known, and resveratrol's presence has also been linked to the antioxidant potential of the Japanese knotweed rhizome [8,73]. Resveratrol may cause synergistic or additive antioxidant effects in combination with epicatechin or other extract constituents (Table 3). Recently, an important contribution to the high antioxidant potential of this plant material was attributed to flavan-3-ols and proanthocyanidins [10]. Epicatechin was confirmed in the antioxidant fraction by three orthogonal methods, SEC-HPLC, RP-HPLC-MS, and HPTLC, among which the latter enabled the identification of (−)-epicatechin, which was already recognized as an antioxidant [18,29,42].

We also compared the antioxidant activities of (−)-epicatechin and *trans*-resveratrol standards by DPPH assay. The results showed that (−)-epicatechin is a stronger DPPH radical scavenger than *trans*-resveratrol (higher IC$_{50}$; 7.08 μg/mL or 31.02 μM). Moreover, (−)-epicatechin was shown to be present in higher quantities in Japanese knotweed rhizome bark in comparison to *trans*-resveratrol [11].

Table 3. RP-HPLC-MS analysis of the compounds in the SEC-HPLC-UV fractions (FR 1–FR 14), corresponding to the SEC t_R ranges (FR 1: 7.7–8.0, FR 2: 8.3–8.6, FR 3: 9.3–9.8, FR 4: 11.0–11.7, FR 5: 13.0–13.4, FR 6: 13.6–15.0, FR 7: 16.1–16.6, FR 8: 16.8–18.0, FR 9: 19.4–19.8, FR 10: 20.8–22.9, FR 11: 24.0–25.5, FR 12: 26.4–27.8, FR 13: 28.7–30.2, and FR 14: 32.0–32.9). Different numbers of collection runs were performed to isolate the SEC fractions: 122 (FRs 1–7, 9, 14), 96 (FRs 10–13), and 77 (FR 8). Fractions were dissolved in different volumes of water:ethanol (3:1, v/v): 150 (FRs 2, 5, 7), 200 (FRs 1, 3, 4), 250 (FRs 6, 9), 300 (FR 8), 500 (FR 14), and 1000 µL (FRs 10–13) and injected in different volumes (5 (FRs 10–13), 10 (FRs 1, 6, 9, 14), and 15 µL (FRs 2–5, 7, 8)) into the RP-HPLC-MS system.

FR	t_R [min] [a]	MS [M-H]⁻	MS² and MS³ [b]	Tentatively Identified Compounds
1	6.9	395	[395]: 215	derivative of emodin bianthrone-hexose-malonic acid [10] [c]
	10.2, 9.4	1005	[1005]: 713, 917, 961, 458	[c]
	7.3	521	[521]: 359	[c]
2	7.3	581	[581]: 521, 522, 544, 563, 499, 483, 417	[c]
	7.3	603	[603]: 543, 521	[c]
	10.2	919	[919]: 713, 671, 875, 458, 509, 416	emodin bianthrone-hexose-(malonic acid)-hexose [10]
	10.2	941	No data	[c]
3	11.4, 12.2	933	[933]: 889, 458, 727	methyl derivative of emodin bianthrone-hexose-(malonic acid)-hexose [10]
	10.2	919	[919]: 713, 671, 875, 458, 416, 509	emodin bianthrone-hexose-(malonic acid)-hexose [10]
	10.2	1005	[1005]: 917, 961, 875, 713, 458	derivative of emodin bianthrone-hexose-malonic acid [10]
	10.2, 12.0	1027	[1027]: 939, 983, 735 (10.2 min) [1027]: 389, 489, 533, 449, 744, 862, 939, 983, 994 (12.0 min)	[c]
4	12.3	1009	[1009]: 471, 389, 515, 921, 965	[c]
	12.3	987	[987]: 449, 943	[c]
	12.3	449	[449]: 245	torachrysone 8-O-(6'-O-acetyl)-glucoside [67]
	6.6, 10.6	473	[473]: 455, 413 (6.6 min) [473]: 269 (10.6 min)	emodin-O-(acetyl)-hexoside [67]
5	6.6, 10.6	605	[605]: 587	[c]
	6.6, 10.6	665	[665]: 647, 605, 589, 545, 501, 567	[c]
	10.6, 20.6	269	[269]: 225, 269, 251, 241, 187	emodin [67,74]
	11.2	265	No data	[c]
	11.2	297	No data	[c]
6	11.2, 11.8	1005, 502, 458	[1005]: 713, 917, 458	derivative of emodin bianthrone-hexose-malonic acid [10]
	11.2, 11.8	1027	[1027]: 781, 863, 699, 715, 945, 617	[c]
	13.7	1019, 975	[1019]: 691, 773, 855, 609, 527, 937	derivative of bianthrone [10]
	11.2	265	No data	[c]
7	11.6	407	[407]: 245	torachrysone-8-O-glucoside/procyanidin degradation product [67]
	13.5	933	[933]: 889, 685, 416	methyl derivative of emodin bianthrone-hexose-(malonic acid)-hexose [10]
	13.5	1019	No data	[c]

Table 3. Cont.

FR	t_R [a] [min]	MS [M-H]−	MS[2] and MS[3] [b]	Tentatively Identified Compounds
	5.6, 6.3	289	[289]: 245, 205, 179, 203; [289→245] b: 203, 227, 161, 175, 187, 217, 245	(−)-epicatechin (6.32 min) [67], (−)-epicatechin standard
	9.2, 8.3	431	[431]: 227, 389	resveratrol acetyl hexoside [67]
	9.7, 9.0, 8.3	445	[445]: 385 (9.7 min)	c
8			[445]: 281, 325, 369, 427, 263, 211 (9.0, 8.3 min)	c
	9.2, 8.3	475	[475]: 431	resveratrol malonyl hexoside [67]
	9.2, 8.3	491	[491]: 431	c
	9.2, 8.3	227	[227]: 185, 183, 159, 157, 227, 209, 143	resveratrol [52,67]
	5.6, 6.3	289	[289]: 245, 205, 179, 203;	(−)-epicatechin (6.32 min) [67], (−)-epicatechin standard
	5.6	289	[289]: 245, 205, 203, 179	catechin [67]
	9.9	431	[431]: 269	emodin-O-hexoside [67]
9	9.9, 20.5	269	[269]: 269, 225, 241, 251, 209, 271	emodin [67,74]
	9.9	385	No data	c
	7.1, 8.9	389	[389]: 227	polydatin (piceid)/resveratroloside [67]
	7.1, 8.9	425d	[425]: 389	polydatin (piceid) (dihydrate)/resveratroloside (dihydrate) [67]
	7.1	449d	[449]: 389, 227	resveratrol acetyl hexoside (hydrate) [67]
10	7.1, 8.9	227	[227]: 185, 183, 159, 157, 209, 143, 165	resveratrol [67]
	10.8	473	[473]: 269, 311	emodin-O-(acetyl)-hexoside [67]
	10.8	517	[517]: 473, 431	emodin-O-(6′-O-malony)-hexoside [67]
	6.6, 8.3	405	[405]: 243	piceatannol-3-O-glucoside [10]
11	6.6, 8.3	243	[243]: 225, 201, 199, 175, 215, 159	piceatannol [75]
	7.9, 9.1	389	[389]: 227	polydatin (piceid)/resveratroloside [67]
	7.9, 9.1	227	[227]: 185, 183, 209, 159, 157, 165, 143	resveratrol [67]
12	7.9, 9.1	425 d	[425]: 389, 227	polydatin (piceid) (dihydrate)/resveratroloside (dihydrate) [67]
	11.6	431	[431]: 269, 311, 413	emodin-O-hexoside [67]
13	11.6	269	[269]: 225, 269, 241, 251	emodin [67,74]
	4.9	565	No data	c
	7.2, 9.5	245	[245]: 230 (7.2 min)	c [67]
			[245]: 229 (230) (9.5 min)	c [67]
14	7.2, 9.5	325 d	[325]: 245 (7.2 min)	catechin dihydrate/unknown [67]
	7.2, 9.5	245	[325]: 244 (245), 203, 283 (9.5 min)	catechin dihydrate/unknown [67]

[a] t_R obtained by RP-HPLC-ESI-MS; [b] MS[3]; [c] Not identified; [d] [M-H+(2)H$_2$O].

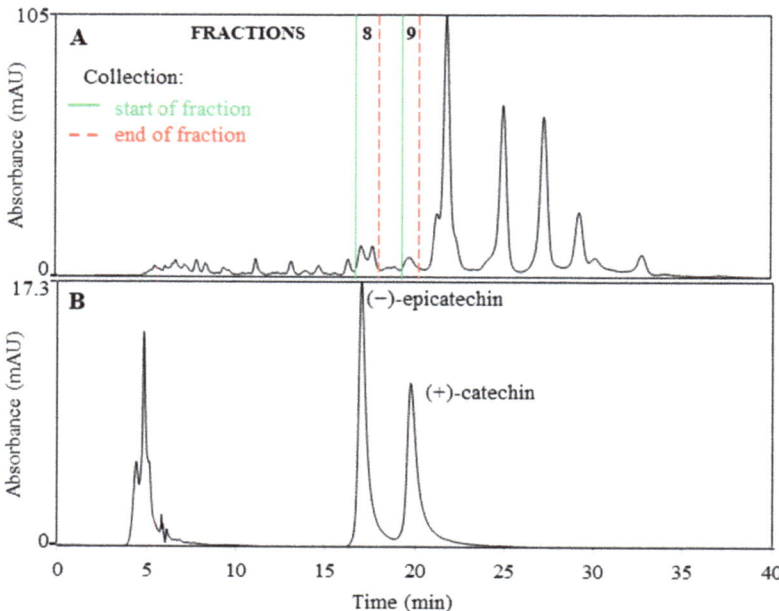

Figure 7. Matching the t_{RS} of the antioxidant fraction FR 8 (**A**) and (−)-epicatechin (**B**), and the t_{RS} of FR 9 (**A**) and (+)-catechin (**B**). Chromatograms were acquired at 280 nm using the SEC-HPLC method.

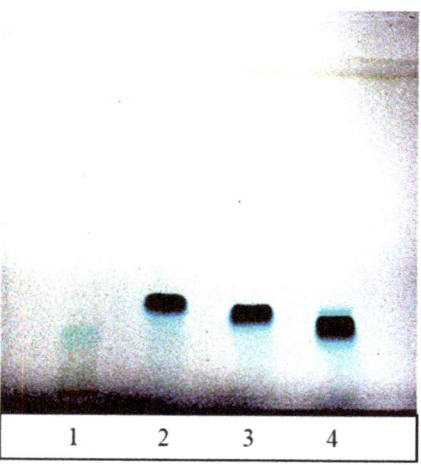

Figure 8. Chromatogram of FR 8 (**track 1**, 40 μL), (+)-catechin (**track 2**, 400 ng), (−)-catechin (**track 3**, 400 ng), and (−)-epicatechin (**track 4**, 400 ng) applied as 8 mm bands on the HPTLC cellulose plate developed with water, derivatized with DMACA reagent, and documented with illumination with white light.

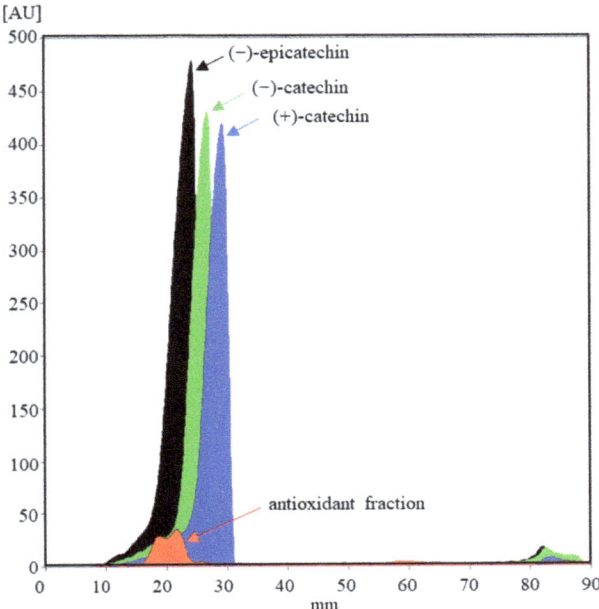

Figure 9. Densitograms of FR 8 (40 µL) and monomeric flavan-3-ol standards (400 ng) scanned at 655 nm in the absorption/reflectance mode on the HPTLC cellulose plate developed with water and derivatized with DMACA.

As in previous experiments with 70% ethanolic$_{(aq)}$ JKRB extract and ascorbic acid methanolic solutions (Sections 3.1 and 3.2), a spectrophotometric DPPH assay was performed to determine the IC$_{50}$ value of the free radical scavenging potential of the methanolic solutions of (−)-epicatechin and to test the stability of its antioxidant activity over time (t = 0, 2, 4, 6, 8, 24, and 50 h, and 7 and 14 d). The IC$_{50}$ value of the radical scavenging of (−)-epicatechin was ~1.56 µg mL^{-1}, which indicated a higher antioxidant activity compared to that of ascorbic acid. Surprisingly, the antioxidant activity of the (−)-epicatechin standard remained constant over time (0 h to 14 days; ~1.56 µg mL^{-1}) (Figure 10, Table 4).

The low IC$_{50}$ value of (−)-epicatechin's radical scavenging potential and the stability of its antioxidant activity for at least 14 days indicated that (−)-epicatechin could represent one of the most important contributors to the antioxidant activity of the JKRB extract. The reaction of antioxidants with DPPH is influenced by steric hindrance, with a preference for small antioxidant molecules [18]. Therefore, the antioxidant potential of fractions composed of different molecules is only indicative [18]. The results of the radical scavenging activity of JKRB extract, ascorbic acid, and (−)-epicatechin could not be directly compared to the results of other antioxidant assays.

The antioxidant potential of the whole extract may be the result of a synergistic or additive effect of different matrix compounds, which may be even more potent compared to the isolated single compounds' effect either in the human body [18] or as food antioxidants [76,77]. In the current study, a high time-dependent stability (up to 14 days) of the antioxidant activities of the JKRB extract and (−)-epicatechin (standard solution) was observed.

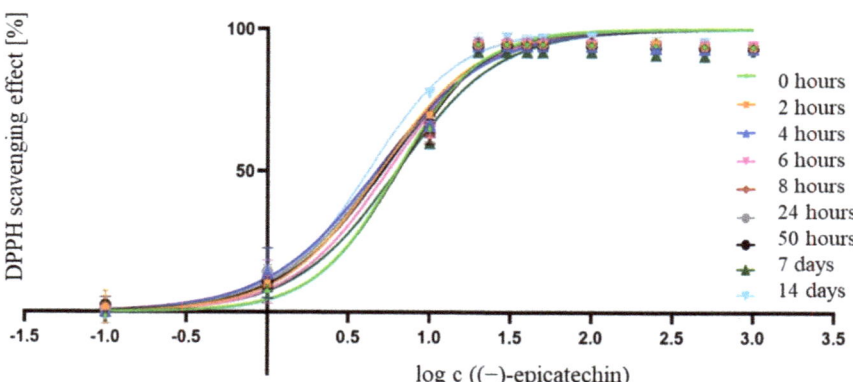

Figure 10. Logarithmic curves plotting the DPPH scavenging effect (%) of (−)-epicatechin against the concentration, measured over time.

Table 4. The calculated IC_{50} values of the antioxidant activity of (−)-epicatechin tested in the range of 0.1–1000 μM or 0.029–290 μg mL^{-1} over time.

	0 h	2 h	4 h	6 h	8 h	24 h	50 h	7 d	14 d
IC_{50} (μM)	6.298	4.967	4.738	5.539	6.393	4.949	5.129	6.280	4.190
IC_{50} (μg mL^{-1})	1.828	1.442	1.375	1.608	1.856	1.436	1.489	1.823	1.216
LogIC_{50}	0.799	0.696	0.676	0.744	0.806	0.695	0.710	0.798	0.622
LogIC_{50} std. error	0.039	0.040	0.047	0.045	0.043	0.044	0.041	0.052	0.039
Hillslope	1.690	1.427	1.282	1.441	1.669	1.315	1.367	1.375	1.538
Hillslope std. error	0.176	0.110	0.106	0.134	0.188	0.107	0.109	0.153	0.112

4. Conclusions

Antioxidant activities of Japanese knotweed rhizome bark extracts prepared with water, methanol, 80% methanol$_{(aq)}$, acetone, 70% acetone$_{(aq)}$, ethanol, 70% ethanol$_{(aq)}$, and 90% ethyl acetate$_{(aq)}$ were measured using a DPPH free radical-scavenging assay (IC_{50} = 3.561, 3.715, 3.469, 2.632, 3.350, 2.893, 3.503, and 2.786 μg mL^{-1}, respectively). Due to the highest extraction yield, the 70% ethanol$_{(aq)}$ extract was selected for further fractionation.

A SEC method was developed for the first time for fractionation of the Japanese knotweed rhizome (bark) extract. Its antioxidant potential was tested for the first time using the SEC-HPLC-UV/Vis method with an on-line post-column DPPH assay. This approach can also be used for the isolation of other plant bioactive constituents. The compounds in the isolated SEC fractions were determined with a new RP-HPLC-UV-MS^n method. Epicatechin was confirmed in the antioxidant fraction by three orthogonal methods, SEC-HPLC-UV, RP-HPLC-MS, and HPTLC, among which the latter enabled the identification of (−)-epicatechin. The antioxidant activity of the (−)-epicatechin standard was additionally proven with a DPPH free radical-scavenging assay.

The IC_{50} values of the antioxidant activity of the selected extract (~3.7 μg mL^{-1}) and of (−)-epicatechin (~1.6 μg mL^{-1}) remained constant for 14 days, while the IC_{50} values of ascorbic acid increased over time (3.115–62.787 μg mL^{-1}). The antioxidant activity of the extract was comparable to that of ascorbic acid at t_0, while the antioxidant activity of (−)-epicatechin was even higher.

Author Contributions: Conceptualization, U.J. and K.N.; methodology, U.J. and K.N.; validation, U.J. and K.N.; formal analysis, U.J.; investigation, U.J. and K.N.; resources, I.V.; data curation, U.J.; writing—original draft preparation, U.J.; writing—review and editing, K.N. and I.V.; visualization, U.J.; supervision, K.N. and I.V.; project administration, I.V.; funding acquisition, I.V. All authors have read and agreed to the published version of the manuscript.

Funding: This research was funded by the Slovenian Research Agency (research core funding No. P1-0005 and "Young Researchers" program).

Institutional Review Board Statement: Not applicable.

Informed Consent Statement: Not applicable.

Data Availability Statement: The data presented in this study are available in this article.

Acknowledgments: The authors would like to thank the Slovenian Research Agency (research core funding No. P1-0005 and "Young Researchers" program), Kaja Loboda Bergant for the help with the preparation of graphics in GraphPad Prism 7, Andreja Krušič and Tinka Palkovič for their help with the experimental work, and Jure Zekič for the discussions regarding the protocol for the analysis of ascorbic acid.

Conflicts of Interest: The authors declare no conflict of interest. The funders had no role in the design of the study; in the collection, analyses, or interpretation of data; in the writing of the manuscript, or in the decision to publish the results.

References

1. Balogh, L. Japanese, Giant and Bohemian knotweed. In *The Most Important Invasive Plants in Hungary*; Botta-Dukat, Z., Balogh, L., Eds.; HAS Institute of Ecology and Botany: Budapest, Hungary, 2008; pp. 13–33.
2. Zhang, H.; Li, C.; Kwok, S.-T.; Zhang, Q.-W.; Chan, S.-W. A review of the pharmacological effects of the dried root of *Polygonum cuspidatum* (Hu Zhang) and its constituents. *Evid. Based Complementary Altern. Med.* **2013**. [CrossRef] [PubMed]
3. Lin, Y.-W.; Yang, F.-J.; Chen, C.-L.; Lee, W.-T.; Chen, R.-S. Free radical scavenging activity and antiproliferative potential of *Polygonum cuspidatum* root extracts. *J. Nat. Med.* **2010**, *64*, 146–152. [CrossRef] [PubMed]
4. Hsu, C.-Y.; Chan, Y.-P.; Chang, J. Antioxidant activity of extract from *Polygonum cuspidatum*. *Biol. Res.* **2007**, *40*, 13–21. [CrossRef] [PubMed]
5. Pogačnik, L.; Rogelj, A.; Ulrih, N.P. Chemiluminescence method for evaluation of antioxidant capacities of different invasive knotweed species. *Anal. Lett.* **2015**, *49*, 350–363. [CrossRef]
6. Lachowicz, S.; Oszmianski, J. Profile of bioactive compounds in the morphological parts of wild *Fallopia japonica* (Houtt) and *Fallopia sachalinensis* (F. Schmidt) and their antioxidative activity. *Molecules* **2019**, *24*, 1436. [CrossRef]
7. Ardelean, F.; Moacă, E.A.; Păcurariu, C.; Antal, D.S.; Dehelean, C.; Toma, C.-C.; Drăgan, S. Invasive *Polygonum cuspidatum*: Physico-chemical analysis of a plant extract with pharmaceutical potential. *Stud. Univ. Vasile Goldis Arad Seria Stiintele Vietii* **2016**, *26*, 415–421.
8. Kurita, S.; Kashiwagi, T.; Ebisu, T.; Shimamura, T.; Ukeda, H. Content of resveratrol and glycoside and its contribution to the antioxidative capacity of *Polygonum cuspidatum* (Itadori) harvested in Kochi. *Biosci. Biotechnol. Biochem.* **2014**, *78*, 499–502. [CrossRef]
9. Chan, C.-L.; Gan, R.-Y.; Corke, H. The phenolic composition and antioxidant capacity of soluble and bound extracts in selected dietary spices and medicinal herbs. *Int. J. Food Sci. Technol.* **2016**, *51*, 565–573. [CrossRef]
10. Nawrot-Hadzik, I.; Ślusarczyk, S.; Granica, S.; Hadzik, J.; Matkowski, A. Phytochemical diversity in rhizomes of three *Reynoutria* species and their antioxidant activity correlations elucidated by LC-ESI-MS/MS analysis. *Molecules* **2019**, *24*, 1136. [CrossRef]
11. Pogačnik, L.; Bergant, T.; Skrt, M.; Poklar Ulrih, N.; Viktorová, J.; Ruml, T. In vitro comparison of the bioactivities of Japanese and Bohemian knotweed ethanol extracts. *Foods* **2020**, *9*, 544. [CrossRef]
12. Zhang, C.; Zhang, X.; Zhang, Y.; Xu, Q.; Xiao, H.; Liang, X. Analysis of estrogenic compounds in *Polygonum cuspidatum* by bioassay and high performance liquid chromatography. *J. Ethnopharmacol.* **2006**, *105*, 223–228. [CrossRef] [PubMed]
13. Shan, B.; Cai, Y.-Z.; Brooks, J.D.; Corke, H. Antibacterial properties of *Polygonum cuspidatum* roots and their major bioactive constituents. *Food Chem.* **2008**, *109*, 530–537. [CrossRef]
14. Lin, H.-W.; Sun, M.-X.; Wang, Y.-H.; Yang, L.-M.; Yang, Y.-R.; Huang, N.; Xuan, L.-J.; Xu, Y.-M.; Bai, D.-L.; Zheng, Y.-T.; et al. Anti-HIV activities of the compounds isolated from *Polygonum cuspidatum* and *Polygonum multiflorum*. *Planta Med.* **2010**, *76*, 889–892. [CrossRef] [PubMed]
15. Fan, P.; Zhang, T.; Hostettmann, K. Anti-inflammatory activity of the invasive neophyte *Polygonum cuspidatum* Sieb. and Zucc. (*Polygonaceae*) and the chemical comparison of the invasive and native varieties with regard to resveratrol. *J. Tradit. Complement. Med.* **2013**, *3*, 182–187. [CrossRef] [PubMed]
16. Xue, Y.; Liang, J. Screening of bioactive compounds in rhizoma *Polygoni cuspidati* with hepatocyte membranes by HPLC and LC-MS. *J. Sep. Sci.* **2014**, *37*, 250–256. [CrossRef]

17. Cos, P.; De Bruyne, T.; Hermans, N.; Apers, S.; Vanden Berge, D.; Vlietinck, A.J. Proanthocyanidins in health care: Current and new trends. *Curr. Med. Chem.* **2004**, *11*, 1345–1359. [CrossRef]
18. Apak, R.; Gorinstein, S.; Böhm, V.; Schaich, K.M.; Özyürek, M.; Güçlü, K. Methods of measurement and evaluation of natural antioxidant capacity/activity (IUPAC Technical Report). *Pure Appl. Chem.* **2013**, *85*, 957–998. [CrossRef]
19. Alam, M.N.; Bristi, N.J.; Rifiquzzaman, M. Review on in vivo and in vitro methods evaluation of antioxidant activity. *Saudi Pharm. J.* **2013**, *21*, 143–152. [CrossRef]
20. Pisoschi, A.M.; Negulescu, G.P. Methods for total antioxidant activity determination: A review. *Biochem. Anal. Biochem.* **2011**, *1*. [CrossRef]
21. Ojha, K.; Dubey, S.; Chandrakar, J.; Minj, R.A.; Dehariya, R.; Dixit, A.K. A review on different methods of determination of antioxidant activity assay of herbal plants. *Res. J. Life Sci. Bioinf. Pharm. Chem. Sci.* **2018**, *4*, 707–730. [CrossRef]
22. Koleva, I.I.; Van Beek, T.A.; Linssen, J.P.H.; De Groot, A.; Evstatieva, L.N. Screening of Plant Extracts for Antioxidant Activity: A Comparative Study on Three Testing Methods. *Phytochem. Anal.* **2002**, *13*, 8–17. [CrossRef] [PubMed]
23. Vovk, I.; Simonovska, B.; Andrenšek, S.; Vuorela, H.; Vuorela, P. Rotation planar extraction and rotation planar chromatography of oak (*Quercus robur* L.) bark. *J. Chromatogr. A* **2003**, *991*, 267–274. [CrossRef]
24. Orsini, F.; Vovk, I.; Glavnik, V.; Jug, U.; Corradini, D. HPTLC, HPTLC-MS/MS and HPTLC-DPPH methods for analyses of flavonoids and their antioxidant activity in *Cyclanthera pedata* leaves, fruits and dietary supplement. *J. Liq. Chromatogr. Relat. Technol.* **2019**, *42*, 290–301. [CrossRef]
25. Simonovska, B.; Vovk, I.; Andrenšek, S.; Valentova, K.; Ulrichová, J. Investigation of phenolic acids in yacon (*Smallanthus sonchifolius*) leaves and tubers. *J. Chromatogr. A* **2003**, *1016*, 89–98. [CrossRef]
26. Cieśla, Ł.; Kryszeń, J.; Stochmal, A.; Oleszek, W.; Waksmundzka-Hajnos, M. Approach to develop a standardized TLC-DPPH test for assessing free radical scavenging properties of selected phenolic compounds. *J. Pharm. Biomed. Anal.* **2012**, *70*, 126–135. [CrossRef]
27. Meda, N.R.; Fraisse, D.; Gnoula, C.; Vivier, M.; Felgines, C.; Senejoux, F. Characterization of antioxidants from *Detarium microcarpum* Guill. et Perr. leaves using HPLC-DAD coupled with pre-column DPPH assay. *Eur. Food Res. Technol.* **2017**, *243*, 1659–1666. [CrossRef]
28. Wu, J.-H.; Huang, C.-Y.; Tung, Y.-T.; Chang, S.-T. On-line RP-HPLC-DPPH screening method for detection of radical-scavenging phytochemicals from flowers of *Acacia confuse*. *J. Agric. Food Chem.* **2008**, *56*, 328–332. [CrossRef]
29. Zhang, Y.; Li, Q.; Xing, H.; Lu, X.; Zhao, L.; Qu, K.; Bi, K. Evaluation of antioxidant activity of ten compounds in different tea samples by means of an on-line HPLC-DPPH assay. *Food Res. Int.* **2013**, *53*, 847–856. [CrossRef]
30. Koleva, I.I.; Niederländer, H.A.G.; Van Beek, T.A. An on-line HPLC method for detection of radical scavenging compounds in complex mixtures. *Anal. Chem.* **2000**, *72*, 2323–2328. [CrossRef]
31. Bandoniene, D.; Murkovic, M. On-line HPLC-DPPH screening method for evaluation of radical scavenging phenols extracted from apples (*Malus domestica* L.). *J. Agric. Food Chem.* **2002**, *50*, 2482–2487. [CrossRef]
32. Burnaz, N.A.; Küçük, M.; Akar, Z. An on-line HPLC system for detection of antioxidant compounds in some plant extracts by comparing three different methods. *J. Chromatogr. B* **2017**, *1052*, 66–72. [CrossRef] [PubMed]
33. Pravadali-Cekic, S.; Kocic, D.; Hua, S.; Jones, A.; Dennis, G.R.; Shalliker, R.A. Tuning a parallel segmented flow column and enabling multiplexed detection. *J. Visualized Exp.* **2015**. [CrossRef] [PubMed]
34. Sharma Avasthi, A.; Bhatnagar, M.; Sarkar, N.; Kitchlu, S.; Ghosal, S. Bioassay guided screening, optimization and characterization of antioxidant compounds from high altitude wild edible plants of Ladakh. *J. Food Sci. Technol.* **2016**, *53*, 3244–3252. [CrossRef] [PubMed]
35. Sudha, A.; Srinivasan, P. Bioassay-guided isolation and antioxidant evaluation of flavonoid compound from aerial parts of *Lippia nodiflora* L. *BioMed Res. Int.* **2014**. [CrossRef] [PubMed]
36. Jothy, S.L.; Saito, T.; Kanwar, J.R.; Kavitha, S.; Herng, L.C.; Chen, Y.; Yin-Hui, L.; Sasidharan, S. Bioassay-guided isolation and antioxidant evaluation of rutin from leaf of *Polyalthia longifolia*. *Asian J. Appl. Sci.* **2017**, *5*, 138–148.
37. Lin, H.-Y.; Kuo, Y.-H.; Lin, Y.-L.; Chiang, W. Antioxidative effect and active components from leaves of lotus (*Nelumbo nucifera*). *J. Agric. Food Chem.* **2009**, *57*, 6623–6629. [CrossRef]
38. Chin, Y.-W.; Chai, H.-B.; Keller, W.J.; Douglas Kinghorn, A. Lignans and other constituents of the fruits of *Euterpe oleracea* (Açai) with antioxidant and cytoprotective activities. *J. Agric. Food Chem.* **2008**, *56*, 7759–7764. [CrossRef] [PubMed]
39. Sunil, J.; Janapati, Y.K.; Bramhachari, P.V. Bioassay guided isolation and identification of the antioxidant constituent from *Holostemma ada-kodien* shcult. *Int. J. Pharma Bio Sci.* **2017**, *8*, 1–10. [CrossRef]
40. Lelono, R.A.A.; Tachibana, S. Bioassay-guided isolation and identification of antioxidative compounds from the bark of *Eugenia polyantha*. *Pak. J. Biol. Sci.* **2013**, *16*, 812–818. [CrossRef]
41. Luo, Y.; Wang, H.; Li, Y.; He, T.; Wang, D.; Wang, W.; Jia, W.; Lin, Z.; Chen, S. One injection to profile the chemical composition and dual-antioxidation activities of *Rosa chinensis* Jacq. *J. Chromatogr. A* **2000**, *1613*. [CrossRef]
42. Soobrattee, M.A.; Neergheen, V.S.; Luximon-Ramma, A.; Aruoma, O.I.; Bahorun, T. Phenolics as potential antioxidant therapeutic agents: Mechanism and actions. *Mutat. Res.* **2005**, *579*, 200–213. [CrossRef] [PubMed]
43. Proteggente, A.R.; Pannala, A.S.; Paganga, G.; Van Buren, L.; Wagner, E.; Wiseman, S.; Van de Put, F.; Dacombe, C.; Rice-Evans, C.A. The antioxidant activity of regularly consumed fruit and vegetables reflects their phenolic and vitamin C composition. *Free Radic. Res.* **2002**, *36*, 217–233. [CrossRef] [PubMed]

44. Liang, T.; Yue, W.; Li, Q. Comparison of the phenolic content and antioxidant activities of *Apocynum venetum* L. (Luo-Bu-Ma) and two of its alternative species. *Int. J. Mol. Sci.* **2010**, *11*, 4452–4464. [CrossRef] [PubMed]
45. Yi, T.; Zhang, H.; Cai, Z. Analysis of rhizoma *Polygoni cuspidati* by HPLC and HPLC-ESI/MS. *Phytochem. Anal.* **2007**, *18*, 387–392. [CrossRef]
46. Fan, P.; Hay, A.-E.; Marston, A.; Lou, H.; Hostettmann, K. Chemical variability of the invasive neophytes *Polygonum cuspidatum* Sieb. and Zucc and *Polygonum sachalinensis* F. Schmidt ex Maxim. *Biochem. Syst. Ecol.* **2009**, *37*, 24–34. [CrossRef]
47. Beňová, B.; Adam, M.; Pavlíková, P.; Fischer, J. Supercritical fluid extraction of piceid, resveratrol and emodin from Japanese knotweed. *J. Supercrit. Fluids* **2010**, *51*, 325–330. [CrossRef]
48. Zhao, Y.; Chen, M.X.; Kongstad, K.T.; Jäger, A.K.; Staerk, D. Potential of *Polygonum cuspidatum* root as an antidiabetic food: Dual high-resolution α-glucosidase and PTP1B inhibition profiling combined with HPLC-HRMS and NMR for identification of antidiabetic constituents. *J. Agric. Food. Chem.* **2017**, *65*, 4421–4427. [CrossRef]
49. Fu, J.; Wang, M.; Guo, H.; Tian, Y.; Zhang, Z.; Song, R. Profiling of components of rhizoma et radix *Polygoni cuspidati* by high-performance liquid chromatography with ultraviolet diode-array detector and ion trap/time-of-flight mass spectrometric detection. *Pharmacogn. Mag.* **2015**, *11*, 486–501. [CrossRef]
50. Nawrot-Hadzik, I.; Granica, S.; Domaradzki, K.; Pecio, Ł.; Matkowski, A. Isolation and determination of phenolic glycosides and anthraquinones from rhizomes of various *Reynoutria* species. *Planta Med.* **2018**, *84*, 1118–1126. [CrossRef]
51. Lachowicz, S.; Oszmiański, J.; Wojdyło, A.; Cebulak, T.; Hirnle, L.; Siewiński, M. UPLC-PDA-Q/TOF-MS identification of bioactive compounds and on-line UPLC-ABTS assay in *Fallopia japonica* Houtt and *Fallopia sachalinensis* (F. Schmidt) leaves and rhizomes grown in Poland. *Eur. Food. Res. Technol.* **2019**, *245*, 691–706. [CrossRef]
52. Glavnik, V.; Vovk, I.; Albreht, A. High performance thin-layer chromatography-mass spectrometry of Japanese knotweed flavan-3-ols and proanthocyanidins on silica gel plates. *J. Chromatogr. A* **2017**, *1482*, 97–108. [CrossRef]
53. Glavnik, V.; Vovk, I. High performance thin-layer chromatography-mass spectrometry methods on diol stationary phase for the analyses of flavan-3-ols and proanthocyanidins in invasive Japanese knotweed. *J. Chromatogr. A* **2019**, *1598*, 196–208. [CrossRef] [PubMed]
54. Zhao, R.-Z.; Liu, S.; Zhou, L.-L. Rapid quantitative HPTLC analysis, on one plate, of emodin, resveratrol, and polydatin in the Chinese herb *Polygonum cuspidatum*. *Chromatographia* **2005**, *61*, 311–314. [CrossRef]
55. Hawryl, M.A.; Waksmundzka-Hajnos, M. Two-dimensional thin-layer chromatography of selected *Polygonum* sp. extracts on polar-bonded stationary phases. *J. Chromatogr. A* **2011**, *1218*, 2812–2819. [CrossRef] [PubMed]
56. Vaher, M.; Koel, M. Separation of polyphenolic compounds extracted from plant matrices using capillary electrophoresis. *J. Chromatogr. A* **2003**, *990*, 225–230. [CrossRef]
57. Koyama, J.; Morita, I.; Kawanishi, K.; Tagahara, K.; Kobayashi, N. Capillary electrophoresis for simultaneous determination of emodin, chrysophanol, and their 8-β-D-glucosides. *Chem. Pharm. Bull.* **2003**, *51*, 418–420. [CrossRef]
58. Sharma, O.P.; Bhat, T.K. DPPH antioxidant assay revisited. *Food Chem.* **2009**, *113*, 1202–1205. [CrossRef]
59. Oldoni, T.L.C.; Melo, P.S.; Massarioli, A.P.; Moreno, I.A.M.; Bezerra, R.M.N.; Rosalen, P.L.; Da Silva, G.V.J.; Nascimento, A.M.; Alencar, S.M. Bioassay-guided isolation of proanthocyanidins with antioxidant activity from peanut (*Arachis hypogaea*) skin by combination of chromatography techniques. *Food Chem.* **2016**, *192*, 306–312. [CrossRef]
60. *GraphPad Prism*; Version 700 for Windows; GraphPad Software: La Jolla/San Diego, CA, USA, 2016.
61. Glavnik, V.; Simonovska, B.; Vovk, I. Densitometric determination of (+)-catechin and (−)-epicatechin by 4-dimethylaminocinnamaldehyde reagent. *J. Chromatogr. A* **2009**, *1216*, 4485–4491. [CrossRef]
62. Vovk, I.; Simonovska, B.; Vuorela, H. Separation of eight selected flavan-3-ols on cellulose thin-layer chromatographic plates. *J. Chromatogr. A* **2005**, *1077*, 188–194. [CrossRef]
63. Glavnik, V.; Vovk, I. Analysis of dietary supplements. In *Instrumental Thin-Layer Chromatography*; Poole, C., Ed.; Elsevier: Amsterdam, The Netherlands, 2015; pp. 589–635.
64. Akar, Z.; Küçük, M.; Doğan, H. A new colorimetric DPPH scavenging activity method with no need for a spectrophotometer applied on synthetic and natural antioxidants and medicinal herbs. *J. Enzyme Inhib. Med. Chem.* **2017**, *32*, 640–647. [CrossRef] [PubMed]
65. Brand-Williams, W.; Cuvelier, M.E.; Berset, C. Use of a free radical method to evaluate antioxidant activity. *LWT Food Sci. Technol.* **1995**, *28*, 25–30. [CrossRef]
66. Kurechi, T.; Kikugawa, K.; Kato, T. Studies on the antioxidants. XIII. Hydrogen donating capability of antioxidants to 2,2-diphenyl-1-picrylhydrazyl. *Chem. Pharm. Bull.* **1980**, *28*, 2089–2093. [CrossRef]
67. Jug, U.; Glavnik, V.; Vovk, I.; Makuc, D.; Naumoska, K. *Off-line* multidimensional high performance thin-layer chromatography for fractionation of Japanese knotweed rhizome bark extract and isolation of flavan-3-ols, proanthocyanidins and anthraquinones. *J. Chromatogr. A* **2021**, *1637*, 461802. [CrossRef]
68. Grodowska, K.; Parczewski, A. Organic solvents in the pharmaceutical industry. *Acta Pol. Pharm.* **2010**, *67*, 3–12. Available online: https://www.ptfarm.pl/wydawnictwa/czasopisma/acta-poloniae-pharmaceutica/110/-/12992 (accessed on 10 September 2020).
69. Wawrzyniak, J.; Ryniecki, A.; Zembrzuski, W. Application of voltammetry to determine vitamin C in apple juices. *Acta Sci. Pol. Technol. Aliment.* **2005**, *4*, 5–16.

70. Adepoju, T.S.; Olasehinde, E.F.; Aderibigbe, A.D. Effect of sodium metabisulphite and disodium ethylenediaminetetraacetic acid (EDTA) on the stability of ascorbic acid in vitamin C syrup. *Researcher* **2014**, *6*, 6–9.
71. Hider, R.C.; Liu, Z.D.; Khodr, H.H. Metal chelation of polyphenols. *Methods Enzymol.* **2001**, *335*, 190–203. [CrossRef]
72. Yen, G.-C.; Duh, P.-D.; Chuang, D.-Y. Antioxidant activity of anthraquinones and anthrone. *Food Chem.* **2000**, *70*, 437–441. [CrossRef]
73. Matkowski, A.; Jamiołkowska-Kozlowska, W.; Nawrot, I. Chinese medicinal herbs as source of antioxidant compounds-where tradition meets the future. *Curr. Med. Chem.* **2013**, *20*, 984–1004. [CrossRef]
74. Glavnik, V.; Vovk, I. Extraction of anthraquinones from Japanese knotweed rhizomes and their analyses by high performance thin-layer chromatography and mass spectrometry. *Plants* **2020**, *9*, 1753. [CrossRef] [PubMed]
75. Ha Lai, T.N.; Herent, M.-F.; Quetin-Leclercq, J.; Thuy Nguyen, T.B.; Rogez, H.; Larondelle, Y.; André, C.M. Piceatannol, a potent bioactive stilbene, as major phenolic component in *Rhodomyrtus tomentosa*. *Food Chem.* **2013**, *138*, 1421–1430. [CrossRef] [PubMed]
76. Kranl, K.; Schlesier, K.; Bitsch, R.; Hermann, H.; Rohe, M.; Böhm, V. Comparing antioxidative food additives and secondary plant products—Use of different assays. *Food Chem.* **2005**, *93*, 171–175. [CrossRef]
77. Miguel, M.G. Antioxidant activity of medicinal and aromatic plants. A review. *Flavour Fragrance J.* **2010**, *25*, 291–312. [CrossRef]

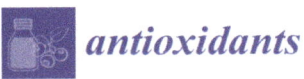

Article

Natural Food Supplements Reduce Oxidative Stress in Primary Neurons and in the Mouse Brain, Suggesting Applications in the Prevention of Neurodegenerative Diseases

Miriam Bobadilla, Josune García-Sanmartín and Alfredo Martínez *

Oncology Area, Center for Biomedical Research of La Rioja (CIBIR), 26006 Logroño, Spain; mbobadilla@riojasalud.es (M.B.); jgarcias@riojasalud.es (J.G.-S.)
* Correspondence: amartinezr@riojasalud.es; Tel.: +34-941-278-775

Abstract: Neurodegenerative diseases pose a major health problem for developed countries, and stress has been identified as one of the main risk factors in the development of these disorders. Here, we have examined the protective properties against oxidative stress of several bioactive natural food supplements. We found that MecobalActive®, Olews®, and red and white grape seed polyphenol extracts may have a neuroprotective effect in vitro, both in the SH-SY 5Y cell line and in hippocampal neuron cultures, mainly by reducing reactive oxygen species levels and decreasing caspase-3 activity. In vivo, we demonstrated that oral administration of the supplements reduces the expression of genes involved in inflammation and oxidation mechanisms, whereas it increments the expression of genes related to protection against oxidative stress. Furthermore, we found that preventive treatment with these natural extracts increases the activity of antioxidant enzymes and prevents lipid peroxidation in the brain of stressed mice. Thus, our results indicate that some natural bioactive supplements may have important protective properties against oxidative stress processes occurring in the brain.

Keywords: oxidative stress; ROS; neurodegenerative diseases; red grape polyphenol extract; white grape seed polyphenol extract; MecobalActive®; Olews®

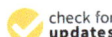

Citation: Bobadilla, M.; García-Sanmartín, J.; Martínez, A. Natural Food Supplements Reduce Oxidative Stress in Primary Neurons and in the Mouse Brain, Suggesting Applications in the Prevention of Neurodegenerative Diseases. *Antioxidants* **2021**, *10*, 46. https://doi.org/10.3390/antiox10010046

Received: 4 December 2020
Accepted: 24 December 2020
Published: 2 January 2021

Publisher's Note: MDPI stays neutral with regard to jurisdictional claims in published maps and institutional affiliations.

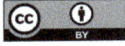

Copyright: © 2021 by the authors. Licensee MDPI, Basel, Switzerland. This article is an open access article distributed under the terms and conditions of the Creative Commons Attribution (CC BY) license (https://creativecommons.org/licenses/by/4.0/).

1. Introduction

The increasing population lifespan in developed countries is leading to a higher incidence of age-related illnesses, including neurodegenerative diseases (ND) [1]. NDs are characterized by a progressive loss of selectively vulnerable neuron populations in specific brain areas [2]. NDs encompass a heterogeneous group of chronic disorders that include, among others, Alzheimer's disease (AD) and other dementias, Huntington´s disease, Parkinson´s disease, multiple sclerosis, human prion, and motoneuron diseases [3–6]. Unfortunately, all these diseases are untreatable at the moment, and, in terms of human suffering and economic and social costs, they represent the fourth cause of global disease burden in developed countries [1].

The current literature clearly shows that oxidative stress is one of the main risk factors for AD [7]. The balance between the production of reactive oxygen species (ROS) and reactive nitrogen species (RNS), on the one hand, and of antioxidant substances on the other, is critical for a correct cell function [8]. When unbalanced, the overproduction of ROS and RNS, combined with failing antioxidant defenses, causes oxidative stress [9]. For instance, in AD, a clear diminution of antioxidant activity occurs, which leads to the accumulation of oxidative damage [10]. Additionally, decreased levels of antioxidants such as vitamin C and E and uric acid are observed in AD patients. Many studies have demonstrated that the production of excessive ROS and signs of oxidative stress were detected in the brains of these patients [11,12]. Furthermore, there is evidence that mitochondrial damage resulting in an increased production of ROS contributes to the early stages of the disease prior to the onset of clinical symptoms [9,13]. For these reasons, numerous scientific studies suggest that diets rich in antioxidants may be helpful in preventing, postponing, or controlling the progression of AD [14,15].

To date, there is no effective treatment for these degenerative diseases. Some drugs are used for relieving the symptoms, although they usually generate many side effects and have limited efficacy [16]. Therefore, in order to develop novel preventive therapies, a large number of natural plant extracts have been tested as neuroprotective agents [17]. In nature, there are multiple compounds, including polyphenols, flavonoids, and vitamins, which are capable of counteracting the harmful effects of oxidative stress and reducing the risk of developing NDs [7,18]. Special attention has been paid to flavonoids, a type of polyphenolic compounds that are abundantly present in fruits, vegetables, red and white grapes, and green tea [1]. Flavonoids are nutrients with beneficial health effects derived from their antioxidant and anti-inflammatory properties [19,20]. There is now extensive scientific literature describing the beneficial effects of flavonoids in disease prevention [21,22].

The purpose of the present study was to investigate the protective properties against oxidative stress of several bioactive natural food supplements in vitro and in vivo. The addition of these supplements to commonly used food staples may provide a new and affordable strategy for the prevention of NDs.

2. Materials and Methods

2.1. Cell Culture

Human neuroblastoma SH-SY 5Y cell line was obtained from the American Tissue Culture Collection (ATCC, Manassas, VA, USA). Cells were grown in Dulbecco's Modified Eagle's Medium (DMEM)-F12 medium (Hyclone, Logan, UT, USA) with 10% fetal bovine serum (Gibco, Carlsbad, CA, USA), 1% penicillin/streptomycin (Gibco), and maintained at 37 °C, 5% CO_2. Cell culture medium was changed thrice a week.

The cell line was authenticated by STR profiling (IDEXX BioAnalytics, Kornwestheim, Germany).

2.2. Primary Hippocampal Neuron Isolation and Culture

Mouse hippocampal neurons were isolated from postnatal day 1 (P1) C57BL/6J mice, as described [23], with slight modifications. Briefly, the hippocampus was dissected in Hank's balanced salt solution (HBSS) and incubated at 37 °C for 15 min with trypsin/ethylenediaminetetraacetic acid (EDTA) (Sigma-Aldrich, St. Louis, MO, USA). After 3 washes in HBSS, tissue was triturated using a sterile 9-inch Pasteur pipette. HBSS was replaced with Neurobasal plating medium (neurobasal medium, Gibco) containing B27 supplement (1:50) (Gibco), 0.5-mM glutamine solution (Gibco), penicillin/streptomycin (Gibco), 1-mM 4-(2-hydroxyethyl)-1-piperazineethanesulfonic acid (HEPES) (Hyclone), and 10% heat-inactivated donor horse serum (Gibco). Neuroblasts were plated on poly-D-lysine-coated glass coverslips (p96) at a density of 3×10^4 cells/well and placed in a 37 °C, 5% CO_2 incubator overnight. Next day, in vitro neurobasal plating medium was replaced with neurobasal feeding medium (neurobasal medium containing B27 Supplement (1:50), 0.5-mM glutamine solution, penicillin/streptomycin (1:200), and 1-mM HEPES). Half of the feeding medium was replaced with fresh medium every 4 days.

2.3. Natural Extracts

Six commercial natural food supplements were used in this study. They included red grape polyphenol and white grape seed polyphenol extracts (generously provided by Alvinesa Natural Ingredients, Daimiel, Ciudad Real, Spain), extracts from the olive tree (Olews®), citicoline, MecobalActive®, and Cardiose® (all generously provided by HealthTech Bio Actives, Barcelona, Spain).

Red grape polyphenol and grape seed polyphenol extracts, from Alvinesa Natural Ingredients, are entirely constituted by phenolic compounds (premium selected blending of monomers, dimers, oligomers, and polymers) and have a unique formulation that facilitates direct absorption of the phenolic compounds by the small intestine. All these extracts are currently used as commercial supplements approved for human consumption. Some of these extracts have demonstrated their antioxidant properties in other contexts [24].

2.4. Preparation of Aluminum Maltolate

Aluminum maltolate (Al(mal)$_3$) was prepared according to published procedures [25]. AlCl$_3$·6H$_2$O was dissolved in distilled water to a final concentration of 80 mM. Maltolate was dissolved in phosphate-buffered saline (PBS) to a final concentration of 240 mM. The solutions were mixed in equal volumes, and pH was adjusted to 7.4, inducing the precipitation of Al(mal)$_3$ crystals. All solutions were filtered using 0.22-μm syringe filters just before use.

2.5. Cell Proliferation Assay

Cell proliferation was analyzed using the Cell Titer 96 Aqueous One Solution Cell Proliferation Assay (Promega, Madison, WI, USA), following the manufacturer's instructions. Cells were seeded in 96-well plates at a density of 3×10^4 cells per well, allowed to attach for 24 h, and exposed to different concentrations of natural bioactive extracts with or without 125-μM Al(mal)$_3$ for 72 h. The MTS reagent (3-(4,5-dimethylthiazol-2-yl)-5-(3-carboxymethoxyphenyl)-2-(4-sulfophenyl)-2H-tetrazolium) was added for 4 h, and absorbance was examined at 490 nm using a microplate reader (POLARstar Omega, BMG Labtech, Ortenberg, Germany). The GI$_{50}$ (growth inhibition of 50% of cells) values of the different compounds were determined using nonlinear regression plots with Prism 8.3.0 (GraphPad Software, San Diego, CA, USA).

2.6. Measurement of Intracellular ROS Levels

The levels of ROS were determined in cell cultures by using the cellular ROS assay kit (ab113851, Abcam, Cambridge, UK), following the manufacturer's instructions. Briefly, SH-SY 5Y cells (8×10^3 cell/well) were incubated with different concentrations of natural bioactive extracts with or without 125-μM Al(mal)3 for 48 h, followed by an incubation with 25-μM 2'-7'dichlorofluorescin diacetate (DCFH-DA) for 45 min at 37 °C in the dark. After two washes with PBS, DCFH-DA was detected by fluorescence spectroscopy, with excitation/emission at 485/535 nm in a microplate reader (POLARstar Omega).

2.7. Caspase-3 Activation Assay

Levels of caspase-3 were determined in cell cultures by using the caspase-3 colorimetric assay kit (K106-100; BioVision Inc., Milpitas, CA, USA), following the manufacturer's instructions and previous studies [26]. Briefly, enzyme reactions were performed in 96-well microplates, and 50 μL of cell lysate was added to each reaction mixture. Absorbance at 405 nm was measured using a plate reader (POLARstar Omega).

2.8. Measurement of Nitrite and Nitrate Concentrations

Cell media were collected and analyzed for their nitrite and nitrate contents by using the nitrite/nitrate colorimetric assay (780001, Cayman Chemicals, Ann Arbor, MI, USA), following the manufacturer's instructions. NO$_X$ (nitrite + nitrate) concentrations were determined by measuring absorbance at 540 nm using a microplate reader (POLARstar Omega). Cell media nitrate concentrations were calculated by subtracting the concentrations of cell media nitrite from the NO$_X$ concentrations.

2.9. Restrain Stress and In Vivo Treatments

Six-week-old C57BL/6J mice (Charles-River) were used for this assay. Mice were housed under standard conditions at a temperature of 22 °C (± 1 °C) and a 12-h light/dark cycle with free access to food and water.

Mice were subjected to an acute model of stress by immobilization, as previously described [4,27], by placing them inside 50-mL conical tubes with no access to food or water for the indicated periods of time. Adequate ventilation was provided by several air holes (0.5 cm in diameter) drilled into the conical end of the tube and at its sides. The tubes prevented forward, backward, or rotational movements of the mice. Due to the corticosterone circadian rhythm [28], restraint stress was started at the same time of the day (9:00 a.m.) in all experiments.

In a pilot study, mice were subjected to restraint for 0, 2, 4, or 6 h, and stress markers were measured (see below). A period of 6h was chosen as the optimal time of restraint for further experiments.

Mice were randomly divided into different experimental groups (n = 8 per group) and received different doses of the natural extracts (or PBS as a control) in 200 μL by oral gavage during 5 consecutive days (Table 1). On the 6th day, mice were subjected to 6 h of restraint stress and immediately sacrificed. The whole brain was dissected out. The olfactory bulbs and the cerebellum were removed, and the remaining tissue was divided into two equal halves by a sagittal section. Each half was frozen separately in liquid N_2 and stored at −80 °C. One side was used for RNA extraction and the other one for antioxidant enzyme analysis (see below).

Table 1. Food supplements and concentrations used for the in vivo study.

Natural Extract	Dose	References
Red grape	100 mg/kg 300 mg/kg	[29,30]
White grape	100 mg/kg 300 mg/kg	[29,30]
MecobalActive®	65 μg/kg 135 μg/kg	[31]
Olews®	300 mg/kg 600 mg/kg	[32,33]

2.10. Quantitative Real-Time PCR

Total RNA was isolated from mouse brains and purified as described [34]. Briefly, total RNA was isolated using Trizol reagent (Invitrogen, Carlsbad, CA, USA), with the DNase digestion step performed (Qiagen, Hilden, Germany) according to the manufacturer's instructions. Resulting RNA (5 μg) was reverse-transcribed using the Superscript III First-Strand Synthesis System for RT-PCR (Invitrogen), and the synthesized cDNA was amplified using SYBR Green PCR Master Mix (Applied Biosystems, Foster City, CA, USA). Transcripts were amplified by real-time PCR (7300 Real-Time PCR System, Applied Biosystems). At the end, a dissociation curve was implemented from 60 to 95 °C to validate the amplicon specificity. For each transcript, a specific calibration curve of cDNA was included to analyze the expression of NADPH oxidase 2 (NOX-2), heme oxygenase (decycling) 1 (HMOX-1), interleukin 6 (IL-6), tumor necrosis factor alpha (TNF-alpha), and nuclear factor erythroid 2-related factor 2 (Nrf-2). All measurements were normalized to glyceraldehyde-3-phosphate dehydrogenase (GAPDH) as a housekeeping gene. Specific primers are shown in Table 2.

Table 2. Primers used in this study. Annealing temperature was 60 °C for all transcripts.

Gene	Forward Primer (5'-3')	Reverse Primer (5'-3')
NOX-2	GCTGGGATCACAGGAATTGT	CTTCCAAACTCTCCGCAGTC
HMOX-1	TGCTCGAATGAACACTCTGG	TAGCAGGCCTCTGACGAAGT
IL-6	ATGGATGCTACCAAACTGGAT	TGAAGGACTCTGGCTTTGTCT
TNF-alpha	CCACCACGCTCTTCTGTCTA	CACTTGGTGGTTTGCTACGA
Nrf-2	AGCGAGCAGGCTATCTCCTA	TCTTGCCTCCAAAGGATGTC
GAPDH	CATGGCCTTCCGTGTTCCTA	GCGGCACGTCAGATCCA

2.11. Thiobarbituric Acid Reactive Substances (TBARS), Superoxide Dismutase (SOD), and Catalase Activity

For the determination of oxidative stress parameters and antioxidant components in the brain, frozen tissues were homogenized in radioimmunoprecipation assay (RIPA) buffer (Thermo Scientific, Waltham, MA, USA) supplemented with complete and phospho STOP (Roche, Basel, Switzerland) protease inhibitors. Lipid peroxidation was determined using a commercial TBARS assay kit (CA995, Canvax, Córdoba, Spain). The final malondialdehyde (MDA) products were detected by fluorescence spectroscopy, with excitation/emission at 530/590 nm in a microplate reader (POLARstar Omega). Levels of superoxide dismutase (SOD) activity were determined using an SOD assay kit (CA061, Canvax), according to the manufacturer's protocols. Absorbance at 450 nm was measured using a POLARstar Omega plate reader. Catalase activities were determined using a commercial catalase activity assay kit (CA063, Canvax) following the manufacturer's instructions. Enzyme activity was detected by fluorescence spectroscopy, with excitation/emission at 530/590 nm in a microplate reader (POLARstar Omega).

2.12. Statistical Analysis

All datasets were analyzed for normalcy and homoscedasticity. Normal data were analyzed by one-way ANOVA and Dunnett's multiple comparison post-hoc test. Data that did not follow a normal distribution were compared by the Kruskal-Wallis test, followed by the Mann Whitney post-hoc test. Analyses were performed with GraphPad Prism version 8.3.0 (GraphPad Software). A *p*-value < 0.05 was considered statistically significant.

3. Results

3.1. Olews® and Red and White Grape Extracts Have Neuroprotective Effects on the SH-SY 5Y Cell Line

To test whether the natural extracts used in this study have an antioxidant capacity, in a first approach, we tested them in vitro on the human neuroblastoma cell line SH-SY 5Y.

First, we tested the activity of the chosen supplements (Cardiose®, Olews®, citicoline, MecobalActive®, and red and white grape extracts) on the SH-SY 5Y cell line to study their potential toxicity. The cells were exposed to increasing concentrations of extracts for 72 h, and the cell number was determined by colorimetric methods.

Interestingly, two different behaviors were observed: (A) extracts that did not elicit significant changes in the number of cells, as with Cardiose® and citicoline (Figure 1A,C), and (B) extracts that induced a dose-dependent toxicity, as observed with MecobalActive®, Olews®, and red grape and white grape seed extracts. The GI_{50} for these substances were 126, 73, 76, and 134 µg/mL, respectively (Figure 1B,D–F).

Then, we introduced a chemical inducer of cellular stress to assess the neuroprotective effects of the natural extracts. Al(mal)$_3$ is a compound that elicits neurotoxicity by inducing mitochondrial membrane potential changes, elevated reactive oxygen species, DNA damage, and apoptosis in SH-SY 5Y cells [35]. Before checking the food supplements, we established the time and concentration curves of Al(mal)$_3$ toxicity on the SH-SY 5Y cells. The concentration course studies were carried out at 24 h, 48 h, and 72 h after starting treatment with Al(mal)$_3$. We observed that cell death was dose and time-dependent. The GI_{50} concentrations for 24 h, 48 h, and 72 h were 482.60, 85.20, and 53.78 µM, respectively (Figure 2).

Given these results, we chose 72 h and 125-µM Al(mal)$_3$ to perform all in vitro studies involving the stressor. For this, we pretreated the SH-SY 5Y cells with the extracts for 1 h and then exposed them to Al(mal)$_3$. After 72 h of incubation, the cell number was assessed.

In the presence of Al(mal)$_3$, Cardiose®, citicoline, and MecobalActive® did not significantly improve cell survival (Figure 1A′,C′,D′). On the other hand, Olews® and red and white grape extracts presented a slight recovery of cell proliferation at the highest doses, with GI_{50} values of 47, 930, and 1598 µg/mL, respectively (Figure 1B′,E′,F′).

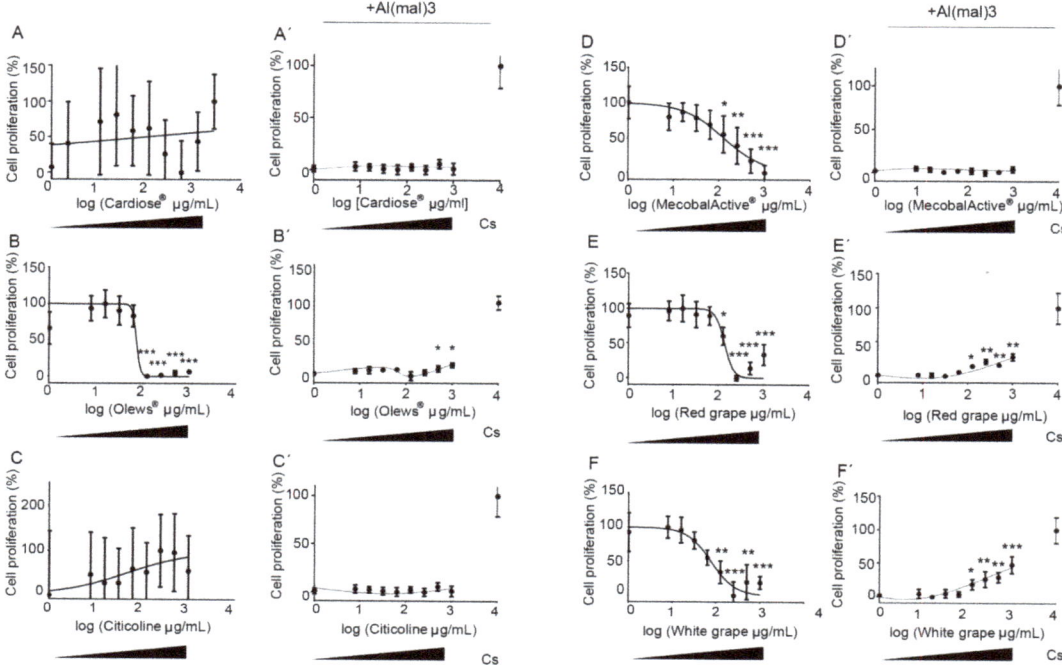

Figure 1. Neuroprotective effects of the extracts on the SH-SY 5Y cell line. Dose-response curve effects of the extracts on the SH-SY 5Y cell line. Cells were incubated with different concentrations of Cardiose® (**A**), Olews® (**B**), citicoline (**C**), MecobalActive® (**D**), red grape (**E**), or white grape extracts (**F**) for 72 h in the absence (**A–F**) or presence (**A′–F′**) of 125-μM Al(mal)$_3$. Data are normalized and expressed as a percentage of the over-basal response (mean ± SEM). Significant differences were analyzed on data from eight different experiments; one-way ANOVA and Dunnett's multiple comparison post-hoc test were used for statistical analysis. * $p < 0.05$, ** $p < 0.01$, and *** $p < 0.001$ versus cells or Al(mal)$_3$ treatment. Cs: control cells, not exposed to Al(mal)$_3$.

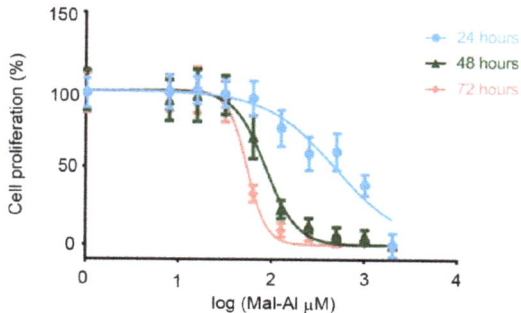

Figure 2. Dose-response curves of the stressor on the SH-SY 5Y cell line. Cells were incubated with different concentrations of Al(mal)$_3$ for 24, 48, or 72 h. Data are normalized and expressed as a percentage of the over-basal response (mean ± SEM). Significant differences were analyzed on data from eight different experiments; one-way ANOVA and Dunnett's multiple comparison post-hoc test were used for statistical analysis; 24 h, $p < 0.00001$; 48 h, $p < 0.0001$; and 72 h, $p < 0.0001$.

3.2. Olews®, MecobalActive®, and Red and White Grape Extracts Have Neuroprotective Effects on Neuroblasts In Vitro

The cytotoxic activity shown for some of the extracts on the tumor cell line led us to ask whether this was specifically an antitumor effect or was due to a broader toxicity. To answer this question, we repeated the experiments using primary cultures of mouse hippocampal neuroblasts.

As with the tumor cells, we first tested the activity of the food supplements on hippocampal neuron cultures. As with the SH-SY 5Y cells, we observed a potent and dose-independent toxicity when we added Cardiose® and citicoline to the cell cultures (Figure 3A,C). However, the toxicity was dose-dependent after adding Olews®, MecobalActive®, and red grape and white grape seed extracts, with EC_{50} values of 16.8, 28.5, 18.2, and 259 µg/mL, respectively (Figure 3B,D–F).

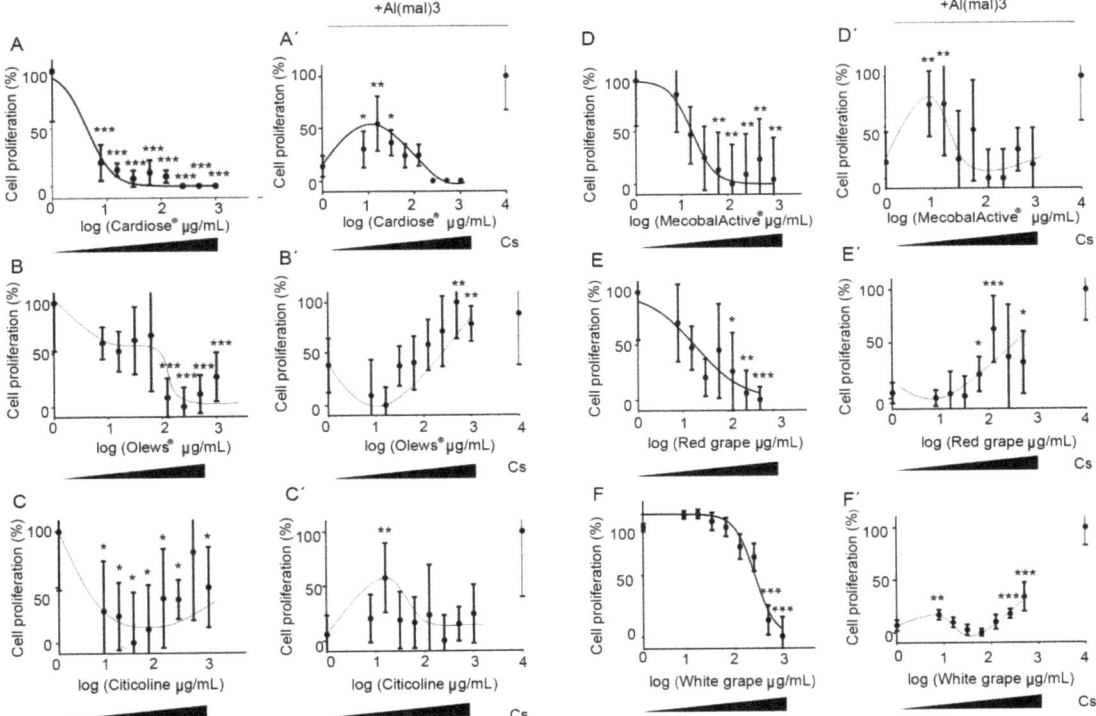

Figure 3. Neuroprotective effects of the extracts on hippocampal neuron cultures. Dose-response curves of the extracts on hippocampal neuron cultures. Cells were incubated with different concentrations of Cardiose® (**A**), Olews® (**B**), citicoline (**C**), MecobalActive® (**D**), red grape (**E**), or white grape extracts (**F**) for 72 h in the absence (**A–F**) or presence (**A′–F′**) of 125-µM Al(mal)$_3$. Data are normalized and expressed as a percentage of the over-basal response (mean ± SEM). Significant differences were analyzed on data from eight different experiments; one-way ANOVA and Dunnett's multiple comparison post-hoc test were used for statistical analysis. * $p < 0.05$, ** $p < 0.01$, and *** $p < 0.001$ versus cells or Al(mal)$_3$ treatment. Cs: control cells, not exposed to Al(mal)$_3$.

Next, to study the neuroprotective effects of the natural extracts, we pretreated hippocampal cells with the extracts, and then, we exposed them to Al(mal)$_3$. Seventy-two h later, the cell numbers were assessed for all experimental conditions. Olews® and red and white grape extracts presented a slight but significant recovery of the number of cells with the highest doses, with GI_{50} values of 85, 400, and 800 µg/mL, respectively

(Figure 3B′,E′,F′). In the case of Cardiose®, citicoline, and MecobalActive®, there was higher protection by the lower concentrations (7.8 to 15.6 µg/mL) (Figure 3A′,C′,D′). Taken together, these results suggest that Cardiose®, Olews®, citicoline, MecobalActive®, and red and white grape extracts may have certain neuroprotective roles on neuroblasts in vitro.

3.3. MecobalActive®, Olews®, and Red and White Grape Extracts Treatment Reduces ROS Levels and Caspase-3 Activity

Previous studies found that Al(mal)$_3$ induces neurotoxicity in SH-SY 5Y cells by disrupting the levels of ROS and by inducing apoptosis [35]. To find out the mechanisms mediating the neuroprotection role in vitro of Olews®, MecobalActive®, and red and white grape extracts, we studied both mechanisms in depth. For each extract, we selected a concentration closer to its GI$_{50}$.

The ROS measurements indicated that there were no increases in ROS activity elicited by the supplements (Figure 4A). On the other hand, Al(mal)$_3$ produced a four-fold increase in ROS activity, as expected (Figure 4A). The ROS levels decreased very significantly when any of the supplements were added in combination with Al(mal)$_3$ (Figure 4A).

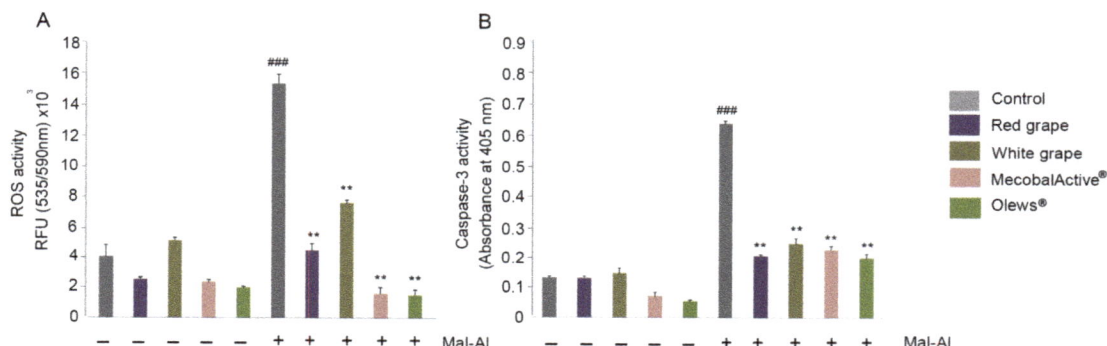

Figure 4. Reactive oxygen species (ROS) levels (**A**) and caspase-3 activity (**B**) on SH-SY 5Y cells after extract treatment. Cells were treated with red grape, white grape, MecobalActive®, or Olews® for 48 h in the absence or presence of 125-µM Al(mal)$_3$. ROS activity (**A**) was quantified by measuring the fluorescence at 535/590 nm. Caspase-3 activity (B) was quantified by measuring the absorbance at 405 nm. Values are presented as mean ± SEM from at least three independent experiments; Kruskal-Wallis test followed by Mann Whitney post-hoc test were used for statistical analysis. ### $p < 0.001$ versus untreated cells and ** $p < 0.01$ versus Al(mal)3. Abbreviations: Mal-Al: Al(mal)$_3$.

In a similar way, the supplements had no effect on the caspase-3 levels of the treated cells, but they greatly and significantly reduced the Al(mal)$_3$-induced caspase-3 levels (Figure 4B). No differences were found in the nitrite or nitrate levels (data not shown), indicating that Al(mal)$_3$ does not influence the RNS.

3.4. Immobilization for Six h Causes Oxidative Stress in Mouse Brains

Based on our previous findings, we hypothesized that the oral administration of these natural supplements could prevent the appearance of oxidative stress in the brain. Before starting the formal experiments, we investigated which was the shortest period of immobilization needed to cause detectable stress in the mouse brain. For this, the animals were immobilized for zero (control), two, four, or six h, and the mRNA expression of the inflammatory markers IL-6 and TNF-alpha, as well as the oxidation marker NOX-2, were determined in the brain tissue.

We observed a statistically significant increase in the expression of IL-6 (1.7-fold) (Figure 5A), NOX-2 (two-fold) (Figure 5B), and TNF-alpha (2.2-fold) (Figure 5C) only after six h of immobilization. Shorter immobilization times did not result in the significant modification of these markers (Figure 5). For this reason, we chose six h as the optimal immobilization time for further experiments.

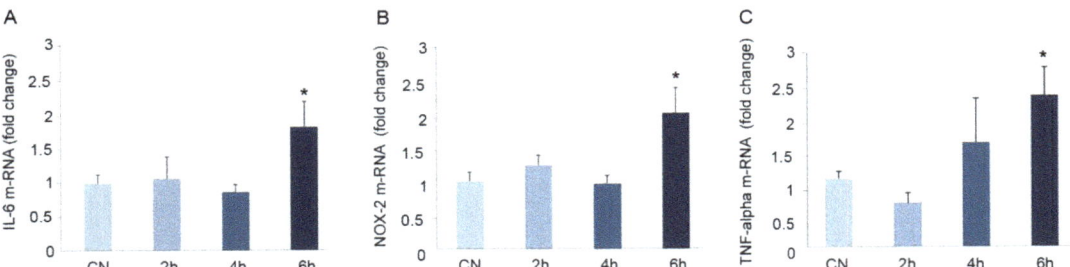

Figure 5. Immobilization causes oxidative stress in mouse brains. Mice were immobilized for different times: 0 (CN), 2, 4, or 6 h. The mRNA expression of IL-6 (**A**), NOX-2 (**B**), and TNF-alpha (**C**) were quantified by real-time (RT)-PCR. The mRNA expression was normalized with GAPDH. All data were related to that from the control and are expressed as a fold change. Values are presented as mean ± SEM from at least three independent experiments. Kruskal-Wallis test followed by Mann Whitney post-hoc test were used for statistical analysis. * $p < 0.05$ versus CN. Abbreviations: CN: control.

3.5. Oral Administration of Natural Extracts Provides Protection against Oxidative Stress

Four natural extracts were selected based on their in vitro behavior and inoculated: red grape, white grape, MecobalActive®, and Olews®, each of them at two different concentrations (Table 1). In agreement with our previous results (Figure 5), immobilization stress significantly increased the expression of IL-6 and TNF-alpha when compared to the control (2.5-fold and two-fold respectively) (Figure 6A,B). The administration of the extracts resulted in a statistically significant diminution of the expression of both genes in all used conditions (Figure 6A,B). For some of the extracts, specifically red grape, MecobalActive®, and Olews®, we found values very close to those obtained in the control animals. In addition, we also studied the expressions of NOX-2 and HMOX-1. These genes are involved in oxidation mechanisms, and they increase in the brain of mice subjected to stress [4]. The administration of natural extracts significantly decreased the immobilization-increased expression of both NOX-2 and HMOX-1 (Figure 6C,D). In the same way that occurred with inflammatory cytokines, the extracts brought the expression of both genes to levels very similar to those found in the animals without stress. Finally, we also analyzed Nrf-2 expression. This molecule is a transcription factor that regulates the expression of numerous antioxidant genes. Numerous authors have described Nrf-2 expression as a protective mechanism for oxidative stress [36–38]. As expected, immobilization stress reduced Nrf-2 expression (Figure 6E), and all extracts restored Nrf-2 expression to control or even to higher levels, indicating a potent antioxidant effect (Figure 6E).

3.6. Preventive Treatment with Natural Extracts Increases Antioxidant Enzyme Activity in the Brain

To verify the possible protective role of these extracts in oxidative stress, we studied the activity of two antioxidant enzymes, catalase and superoxide dismutase (SOD), in the mouse brains.

It has been described that stress causes a decrease in catalase activity in the mouse brain [4]. First, we confirmed that our experimental model of acute stress was able to reproduce these results. Indeed, we observed a significant reduction in catalase activity in stressed mice compared to nonstressed animals (Figure 7A). Furthermore, the administration of natural extracts led to a statistically significant increase in the levels of catalase activity after the addiction of the red grape extract, MecobalActive®, and Olews®. No differences were seen after the treatment with white grape extracts (Figure 7A). SOD is one of the most important antioxidant enzymes in cells. It catalyzes the dismutation of the superoxide anion into hydrogen peroxide and molecular oxygen [39]. As with catalase activity, stress caused a significant decrease in SOD activity in the mouse brains (Figure 7B). Interestingly, the administration of natural extracts: red grape, white grape, MecobalActive®, and Olews® significantly increased the activity of the SOD enzyme in all used conditions (Figure 7B).

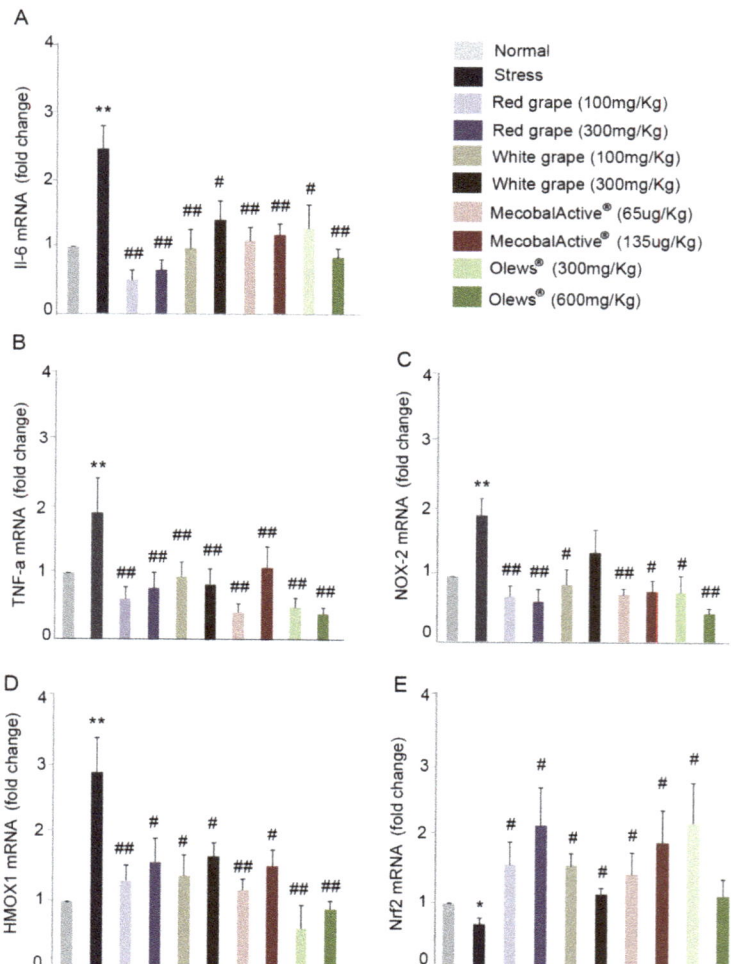

Figure 6. Natural extracts protect against oxidative stress. Red and white grape seed extracts, MecobalActive®, and Olews® were administered orally during 5 consecutive days. Then, mice were immobilized for 6 h. The mRNA expressions of IL-6 (**A**), TNF-alpha (**B**), NOX-2 (**C**), HMOX1 (**D**), and Nrf2 (**E**) were quantified in mouse brains by RT-PCR. Gene expression was normalized with GAPDH. All data were normalized to levels found in nonstressed mice (normal) and are expressed as a fold change. Values are presented as mean ± SEM from eight experimental animals. One-way ANOVA and Dunnett's multiple comparison post-hoc test were used for statistical analysis. * $p < 0.05$ and ** $p < 0.01$ versus normal mice, and # $p < 0.05$ and ## $p < 0.01$ versus restrained mice (stress).

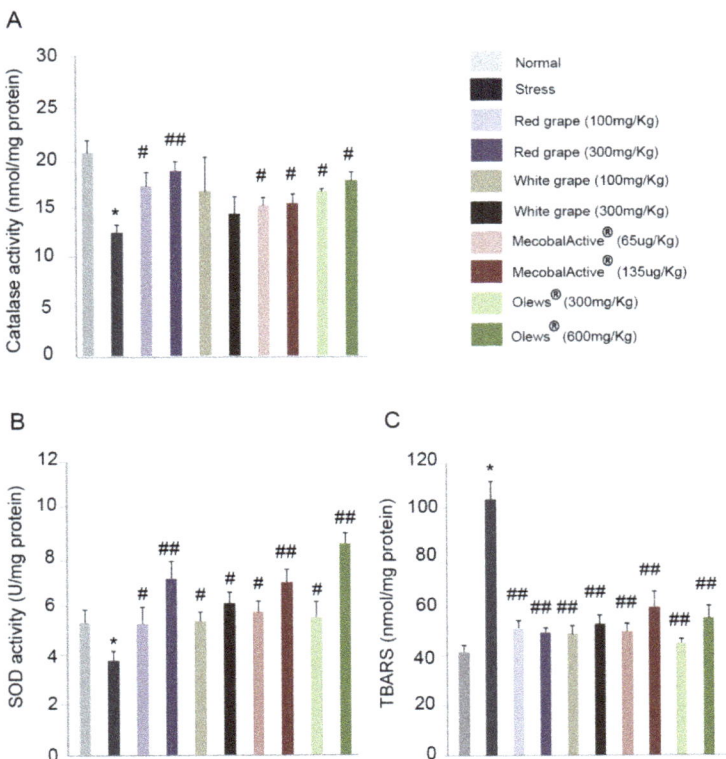

Figure 7. Natural extracts increase the activity of antioxidant enzymes. Mouse brains were isolated, and the catalase activity (**A**), SOD activity (**B**), and TBARS (**C**) were analyzed. The values are presented as mean ± SEM from eight experimental animals. One-way ANOVA and Dunnett's multiple comparison post-hoc test were used for statistical analysis. * $p < 0.05$ versus normal mice, and # $p < 0.05$ and ## $p < 0.01$ versus restrained (stress) mice. Abbreviations: SOD: superoxide dismutase; TBARS: thiobarbituric acid reactive substances.

3.7. Treatment with Natural Extracts Prevents the Formation of Lipid Peroxidation Products in the Brain

Lipid peroxidation, an oxidative degradation of cellular lipids, is another important parameter to take into account when studying oxidative stress [40]. We measured the MDA levels present in the mouse brain. Acute stress more than doubled the MDA levels when compared with the nonstressed control group (Figure 7C). In addition, a treatment with any of the extracts drastically reduced MDA levels in the brain tissue, which reached levels very similar to those found in the animals without stress (Figure 7C).

4. Discussion

NDs pose a major health problem for developed countries, and this situation will progressively worsen due to a rapidly ageing population. Stress is known as the "21st century disease" and has been identified as one of the main risk factors in the development of NDs [41]. In this context, the use of natural bioactive extracts has been postulated as a possible preventive treatment of NDs due to their antioxidant power, which is able to reduce stress efficiently [42].

In this work, we found that natural bioactive supplements such as MecobalActive®, Olews®, and red and white grape seed extracts may have neuroprotective effects in vitro, both in the SH-SY 5Y cell line and in hippocampal neuron cultures, mainly by reducing ROS levels and decreasing caspase-3 activity. In vivo, we demonstrated that oral administration of the supplements for just five days reduces the expression of genes involved in inflammation and oxidation mechanisms, whereas it increments the expression of genes related to protection against oxidative stress. Furthermore, we found that a preventive treatment with these natural extracts increases the activity of antioxidant enzymes and prevents lipid peroxidation in the brains of stressed mice.

We found that Olews®, MecobalActive®, and red and white grape seed extracts show a dose-dependent toxicity in SH-SY 5Y cells. Similar results have been described in previous studies. For instance, grape seed extracts were toxic for cell line PC12 at concentrations higher than 200 µg/mL [12]. Similar extracts exhibited a dose-dependent toxicity for oral cancer cell line Ca9-22, which was very significant at doses higher than 100 µg/mL [43]. All these results have been obtained on tumor cell lines, and some authors have proposed that natural antioxidant extracts have an antitumoral capacity [44]. This is why we decided to test the extracts in a primary culture of mouse neurons. To the best of our knowledge, this is the first time that antioxidant extracts were tested in primary cultures, and we were surprised to find that this cellular toxicity also affected the nontransformed cells. Furthermore, with some extracts, the doses needed to elicit a significant antistress response were higher than the GI_{50} value, suggesting that the same treatment was simultaneously cytotoxic and antioxidant. This can be explained if we realize that these extracts are not constituted by a pure substance, but they are a mixture of several chemicals. It is easy to envision a situation in which one or several of the components are cytotoxic, whereas others are antioxidant and, thus, cytoprotective in the presence of a stressor.

This cytotoxic behavior of the extracts seems to be at odds with the approval of these substances for human consumption and their ample use with no reported side effects. We need to understand that these extracts are approved for oral use (and not as injectable drugs), and therefore, we need to take into consideration the digestive and absorption processes. Digestion could destroy and/or modify some of the extracts´ components, whereas absorption would take only specific substances in such a way that the potentially cytotoxic molecules never reach normal neurons. The vast majority of antioxidant substances need to be fermented by the microbiota of either the small intestine or the colon to achieve optimal absorption [45]. Specifically, Cardiose® contains a flavonoid, diglycoside, that cannot be absorbed in the small intestine. It must proceed to the colon, where it is fermented prior to absorption [46]. Oleuropein, the main component of Olews®, is poorly absorbed in vitro [47], although it is fermented by intestinal bacteria, which facilitates intestinal absorption [48]. MecobalActive® needs a carrier protein that serves as a mediator for its intestinal absorption [49]. In the case of grape seed extracts, they need to be digested before reaching circulation [50]. Furthermore, simulated digestion experiments suggest that grape seed extracts are stable in acid-based environments, such as the stomach, but are processed under a simulation of duodenal conditions [51]. Therefore, we have to be cautious when interpreting in vitro results, paying more attention to in vivo studies, which should be more informative about the antioxidant neuroprotector effects of tested supplements.

Oxidative stress is recognized as a very significant contributor to the pathogenesis of many devastating NDs [52]. In particular, mitochondrial dysfunction leads to the aberrant production of ROS, which are capable of oxidizing lipids and proteins, ultimately causing cell death [53]. We used Al(mal)$_3$ to induce neurotoxicity, because it is able to induce mitochondrial membrane potential changes, elevate the ROS, and promote apoptosis in neuron cells [54]. Here, we found that Olews®, MecobalActive®, and red and white grape extracts reduce Al(mal)$_3$–induced ROS in SH-SY 5Y cells. In addition, Al(mal)$_3$ causes caspase-3 activation, thus inducing apoptosis and, subsequently, cell death [54]. We also demonstrated that Olews®, MecobalActive®, and red and white grape extracts were able to reduce Al(mal)$_3$-induced caspase-3 activity. In summary, our results suggest that these natural extracts may play certain antioxidant neuroprotective roles in vitro.

Excessive stress can provoke oxidative stress damage, and the brain tissue has been described as more susceptible to oxidation than other organs [55]. The use of stress models is supported by substantial evidence implicating stress as a precipitating factor for several neuropsychiatric disorders [56]. Most authors in the field use six h of immobilization for their stress-inducing experiments [4,57], but no information of what happens at shorter times is available. We ran a time course and measured the levels of inflammatory cytokines and NOX-2 in brain tissue after two, four, and six h of immobilization. The differences were statistically significant only after the longest exposure (six h), indicating that shorter times do not generate measurable changes in gene expressions in the mouse brain.

Acute restraint stress stimulates several cellular events, resulting in enhanced ROS production [58]. While intracellular ROS serve mainly for host defense against infectious agents, redox-sensitive signal transduction, and other cellular processes, the extracellular release of ROS damages surrounding tissues and triggers inflammatory processes [59] that finally enhance the lipopolysaccharide (LPS)-mediated production of proinflammatory cytokines IL-1β, IL-6, and TNF-α [60,61]. NOX2 is well-known for generating superoxide molecules under oxidative stress-mediated circumstances. Furthermore, HMOX1 acts as a heat shock protein and is induced by oxidative stress [62]. HMOX1 and NOX-2 expressions are upregulated in the stressed brain [63] and in experimental models of NDs [64]. On the contrary, nuclear factor Nrf-2 induces the expression of antioxidant genes that eventually provoke an anti-inflammatory expression profile that is crucial for the initiation of healing [65]. In accordance with this general pathway, we described that the administration of all extracts used in the study (red grape, white grape, MecobalActive®, and Olews®) prevents the expression of genes involved in inflammation and oxidation mechanisms, while increasing the expression of genes related to protection against oxidative stress, thus identifying them as efficient inhibitors of stress-related cellular damage.

Similarly, restraint stress in rodents precipitates many neurochemical, hormonal, and behavioral abnormalities that are often associated with an imbalance in the brain's intracellular redox state. Numerous studies have reported that restraint stress enhances lipid peroxidation and decreases antioxidant enzyme activities in rodents [58,66]. To prevent oxidative stress damage, most organisms are equipped with antioxidant mechanisms. SOD and catalase are the best-known antioxidant enzymes [4]. We found that a pretreatment with the extracts increased the activity of catalase and SOD when compared to stressed mice. On the other hand, lipid peroxidation is the oxidative degradation of lipids [67]. MDA is one of the final products of polyunsaturated fatty acid peroxidation in cells. An increase in free radicals causes the overproduction of MDA, which is commonly used as a marker of oxidative stress [68]. In agreement with this, we found that MDA levels significantly increased in the brains of stressed animals but were very efficiently normalized by oral administration of the supplements.

5. Conclusions

Taken together, our results suggest that some natural bioactive supplements (specifically, Olews®, MecobalActive®, and red and white grape seed extracts) may have important protective properties against oxidative stress processes occurring in the brain. Since oxidative stress has a critical role in the development of NDs, we propose the addition of these natural supplements to commonly used food staples as a possible global preventive treatment for NDs.

Author Contributions: Conceptualization, M.B. and A.M.; methodology, M.B., J.G.-S.; validation, M.B., J.G.-S., and A.M.; formal analysis, M.B., J.G.-S., and A.M.; investigation, M.B., J.G.-S., and A.M.; writing—original draft preparation, M.B.; writing—review and editing, A.M.; supervision, A.M.; and funding acquisition, A.M. All authors have read and agreed to the published version of the manuscript.

Funding: This research was funded by the Spanish Ministry of Science, Innovation, and Universities (RTC-2017-6424-1) and co-funded by the European Regional Development Fund (FEDER).

Institutional Review Board Statement: All procedures involving animals were carried out in accordance with the European Communities Council Directive (2010/63/EU) and Spanish legislation (RD53/2013) on animal experiments and with approval from the ethical committee on animal welfare of our institution (Órgano Encargado del Bienestar Animal del Centro de Investigación Biomédica de La Rioja, OEBA-CIBIR, procedure number AMR14, date of approval: 24 February 2020).

Informed Consent Statement: Not applicable.

Data Availability Statement: The data presented in this study are available on request from the corresponding author. The data are not publicly available due to their large volume and little interest.

Acknowledgments: We gratefully acknowledge Alvinesa Natural Ingredients and HealthTech Bio Actives for generously providing the food supplements free of charge.

Conflicts of Interest: The authors declare no conflict of interest. The funders had no role in the design of the study; in the collection, analyses, or interpretation of data; in the writing of the manuscript; or in the decision to publish the results.

References

1. Cirmi, S.; Ferlazzo, N.; Lombardo, G.E.; Ventura-Spagnolo, E.; Gangemi, S.; Calapai, G.; Navarra, M. Neurodegenerative Diseases: Might Citrus Flavonoids Play a Protective Role? *Molecules* **2016**, *21*, 1312. [CrossRef]
2. Dugger, B.N.; Dickson, D.W. Pathology of Neurodegenerative Diseases. *Cold Spring Harb. Perspect. Biol.* **2017**, *9*, a028035. [CrossRef] [PubMed]
3. Litvan, I.; Goldman, J.G.; Troster, A.I.; Schmand, B.A.; Weintraub, D.; Petersen, R.C.; Mollenhauer, B.; Adler, C.H.; Marder, K.; Williams-Gray, C.H.; et al. Diagnostic criteria for mild cognitive impairment in Parkinson's disease: Movement Disorder Society Task Force guidelines. *Mov. Disord.* **2012**, *27*, 349–356. [CrossRef] [PubMed]
4. Choi, H.I.; Lee, H.W.; Eom, T.M.; Lim, S.A.; Ha, H.Y.; Seol, I.C.; Kim, Y.S.; Oh, D.S.; Yoo, H.R. A traditional Korean multiple herbal formulae (Yuk-Mi-Jihwang-Tang) attenuates acute restraint stress-induced brain tissue oxidation. *Drug Chem. Toxicol.* **2017**, *40*, 125–133. [CrossRef] [PubMed]
5. Chiurchiu, V.; Maccarrone, M. Chronic inflammatory disorders and their redox control: From molecular mechanisms to therapeutic opportunities. *Antioxid. Redox Signal.* **2011**, *15*, 2605–2641. [CrossRef]
6. Huang, Y.; Mucke, L. Alzheimer mechanisms and therapeutic strategies. *Cell* **2012**, *148*, 1204–1222. [CrossRef]
7. Singh, A.K.; Singh, S.K.; Nandi, M.K.; Mishra, G.; Maurya, A.; Rai, A.; Rai, G.P.; Awasthi, R.; Sharma, B.; Kulkarni, G.T. Berberine: A Plant-derived Alkaloid with Therapeutic Potential to Combat Alzheimer's disease. *Cent. Nerv. Syst. Agents Med. Chem.* **2019**, *19*, 154–170. [CrossRef]
8. Liguori, I.; Russo, G.; Curcio, F.; Bulli, G.; Aran, L.; Della-Morte, D.; Gargiulo, G.; Testa, G.; Cacciatore, F.; Bonaduce, D.; et al. Oxidative stress, aging, and diseases. *Clin. Interv. Aging* **2018**, *13*, 757–772. [CrossRef]
9. Uttara, B.; Singh, A.V.; Zamboni, P.; Mahajan, R.T. Oxidative stress and neurodegenerative diseases: A review of upstream and downstream antioxidant therapeutic options. *Curr. Neuropharmacol.* **2009**, *7*, 65–74. [CrossRef]
10. Kim, M.S.; Kwon, D.Y.; Cho, H.J.; Lee, M.S. Protective effects of Korean herbal remedy against oxidative stress in cardiomyocytes. *Phytother. Res.* **2006**, *20*, 235–236. [CrossRef] [PubMed]
11. Hu, C.W.; Yen, C.C.; Huang, Y.L.; Pan, C.H.; Lu, F.J.; Chao, M.R. Oxidatively damaged DNA induced by humic acid and arsenic in maternal and neonatal mice. *Chemosphere* **2010**, *79*, 93–99. [CrossRef] [PubMed]
12. Lian, Q.; Nie, Y.; Zhang, X.; Tan, B.; Cao, H.; Chen, W.; Gao, W.; Chen, J.; Liang, Z.; Lai, H.; et al. Effects of grape seed proanthocyanidin on Alzheimer's disease in vitro and in vivo. *Exp. Ther. Med.* **2016**, *12*, 1681–1692. [CrossRef] [PubMed]
13. Tonnies, E.; Trushina, E. Oxidative Stress, Synaptic Dysfunction, and Alzheimer's Disease. *J. Alzheimers Dis.* **2017**, *57*, 1105–1121. [CrossRef] [PubMed]
14. Pizzino, G.; Irrera, N.; Cucinotta, M.; Pallio, G.; Mannino, F.; Arcoraci, V.; Squadrito, F.; Altavilla, D.; Bitto, A. Oxidative Stress: Harms and Benefits for Human Health. *Oxid. Med. Cell. Longev.* **2017**, *2017*, 8416763. [CrossRef]
15. Liu, Z.; Ren, Z.; Zhang, J.; Chuang, C.C.; Kandaswamy, E.; Zhou, T.; Zuo, L. Role of ROS and Nutritional Antioxidants in Human Diseases. *Front. Physiol.* **2018**, *9*, 477. [CrossRef]
16. Duraes, F.; Pinto, M.; Sousa, E. Old Drugs as New Treatments for Neurodegenerative Diseases. *Pharmaceuticals* **2018**, *11*, 44. [CrossRef]
17. Rodriguez-Perez, C.; Garcia-Villanova, B.; Guerra-Hernandez, E.; Verardo, V. Grape Seeds Proanthocyanidins: An Overview of In Vivo Bioactivity in Animal Models. *Nutrients* **2019**, *11*, 2435. [CrossRef]
18. Das, V.; Sim, D.A.; Miller, J.H. Effect of taxoid and nontaxoid site microtubule-stabilizing agents on axonal transport of mitochondria in untransfected and ECFP-htau40-transfected rat cortical neurons in culture. *J. Neurosci. Res.* **2014**, *92*, 1155–1166. [CrossRef]
19. Scalbert, A.; Johnson, I.T.; Saltmarsh, M. Polyphenols: Antioxidants and beyond. *Am. J. Clin. Nutr.* **2005**, *81*, 215S–217S. [CrossRef]

20. Perez-Hernandez, J.; Zaldivar-Machorro, V.J.; Villanueva-Porras, D.; Vega-Avila, E.; Chavarria, A. A Potential Alternative against Neurodegenerative Diseases: Phytodrugs. *Oxid. Med. Cell. Longev.* **2016**, *2016*, 8378613. [CrossRef]
21. Dinda, B.; Dinda, M.; Roy, A.; Dinda, S. Dietary plant flavonoids in prevention of obesity and diabetes. *Adv. Protein Chem. Struct. Biol.* **2020**, *120*, 159–235. [PubMed]
22. Ben Youssef, S.; Brisson, G.; Doucet-Beaupre, H.; Castonguay, A.M.; Gora, C.; Amri, M.; Lévesque, M. Neuroprotective benefits of grape seed and skin extract in a mouse model of Parkinson's disease. *Nutr. Neurosci.* **2019**, 1–15. [CrossRef] [PubMed]
23. Seibenhener, M.L.; Wooten, M.W. Isolation and culture of hippocampal neurons from prenatal mice. *J. Vis. Exp.* **2012**, e3634. [CrossRef] [PubMed]
24. Benavente-Garcia, O.; Castillo, J.; Alcaraz, M.; Vicente, V.; Del Rio, J.A. Beneficial action of Citrus flavonoids on multiple cancer-related biological pathways. *Curr. Cancer Drug Targets* **2007**, *7*, 795–809.
25. Bertholf, R.L.; Herman, M.M.; Savory, J.; Carpenter, R.M.; Sturgill, B.C.; Katsetos, C.D.; VandenBerg, S.R.; Wills, M.R. A long-term intravenous model of aluminum maltol toxicity in rabbits: Tissue distribution, hepatic, renal, and neuronal cytoskeletal changes associated with systemic exposure. *Toxicol. Appl. Pharmacol.* **1989**, *98*, 58–74. [CrossRef]
26. Bomfim, L.M.; de Araujo, F.A.; Dias, R.B.; Sales, C.B.S.; Rocha, C.A.G.; Correa, R.S.; Soares, M.B.P.; Batista, A.A.; Bezerra, D.P. Ruthenium(II) complexes with 6-methyl-2-thiouracil selectively reduce cell proliferation, cause DNA double-strand break and trigger caspase-mediated apoptosis through JNK/p38 pathways in human acute promyelocytic leukemia cells. *Sci. Rep.* **2019**, *9*, 11483. [CrossRef]
27. Perez Nievas, B.G.; Hammerschmidt, T.; Kummer, M.P.; Terwel, D.; Leza, J.C.; Heneka, M.T. Restraint stress increases neuroinflammation independently of amyloid beta levels in amyloid precursor protein/PS1 transgenic mice. *J. Neurochem.* **2011**, *116*, 43–52. [CrossRef]
28. Koch, C.E.; Leinweber, B.; Drengberg, B.C.; Blaum, C.; Oster, H. Interaction between circadian rhythms and stress. *Neurobiol. Stress* **2017**, *6*, 57–67. [CrossRef]
29. Chen, C.; Zheng, Y.; Wu, T.; Wu, C.; Cheng, X. Oral administration of grape seed polyphenol extract restores memory deficits in chronic cerebral hypoperfusion rats. *Behav. Pharmacol.* **2017**, *28*, 207–213. [CrossRef]
30. Huang, Y.; Zhao, H.; Cao, K.; Sun, D.; Yang, Y.; Liu, C.; Cui, J.; Cheng, Y.; Li, B.; Cai, J.; et al. Radioprotective Effect of Grape Seed Proanthocyanidins In Vitro and In Vivo. *Oxid. Med. Cell. Longev.* **2016**, *2016*, 5706751. [CrossRef]
31. Gan, L.; Qian, M.; Shi, K.; Chen, G.; Gu, Y.; Du, W.; Zhu, G. Restorative effect and mechanism of mecobalamin on sciatic nerve crush injury in mice. *Neural Regen. Res.* **2014**, *9*, 1979–1984. [CrossRef] [PubMed]
32. Sulaiman, G.M.; Tawfeeq, A.T.; Jaaffer, M.D. Biogenic synthesis of copper oxide nanoparticles using olea europaea leaf extract and evaluation of their toxicity activities: An in vivo and in vitro study. *Biotechnol. Prog.* **2018**, *34*, 218–230. [CrossRef] [PubMed]
33. Sumiyoshi, M.; Kimura, Y. Effects of olive leaf extract and its main component oleuroepin on acute ultraviolet B irradiation-induced skin changes in C57BL/6J mice. *Phytother. Res.* **2010**, *24*, 995–1003. [CrossRef] [PubMed]
34. Ochoa-Callejero, L.; Garcia-Sanmartin, J.; Martinez-Herrero, S.; Rubio-Mediavilla, S.; Narro-Iniguez, J.; Martínez, A. Small molecules related to adrenomedullin reduce tumor burden in a mouse model of colitis-associated colon cancer. *Sci. Rep.* **2017**, *7*, 17488. [CrossRef] [PubMed]
35. Ahmad Rather, M.; Justin Thenmozhi, A.; Manivasagam, T.; Nataraj, J.; Essa, M.M.; Chidambaram, S.B. Asiatic acid nullified aluminium toxicity in in vitro model of Alzheimer's disease. *Front. Biosci.* **2018**, *10*, 287–299.
36. Bellezza, I.; Giambanco, I.; Minelli, A.; Donato, R. Nrf2-Keap1 signaling in oxidative and reductive stress. *Biochim. Biophys. Acta Mol. Cell Res.* **2018**, *1865*, 721–733. [CrossRef]
37. Ma, Q. Role of nrf2 in oxidative stress and toxicity. *Annu. Rev. Pharmacol. Toxicol.* **2013**, *53*, 401–426. [CrossRef]
38. Levonen, A.L.; Inkala, M.; Heikura, T.; Jauhiainen, S.; Jyrkkänen, H.K.; Kansanen, E.; Määttä, K.; Romppanen, E.; Turunen, P.; Rutanen, J.; et al. Nrf2 gene transfer induces antioxidant enzymes and suppresses smooth muscle cell growth in vitro and reduces oxidative stress in rabbit aorta in vivo. *Arterioscler. Thromb. Vasc. Biol.* **2007**, *27*, 741–747. [CrossRef]
39. Fukai, T.; Ushio-Fukai, M. Superoxide dismutases: Role in redox signaling, vascular function, and diseases. *Antioxid. Redox Signal.* **2011**, *15*, 1583–1606. [CrossRef]
40. Su, L.J.; Zhang, J.H.; Gomez, H.; Murugan, R.; Hong, X.; Xu, D.; Jiang, F.; Peng, Z.Y. Reactive Oxygen Species-Induced Lipid Peroxidation in Apoptosis, Autophagy, and Ferroptosis. *Oxid. Med. Cell Longev.* **2019**, *2019*, 5080843. [CrossRef]
41. Deshmukh, V.D.; Deshmukh, S.V. Stress-adaptation failure hypothesis of Alzheimer's disease. *Med. Hypotheses* **1990**, *32*, 293–295. [CrossRef]
42. Popa-Wagner, A.; Dumitrascu, D.I.; Capitanescu, B.; Petcu, E.B.; Surugiu, R.; Fang, W.H.; Dumbrava, D.A. Dietary habits, lifestyle factors and neurodegenerative diseases. *Neural Regen. Res.* **2020**, *15*, 394–400. [CrossRef] [PubMed]
43. Yen, C.Y.; Hou, M.F.; Yang, Z.W.; Tang, J.Y.; Li, K.T.; Huang, H.W.; Huang, Y.H.; Lee, S.Y.; Fu, T.F.; Hsieh, C.Y.; et al. Concentration effects of grape seed extracts in anti-oral cancer cells involving differential apoptosis, oxidative stress, and DNA damage. *BMC Complement. Altern. Med.* **2015**, *15*, 94. [CrossRef] [PubMed]
44. Dos Santos, D.M.; Rocha, C.V.J.; da Silveira, E.F.; Marinho, M.A.G.; Rodrigues, M.R.; Silva, N.O.; Ferreira, A.S.; Fernandes de Moura, N.; Sagrera Darelli, G.J.; Braganhol, E.; et al. In Vitro Anti/Pro-oxidant Activities of R. ferruginea Extract and Its Effect on Glioma Cell Viability: Correlation with Phenolic Compound Content and Effects on Membrane Dynamics. *J. Membr. Biol.* **2018**, *251*, 247–261. [CrossRef]

45. Nemeth, K.; Plumb, G.W.; Berrin, J.G.; Juge, N.; Jacob, R.; Naim, H.Y.; Williamson, G.; Swallow, D.M.; Kroon, P.A. Deglycosylation by small intestinal epithelial cell beta-glucosidases is a critical step in the absorption and metabolism of dietary flavonoid glycosides in humans. *Eur. J. Nutr.* **2003**, *42*, 29–42. [CrossRef]
46. Jin, H.; Tan, X.; Liu, X.; Ding, Y. The study of effect of tea polyphenols on microsatellite instability colorectal cancer and its molecular mechanism. *Int. J. Colorectal Dis.* **2010**, *25*, 1407–1415. [CrossRef]
47. Corona, G.; Tzounis, X.; Assunta Dessi, M.; Deiana, M.; Debnam, E.S.; Visioli, F.; Spencer, J.P.E. The fate of olive oil polyphenols in the gastrointestinal tract: Implications of gastric and colonic microflora-dependent biotransformation. *Free Radic. Res.* **2006**, *40*, 647–658. [CrossRef]
48. Ciafardini, G.; Marsilio, V.; Lanza, B.; Pozzi, N. Hydrolysis of Oleuropein by Lactobacillus plantarum Strains Associated with Olive Fermentation. *Appl. Environ. Microbiol.* **1994**, *60*, 4142–4147. [CrossRef]
49. Pinto, J.; Paiva-Martins, F.; Corona, G.; Debnam, E.S.; Jose Oruna-Concha, M.; Vauzour, D.; Gordon, M.H.; Spencer, J.P.E. Absorption and metabolism of olive oil secoiridoids in the small intestine. *Br. J. Nutr.* **2011**, *105*, 1607–1618. [CrossRef]
50. Sano, A.; Yamakoshi, J.; Tokutake, S.; Tobe, K.; Kubota, Y.; Kikuchi, M. Procyanidin B1 is detected in human serum after intake of proanthocyanidin-rich grape seed extract. *Biosci. Biotechnol. Biochem.* **2003**, *67*, 1140–1143. [CrossRef]
51. Serra, A.; Macia, A.; Romero, M.P.; Valls, J.; Bladé, C.; Arola, L.; Motilva, M.J. Bioavailability of procyanidin dimers and trimers and matrix food effects in in vitro and in vivo models. *Br. J. Nutr.* **2010**, *103*, 944–952. [CrossRef] [PubMed]
52. Chen, S.D.; Yin, J.H.; Hwang, C.S.; Tang, C.M.; Yang, D.I. Anti-apoptotic and anti-oxidative mechanisms of minocycline against sphingomyelinase/ceramide neurotoxicity: Implication in Alzheimer's disease and cerebral ischemia. *Free Radic. Res.* **2012**, *46*, 940–950. [CrossRef] [PubMed]
53. Ross, E.K.; Gray, J.J.; Winter, A.N.; Linseman, D.A. Immunocal(R) and preservation of glutathione as a novel neuroprotective strategy for degenerative disorders of the nervous system. *Recent Pat. CNS Drug Discov.* **2012**, *7*, 230–235.
54. Rather, H.A.; Thakore, R.; Singh, R.; Jhala, D.; Singh, S.; Vasita, R. Antioxidative study of Cerium Oxide nanoparticle functionalised PCL-Gelatin electrospun fibers for wound healing application. *Bioact. Mater.* **2018**, *3*, 201–211. [CrossRef]
55. Stocchetti, N.; Pagan, F.; Calappi, E.; Canavesi, K.; Beretta, L.; Citerio, G.; Cormio, M.; Colombo, A. Inaccurate early assessment of neurological severity in head injury. *J. Neurotrauma* **2004**, *21*, 1131–1140. [CrossRef]
56. Sathyanesan, M.; Haiar, J.M.; Watt, M.J.; Newton, S.S. Restraint stress differentially regulates inflammation and glutamate receptor gene expression in the hippocampus of C57BL/6 and BALB/c mice. *Stress* **2017**, *20*, 197–204. [CrossRef]
57. Sulakhiya, K.; Patel, V.K.; Saxena, R.; Dashore, J.; Srivastava, A.K.; Rathore, M. Effect of Beta vulgaris Linn. Leaves Extract on Anxiety- and Depressive-like Behavior and Oxidative Stress in Mice after Acute Restraint Stress. *Pharmacognosy Res.* **2016**, *8*, 1–7. [CrossRef]
58. Kumar, A.; Garg, R.; Gaur, V.; Kumar, P. Possible role of NO modulators in protective effect of trazodone and citalopram (antidepressants) in acute immobilization stress in mice. *Indian J. Exp. Biol.* **2010**, *48*, 1131–1135.
59. Duval, C.; Cantero, A.V.; Auge, N.; Mabile, L.; Thiers, J.C.; Negre-Salvayre, A.; Salvayre, R. Proliferation and wound healing of vascular cells trigger the generation of extracellular reactive oxygen species and LDL oxidation. *Free Radic. Biol. Med.* **2003**, *35*, 1589–1598. [CrossRef]
60. Bulua, A.C.; Simon, A.; Maddipati, R.; Pelletier, M.; Park, H.; Kim, K.Y.; Sack, M.N.; Kastner, D.L.; Siegel, R.M. Mitochondrial reactive oxygen species promote production of proinflammatory cytokines and are elevated in TNFR1-associated periodic syndrome (TRAPS). *J. Exp. Med.* **2011**, *208*, 519–533. [CrossRef]
61. Mittal, M.; Siddiqui, M.R.; Tran, K.; Reddy, S.P.; Malik, A.B. Reactive oxygen species in inflammation and tissue injury. *Antioxid. Redox Signal.* **2014**, *20*, 1126–1167. [CrossRef]
62. Agúndez, J.A.; García-Martín, E.; Martínez, C.; Benito-León, J.; Millán-Pascual, J.; Díaz-Sánchez, M.; Calleja, P.; Pisa, D.; Turpín-Fenoll, L.; Alonso-Navarro, H.; et al. Heme Oxygenase-1 and 2 Common Genetic Variants and Risk for Multiple Sclerosis. *Sci. Rep.* **2016**, *6*, 20830. [CrossRef]
63. Emerson, M.R.; LeVine, S.M. Heme oxygenase-1 and NADPH cytochrome P450 reductase expression in experimental allergic encephalomyelitis: An expanded view of the stress response. *J. Neurochem.* **2000**, *75*, 2555–2562. [CrossRef]
64. Van Horssen, J.; Schreibelt, G.; Drexhage, J.; Hazes, T.; Dijkstra, C.D.; van der Valk, P.; de Vries, H.E. Severe oxidative damage in multiple sclerosis lesions coincides with enhanced antioxidant enzyme expression. *Free Radic. Biol. Med.* **2008**, *45*, 1729–1737. [CrossRef]
65. Vomund, S.; Schafer, A.; Parnham, M.J.; Brune, B.; von Knethen, A. Nrf2, the Master Regulator of Anti-Oxidative Responses. *Int. J. Mol. Sci.* **2017**, *18*, 2772. [CrossRef]
66. García-Fernández, M.; Castilla-Ortega, E.; Pedraza, C.; Blanco, E.; Hurtado-Guerrero, I.; Barbancho, M.A.; Chun, J.; Rodríguez-de-Fonseca, F.; Estivill-Torrús, G.; Santín Núñez, L.J. Chronic immobilization in the malpar1 knockout mice increases oxidative stress in the hippocampus. *Int. J. Neurosci.* **2012**, *122*, 583–589. [CrossRef]
67. Dodson, M.; Castro-Portuguez, R.; Zhang, D.D. NRF2 plays a critical role in mitigating lipid peroxidation and ferroptosis. *Redox Biol.* **2019**, *23*, 101107. [CrossRef]
68. Kowalczuk, K.; Stryjecka-Zimmer, M. The influence of oxidative stress on the level of malondialdehyde (MDA) in different areas of the rabbit brain. *Ann. Univ. Mariae Curie Sklodowska Med.* **2002**, *57*, 160–164.

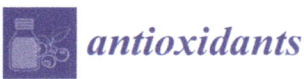

Review

Olive Polyphenols: Antioxidant and Anti-Inflammatory Properties

Monica Bucciantini [1,*], Manuela Leri [1], Pamela Nardiello [2], Fiorella Casamenti [2] and Massimo Stefani [1]

[1] Department of Experimental and Clinical Biomedical Sciences, University of Florence, Florence 50134, Italy; manuela.leri@unifi.it (M.L.); massimo.stefani@unifi.it (M.S.)
[2] Department of Neuroscience, Psychology, Drug Research and Child Health, University of Florence, Florence 50134, Italy; pamela.nardiello@unifi.it (P.N.); fiorella.casamenti@unifi.it (F.C.)
* Correspondence: monica.bucciantini@unifi.it

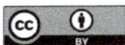

Citation: Bucciantini, M.; Leri, M.; Nardiello, P.; Casamenti, F.; Stefani, M. Olive Polyphenols: Antioxidant and Anti-Inflammatory Properties. *Antioxidants* 2021, 10, 1044. https://doi.org/10.3390/antiox10071044

Academic Editors: Rui F. M. Silva and Lea Pogačnik

Received: 29 May 2021
Accepted: 24 June 2021
Published: 29 June 2021

Publisher's Note: MDPI stays neutral with regard to jurisdictional claims in published maps and institutional affiliations.

Copyright: © 2021 by the authors. Licensee MDPI, Basel, Switzerland. This article is an open access article distributed under the terms and conditions of the Creative Commons Attribution (CC BY) license (https://creativecommons.org/licenses/by/4.0/).

Abstract: Oxidative stress and inflammation triggered by increased oxidative stress are the cause of many chronic diseases. The lack of anti-inflammatory drugs without side-effects has stimulated the search for new active substances. Plant-derived compounds provide new potential anti-inflammatory and antioxidant molecules. Natural products are structurally optimized by evolution to serve particular biological functions, including the regulation of endogenous defense mechanisms and interaction with other organisms. This property explains their relevance for infectious diseases and cancer. Recently, among the various natural substances, polyphenols from extra virgin olive oil (EVOO), an important element of the Mediterranean diet, have aroused growing interest. Extensive studies have shown the potent therapeutic effects of these bioactive molecules against a series of chronic diseases, such as cardiovascular diseases, diabetes, neurodegenerative disorders and cancer. This review begins from the chemical structure, abundance and bioavailability of the main EVOO polyphenols to highlight the effects and the possible molecular mechanism(s) of action of these compounds against inflammation and oxidation, in vitro and in vivo. In addition, the mechanisms of inhibition of molecular signaling pathways activated by oxidative stress by EVOO polyphenols are discussed, together with their possible roles in inflammation-mediated chronic disorders, also taking into account meta-analysis of population studies and clinical trials.

Keywords: EVOO polyphenols; oxidative stress; inflammation

1. Introduction

The increasing extension in life expectancy of humans in advanced countries matches a higher prevalence of a number of lifestyle- and age-associated pathological conditions such as cancer, systemic and neurodegenerative diseases, amyloid diseases, particularly Alzheimer's disease (AD) and Parkinson's (PD) disease, cardiovascular diseases (CVDs) and metabolic diseases including metabolic syndrome (MetS); the latter includes, in addition to type 2 diabetes mellitus (T2DM), CVDs and non-alcoholic hepatitis. These pathologies are characterized by several common features, including, among others, derangement of proteostasis and the redox equilibrium and a remarkable inflammatory response that heavily impair the biochemical and functional features of the affected tissues. Moreover, at present, these pathologies, particularly amyloid diseases, lack effective therapies; it is then evident that, in the light of the latter aspect, prevention appears as the best tool to reduce the risk of these pathological conditions. Accordingly, medical research has progressively focused on the importance of lifestyle. Physical exercise, mental activity and diet, intended as the complex of foods and nutrients taken daily by a person, are three pillars of a healthy lifestyle.

The Mediterranean diet (MD) has been the subject of a huge amount of studies on its properties to prevent different chronic-degenerative diseases from the first evidence from the early 1960s suggesting an association between the alimentation of Mediterranean people and their low cardiovascular mortality [1]. An increasing number of epidemiological and observational studies confirm that the Mediterranean diet (MD) is associated with aging well, a condition where the prevalence of diseases including MetS, CVDs, cancer and cognitive decline appears significantly reduced [2]. The MD can be considered as the heritage of a complex socio-economic development of the Mediterranean populations over past centuries, and includes practices resulting from agricultural, social, territorial and environmental factors intimately associated with the culture and lifestyle of these populations. Recently, modifications of the classical MD have been proposed by the Mediterranean Diet Foundation Expert Group [3]. The new MD pyramid, in addition to the presence of a specific content of characteristic foods (low meat/fish, high fruit, vegetables and carbohydrates, presence of red wine, use of olive oil as main lipid source, moderate caloric intake), also emphasizes the importance of other lifestyle-associated elements, such as moderation, seasonality, adequate rest, conviviality, and physical exercise. The new pyramid also reflects the changes that the MD is undergoing, at the present, within the Mediterranean societies in relation to various geographical, cultural and socio-economic contexts. The high value of the MD and its associated lifestyle was recognized in 2010 by UNESCO, who inscribed the MD in the list of the Intangible Cultural Heritage of Humanity (https://ich.unesco.org/en/RL/mediterranean-diet-00884, accessed on 2013).

An important feature of the MD is the daily consumption of a vast array of phytonutrients including vitamins and plant phenols, which provides its similarities with the Asian diet. In particular, plant polyphenols interfere with multiple signaling pathways involved in protein homeostasis, in the inflammatory response, and in the regulation of both metabolism and the antioxidant defenses [4–6], often recalling a caloric restriction (CR) regimen positively affecting, among others, whole body metabolism, mitochondrial turnover, oxidative stress and the inflammatory and neuroinflammatory response, where autophagy plays an important role [7,8]. Polyphenols can reach these effects by counteracting, at the molecular level, signaling pathways responsible for the cascade reactions involved in aging [9,10]. Overall, present data support the idea that different plant polyphenols, including those from the olive tree, are able to mimic CR effects and to modulate the expression of pro- and anti-apoptotic factors, also through epigenetic modifications [11], thus affecting the same, or very similar, cellular targets. Accordingly, plant polyphenols can be proposed as a useful tool for the prevention and/or treatment of aging-associated diseases connected with chronic inflammation or transcriptional, redox or metabolic derangement [12].

An increasing number of preclinical studies, population studies and clinical trials suggest that adherence to the MD, with particular emphasis on its content of plant polyphenols, often referred to as biophenols, reduces metabolic pathologies and aging-associated deterioration, where derangement of redox homeostasis and an excessive inflammatory response often play pivotal roles. Biophenols are found in many foods of plant origin that play pivotal roles in the MD, including red wine, extra virgin olive oil (EVOO), green tea, spices, berries and aromatic herbs. The content of polyphenols in these foods and their bioavailability are quite low; however, the daily consumption, throughout one's lifetime, of these foods ensures a reduced, yet continuous, intake of polyphenols, providing a rationale for the association between the dietary content of the latter and a significant reduction in the incidence of aging-associated pathologies reported by many population/epidemiological studies and clinical trials [13,14].

A wealth of recent studies has highlighted the fact that, in several aging-associated pathologies such as amyloid diseases, CVDs and MetS, plant polyphenols do not simply interfere with a single step of disease pathogenesis (protein/peptide aggregation, the inflammatory response, the redox/metabolic equilibrium, the proteostasis balance); rather, their positive biological and functional outcomes result from multi-target effects leading to the restoration of altered homeostatic systems in cells and tissues. In addition, the chemical similarities of these structurally distinct molecules can explain why they can induce similar effects. Among others, the importance of natural polyphenols for health has been associated with their remarkable antioxidant power elicited through the modulation of oxidative pathways. The latter can result from interference with enzymes, proteins, receptors, transcription factors and several signaling pathways [4,15]. The ability of plant polyphenols to interfere with biochemical homeostasis has also been taken into consideration [14], and epigenetic modifications of chromatin have been reported to also be involved in these effects [16,17]. Actually, recent research is providing increasing information on the biochemical, cellular and epigenetic modifications induced by several plant polyphenols and the resulting modulation of the homeostasis of key cellular processes such as metabolism, energy balance, redox equilibrium, proteostasis, cell signaling, the inflammatory response, and the control of oxidative stress and of gene expression. The knowledge stemming from these data will allow us to better understand the beneficial effects, for human wellness, of the MD, the importance of its content in plant polyphenols and the role of the latter in disease prevention and, possibly, therapy.

The rising interest in natural polyphenols has resulted in a large number of studies on their medicinal efficacy, carried out not only in cultured cells but also in model organisms and in humans. More recently, an increasing number of studies have also appeared on the biochemical and biological effects of olive polyphenols. The polyphenols elaborated by the olive tree (*Olea europaea*) are present prevalently in the leaves and drupes of the tree and are important as phytoalexins, molecules that the plant elaborates for defense against invasions by microbes and fungi and to discourage leaf-eating insects. EVOO contains over 30 phenolic compounds, including the most represented oleuropein, both in the glycated and in the aglycone (OLE) form, verbascoside, oleocanthal, hydroxytyrosol (HT), tyrosol, and others (see next section). The healthy value of EVOO and olive leaf extracts has been recognized for a long time and scientifically investigated in the last couple of centuries. More recent studies have focused on the biological properties of these molecules, including the antimicrobial, hypoglycemic, vasodilator, antihypertensive, antioxidant and anti-inflammatory ones, whose clinical importance was first reported in 1950 [18]. These properties have led to the inclusion of the alcoholic extract (80%) of olive leaves containing, in addition to minor components, OLE, HT, caffeic acid, tyrosol, apigenin and verbascoside in the European Pharmacopoeia (Ph. Eur.) [19,20].

The molecular determinants of the protection by olive polyphenols against several aging-associated and chronic degenerative conditions, including T2DM [21–23] and non-alcoholic fatty liver disease [24–28], have been extensively investigated in the last 20 years. OLE, HT and other olive polyphenols protect cells against oxidative damage resulting from redox dyshomeostasis [29,30] and an excessive inflammatory response [31], among the main determinants of age-related pathologies such as cancer, T2DM, MetS, osteoporosis and neurological diseases [27,32]. Most of these effects have been associated with the ability of polyphenols to control cell signaling and pathways, to modulate the activity of transcription factors, and to affect gene expression; these nutrigenomic properties of EVOO polyphenols have been recently reviewed [33,34]. Finally, population studies have provided evidence of a significant association between MD, EVOO consumption, and reduced risk of both CVD [35] and cognitive decline [2]. A recent review of the scientific literature focused on clinical trials and population studies has confirmed that the MD and the fortification of the foods with olive leaf extracts protect significantly against several aging-associated degenerative diseases and cancer [36–38]. Accordingly, plant polyphenols are increasingly taken into consideration, as such or their molecular scaffolds, as the starting component to develop new drugs especially designed to combat several chronic degenerative pathologies, including aging-associated neurodegeneration [36,39].

Here, the results of studies on the polyphenols produced by the olive tree and found in EVOO will be reviewed, with a special focus on the antioxidant and anti-inflammatory properties of these molecules. The effects of olive polyphenols in cell and animal models of aging-associated pathologies, including CVDs, MetS and neurodegenerative diseases, the molecular mechanisms underlying these properties, the currently available population studies and clinical trials, and the most recent advances in their possible use to combat neurodegenerative diseases will also be treated.

2. Olive Polyphenols: A Group of Molecules with Shared Chemical and Biological Properties: Structure, Abundance and Bioavailability

Biophenols are a family of over 8000 polyphenolic structures (those presently described) found in almost all plant families mainly as secondary metabolites, including several hundred isolated from edible plants [36,40]. These molecules include non-flavonoids or flavonoids; the latter are further classified as flavonols, flavononols, flavones, anthocyanins, procyanidins, phenolic acids, stilbenes and tannins on the basis of the number of hydroxyls in the molecule and the type and the position of other substituents [41]. The plant sources of plant polyphenols are, among others, bark, leaves, fruits, spices, berries, vegetables, roots, nuts and seeds, herbs, and whole grain products, from which they are transferred in processed foods of plant origin, including EVOO, red wine, green tea, coffee and turmeric. These compounds are characterized by a broad spectrum of biological activities and exert positive effects in a large number of human diseases, including cancer, CVDs, T2DM and neurodegenerative conditions, with molecular mechanisms often related to their antioxidant activity. In the case of EVOO, its healthy properties have been associated with its peculiar chemical composition [42]. EVOO contains both major components (triglycerides and other fatty acid derivatives where mainly monounsaturated fatty acids, in particular oleic acid, are present) and minor components (over 230 different chemicals including aliphatic and triterpenic alcohols, phytosterols, hydrocarbons, tocopherols, and polyphenols) [43]. In the past, the health effects of EVOO were attributed mainly to the presence of oleic acid; however, more recently, attention has been focused on phenolics, a class of bioactive compounds including phenolic acids, phenolic alcohols, flavonoids, secoiridoids and lignans [44].

In particular, olive tree polyphenols include flavonols, lignans and glycosides. Olive glycosides are iridoids, geraniol-derived monoterpenes, whose chemical structure results from a cyclopentane ring fused to a six-member heterocycle with an oxygen atom. In particular, the bicyclic H-5/H-9β, β-*cis*-fused cyclopentanepyran ring system is the most common structural feature and the basic skeletal ring of iridoids. Cleavage of the cyclopentane ring of iridoids produces seco-iridoids, while cleavage of the pyran ring produces iridoid derivatives [45]. Iridoids and secoiridoids, mainly in the glycated form, are found in many medicinal plants belonging to the subclass Asteridae that includes several plant families, particularly Oleaceae.

The polyphenols produced by the olive tree are found in the lipid fraction and in the water fraction (dispersed as minute droplets) of olive oil mainly in the glucose-free form (aglycones), resulting from deglycosylation by plant glycosidases during olive squeezing. The most abundant secoiridoid in olive oil is 3,4-dihydroxyphenylethanol-elenolic acid (3,4-DHPEA-EA), whose glucose-bound form is commonly known as oleuropein; the latter is the main cause of the bitter taste of olive leaves and drupes. Other secoiridoids include oleuropein derivatives, both in the glucose-bound form or as aglycones, such as the dialdehydic form of decarboxymethyl elenolic acid bound to either HT (3,4-dihydroxyphenylethanol-elenolic acid dialdehyde, 3,4-DHPEA-EDA, also known as oleacein) or to tyrosol (p-hydroxyphenylethanol-elenolic acid dialdehyde, p-HPEA-EDA, also known as oleocanthal, or ligstroside aglycone [46,47] (Figure 1). Oleocanthal produces the burning sensation in the back of the throat that accompanies the consumption of freshly squeezed EVOO. Olive oil also has a rich composition in simple phenols; these include tyrosol (p-hydroxyphenylethanol, p-HPEA) and hydroxytyrosol (3,4-dihydroxyphenylethanol, 3,4-DHPEA, DOPET), two phenolic alcohols mostly derived from their secoiridoid precursors. Olive polyphenols also include verbascoside, the caffeoylrhamnosylglucoside of HT, 1-acetoxypinoresinol and pinoresinol (two lignans).

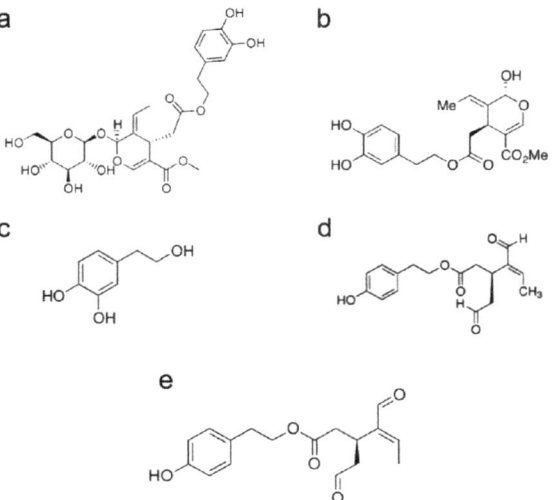

Figure 1. Chemical structure of oleuropein (**a**), oleuropein aglycone (**b**), hydroxytyrosol (**c**), oleacein (**d**), oleocanthal (**e**).

Olive polyphenols are considered to be responsible for some of the recognized pharmacological properties of the olive tree (anti-atherogenic, antihepatotoxic, hypoglycemic, anti-inflammatory, antitumoral, antiviral, analgesic, purgative and immunomodulatory activities) [28,48,49], together with the protection against aging-associated neurodegeneration [29]. For these reasons, the EVOO quality depends not only on the content in free fatty acids resulting from triacylglycerol breakdown (acidity), but also on its content in polyphenols, the molecules responsible for its taste and for many of its healthy properties. Several factors affect the content of polyphenols in olive oil; these include olive cultivar, environmental cues (altitude, meteorological factors and irrigation), cultivation practices, and ripening stage of the fruits [50], together with extraction techniques, systems to separate oil from olive pastes. The conditions of storage (temperature, time) are also of importance, affecting the rate of oxidation/photooxidation reactions and the deposition of suspended water particles rich in polyphenols [51]. Under optimal conditions, the content of polyphenols in EVOO can exceed 60 mg/100 g.

The normal daily dietary intake of plant polyphenols is in the 0.1–1.0 g range; however, the bioavailability of these molecules, including the olive ones, in humans is poor due to reduced intestinal absorption and fast biotransformation that favors their urinary excretion. In addition, in the case of the brain, the circulating polyphenols must also cross the blood–brain barrier before reaching the parenchyma. With few exceptions, polyphenol aglycones can be partially absorbed in the small intestine by passive diffusion [52] much better than their glycated counterparts [53], although important amounts proceed to the large intestine to be eliminated [54]. A review of many studies on polyphenol bioavailability reported a 0 to 4.0 µmol/L plasma concentration of total metabolites produced from the oral administration of 50 mg aglycone equivalents of a polyphenol [55]. After intestinal absorption and passage to the lymph, most polyphenols undergo phase I and phase II metabolism, with substantial biotransformation and production of methylated, sulphated, hydroxylated, thiol-conjugated and glucuronide derivatives and degradation products [56]. These modifications alter the chemical properties of plant polyphenols, favor their excretion and, possibly, provide them new biological activities [57]. The importance of the colonic microflora for polyphenol bioavailability, due to its ability to metabolize and chemically modify polyphenols, has been reported recently [55]. Anyway, recent studies indicate that plant, including olive, polyphenols are absorbed in discrete amounts from the intestine and rapidly distributed through the blood flow to the whole organism, including the brain, both in rats [58,59] and in humans [60,61]. Plant polyphenols do interact with, and cross, synthetic and cell membranes. The interaction of oleuropein aglycone with synthetic phospholipid membranes favored by the presence of anionic lipids has been reported in a very recent study [62]. Another study reported that several polyphenols (the olive ones were not included) protected the mitochondria against membrane permeabilization by amyloid oligomers, suggesting some interference with oligomers' interaction with the membrane [63]. Finally, oleuropein aglycone (OLE) was the main polyphenol found in breast cancer cells treated with an olive leaf extract in a recent metabolite-profiling study, suggesting its ability to cross the plasma membrane of these cells [64].

Due to the rising interest in natural phenols as possible new drugs, strategies to improve their bioavailability are under study, with encapsulation being probably the most actively investigated, in some cases with encouraging results [65,66]. Most of these molecular tools have not been tested in clinical trials, yet this strategy appears promising to improve the efficacy of natural phenols as drugs while reducing the amount of the administered dose. Actually, accurate studies on the effective dose of olive polyphenols to be administered daily to humans to obtain significant protection are still lacking; at any rate, the amount of OLE and other plant polyphenols taken daily in foods appears not adequate to ensure a dose suitable to produce short-term acute effects. However, clinical and experimental evidence indicates that a continuous consumption of moderate amounts of these molecules can be effective in the long term; this can also result in the accumulation in body tissues of these lipophilic molecules, leading to a low-intensity continuous stimulus of cell defenses against amyloid deposition, protein and metabolism dyshomeostasis, oxidative stress and other alterations underlying age-associated pathologies. These effects, although not proven experimentally, could, at least in part, explain the healthy properties of the MD. Nevertheless, the intake of moderate amounts of olive, and other plant, polyphenols provided by a typical MD supports the usefulness of the integration of polyphenol-enriched olive leaf extracts and other polyphenol-enriched nutraceuticals that can intensify, in the short term, the beneficial effects of these molecules.

3. Antioxidant and Anti-Inflammatory Properties of Olive Polyphenols in Animal Models

It is widely recognized that oxidative and nitrosative stress as well as inflammation are the major abnormalities underlying neurodegeneration and that antioxidant molecules, such as olive oil polyphenols, restore neuronal function through the amelioration of the redox status. Some beneficial effects of the MD have been associated with the consumption of EVOO polyphenols; these include antioxidant, hypoglycemic, antimicrobial, antiviral, antitumor, cardioprotective, neuroprotective, antiaging and anti-inflammatory activities [67,68]. It has been reported that EVOO polyphenols are protective against cognitive impairment associated with aging and neurodegenerative diseases due to their ability to protect DNA against oxidative stress, to inhibit mitochondrial dysfunction and to attenuate lipid peroxidation by scavenging free radicals, thus sustaining endogenous antioxidant stability [69,70]. They are also able to inhibit amyloid β (Aβ) and τ protein aggregation and toxicity, the main causes of the neurodegenerative cascade in AD [39,71,72]. EVOO polyphenols participate in the redox balance of the cell as antioxidants and as mild pro-oxidants, with ensuing upregulation of the antioxidant defenses of the cell. Accordingly, they can be considered as hormetic factors. For instance, in the presence of peroxidases, HT can undergo a redox cycling that generates superoxide [70], and tyrosol also increases *C. elegans* lifespan by activating the heat shock response [71]. It was reported that HT reduces brain mitochondrial oxidative stress and neuroinflammation in AD-prone transgenic mice by the induction of Nrf2-dependent gene expression [72]. The eight-week administration of oleuropein (60 mg/kg/day) improved mitochondrial function and reduced oxidative stress by activating the Nrf2 pathway in SHR rats [73]. Furthermore, tyrosol (240 mg/kg) was found to be protective against LPS-induced acute lung injury *through the* inhibition of NF-κB and the activation of AP-1 and of the Nrf-2 pathway [74]. EVOO polyphenols also enhance Nrf-2 activation at the hepatic level and the ensuing release of antioxidant enzymes [75]. Nrf2 is considered the principal regulator of redox homeostasis and its activation inhibits pro-inflammatory mediators such as cytokines, COX-2 and iNOS [76]. EVOO polyphenols limit inflammation by reducing the expression/activity of the transcription factors NF-κB and AP-1 [77] thanks to their free radical scavenging and radical chain breaking capacity and to the reduced formation of ROS and RNS. Moreover, HT inhibits the development of the inflammatory cascade following LPS and carrageenan injection through downregulation of the levels of pro-inflammatory cytokines (TNF-α and IL-1β), COX2, iNOS, NO, PGE2 and NF-kB and reducing DNA damage [78–80]. It was reported that the co-injection of OLE (450 μM) with Aβ42 (50 μM) into the nucleus basalis magnocellularis (NBM) of adult rats interfered with Aβ aggregation and significantly counteracted Aβ toxicity against choline acetyltransferase-positive neurons of the NBM and reduced astrocyte and microglia activation [81]. Another study reported that OLE protects transgenic *C. elegans* strains, constitutively expressing Aβ3-42, by reducing Aβ plaque load and motor deficits [82]. Interestingly, significant anti aggregation and neuroprotective effects of a diet supplemented with OLE, HT or a mix of polyphenols from olive mill wastewater were reported in the TgCRND8 mouse model of Aβ deposition. In these transgenic mice, a significant improvement in cognitive functions and a significant reduction in Aβ plaque number, size, and compactness were found in 3- and 6-month-old mice (at the early and intermediate stage of Aβ deposition, respectively) fed for 8 weeks with the OLE-supplemented diet [83–85]. A significant improvement in synaptic function and a significant reduction in the number, size and compactness of both Aβ42 and its 3-42 pyroglutamylated derivative (pE3-Aβ) deposits occurred even when the treatment was started at 10 months, when these mice display increased brain deposits of Aβ and, in particular, of pE3-Aβ in the cortex and hippocampal areas. These data indicate that oral diet supplementation with OLE not only results in the prevention of amyloid deposition but also in the disaggregation of preformed plaques and in a reduction in pE3-Aβ generation [85]. The effect of OLE against Aβ peptide aggregation was dose-dependent and could be reproduced by diet supplementation with a mix of polyphenols from olive mill wastewater or by HT administered at the same dose as that of pure OLE [84,86]. Interestingly, the treatment with OLE (50 mg/kg of diet for 8 weeks) astonishingly activated neuronal autophagy even in TgCRND8 mice at an advanced stage of pathology. In these animals, histone 3 acetylation on lysine 9 (H3K9) and histone 4 acetylation on lysine 5 (H4K5) were increased in the cortex and the hippocampus; such an increase matched both a decrease in HDAC2 expression and a significant improvement in synaptic function [85].

It is known that abnormal acetylation takes place in memory and learning disorders such as AD, where a significant increase in HDAC2 inhibits gene expression at specific loci, such as those involving autophagy markers [87]. In addition to the induction of an intense and functional autophagic response in the cortex, other relevant biological effects of OLE were uncovered in the TgCRND8 model; these include increased microglia migration to the plaques for phagocytosis, enhanced hippocampal neurogenesis and reduced astrocyte reaction [83,88]. OLE induced autophagy through the increase in cytosolic levels of Ca^{2+} and the subsequent activation of the enzyme complex AMPK by Ca^{2+}/Calmodulin Protein Kinase Kinase β (CaMKKβ) and the ensuing increase in phosphorylation of mammalian target of rapamycin (mTOR) with mTOR inhibition [89]. These data support the idea that autophagy activation by OLE and other olive polyphenols proceeds via modulation of the AMPK–mTOR axis, similarly to data reported for other plant polyphenols [90]. TgCRND8 mice fed with a diet supplemented with OLE or HT (50 mg/kg of food) exhibited increased levels of Beclin-1 and LC3 autophagic markers in the soma and dendrites of neurons of the somatosensory/parietal and entorhinal/piriform cerebral cortex, together with improved autophagosome/lysosome fusion [83,86]. Furthermore, the significant accumulation of PAR polymers and the increase in PARP1 expression found in the cortex at the early (3.5 months) and intermediate (6 months) stage of Aβ deposition in the TgCRND8 mice were rescued to control values by OLE supplementation. OLE-induced reduction in PARP1 activation was paralleled by the overexpression of SIRT1, and by a decrease in the pro-inflammatory NF-κB and the pro-apoptotic p53 marker [88].

The ability of EVOO polyphenols to modulate the action of NF-kB was observed both in vitro and in vivo in different tissues. In vivo, HT attenuated apoptosis in rat brain cells by modulating the levels of caspase-3 and NF-kB p65 subunit [91]; in high-fat diet (HFD)-fed C57BL/6 J male mice, daily doses of HT (5.0 mg/kg) attenuated the increment of NF-κB and SREBP 1c, and increased the activity of Nrf2 and PPAR-γ in the liver [92]. In female BALB/c mice, an EVOO-supplemented diet was protective in the management of induced systemic lupus erythematosus disease, likely through the inhibition of the MAPK, JAK/STAT, and NF-κB pathways in splenocytes [93]. One of the most studied upstream constituents of the NF-κB signaling pathway is the activation of the mitogen-activated protein kinases (MAPKs) [94]. In the TgCRND8 mice, an HT-supplemented diet modulated MAPK signaling by activating ERK and downregulating SAPK/JNK expression, a mechanism that may underlie memory improvements in these mice [86]. These data agree with other findings suggesting an involvement of ERK stimulation in memory formation and synaptic plasticity. In the C57BL/mouse model of AD, the administration of HT and its acetylated derivative significantly improved spatial memory deficits induced by the intracerebral injection of Aβ42 plus ibotenic acid. The latter affected the Bcl-2/Bad levels, activated caspase/cytochrome-dependent apoptosis, and downregulated pro-survival genes also involved in memory functions (Sirt-1, CREB, and CTREB target genes), whereas HT administration alleviated these alterations [95]. Taken together, these data suggest that OLE and/or its metabolite, HT, can be effective to combat cellular alterations underlying AD symptoms in the absence of undesirable side effects.

Finally, HT was shown to inhibit the toxicity associated with α-synuclein aggregation in PD [96]; HT and OLE improved spatial working memory and energetic metabolism in the brain of aged mice [97]; and HT decreased oxidative stress in the brain of *db/db* mice, a widely used human T2DM animal model, by improving mitochondrial function and inducing phase II antioxidative enzymes through the activation of the Nrf2-ARE pathway [98].

To date, less data have been reported for oleocanthal. Recently, in vitro and in vivo studies reported that oleocanthal enhances β-amyloid clearance as a potential neuroprotective mechanism [99,100].

4. Antioxidant Properties of Olive Polyphenols: Molecular Mechanisms

The overproduction of ROS correlates with lipid, protein or DNA damage involved in the onset of degenerative diseases; accordingly, cell defenses against a rise in ROS are fundamental [101]. Antioxidants inhibit oxidation; therefore, to react to oxidative stress, organisms maintain complex systems of antioxidants, primarily glutathione (GSH). Unfortunately, only a few drugs and biological molecules, such as vitamins, have been reported to act as antioxidants, yet with possible side effects [102,103].

Nowadays, researchers are focusing their attention on the antioxidant properties of natural compounds, without relevant side effects. In particular, the importance of the antioxidant activity of lipophilic and hydrophilic phenols in EVOO has emerged [104]. This fraction is physiologically produced by plants to react against the injuries produced by various pathogens or insects [28,105]. The antioxidant activity of the major phenolic components of EVOO, OLE and HT is related to their relative bioavailability with an appreciable level of absorption, fundamental to exert their metabolic and pharmacokinetic properties [49]. In molecular terms, OLE and HT, with their catecholic structure, behave as antioxidants in different ways: (i) by scavenging the peroxyl radicals and breaking peroxidative chain reactions, generating very stable resonance structures [106]; and (ii) by acting as metal chelators, therefore, preventing the copper sulphate-induced oxidation of low-density lipoproteins [107]. The activity of OLE and HT as metal chelators could be attributed to the ability of the hydroxyl groups to behave as electron donors and to the ensuing formation of intramolecular hydrogen bonds with free radicals [32]. However, the scavenging activity of OLE and HT was also assessed in non-metal oxidation systems. Indeed, data obtained in vitro highlight the ability of polyphenols to reduce the inactivation of catalase (CAT) by hypochlorous acid (HOCl); this effect protects against atherosclerosis following LDL oxidation by HOCl through apoB-100 chlorination [108]. Moreover, HT has been reported to improve the redox status of the cell by increasing the levels of GSH [109].

Recently, the oxidative damage in age-related diseases turned out to be primarily caused by reduced levels of the transcriptional Nuclear factor erythroid 2 (NF-E2)-related factor 2 (Nrf2) [110], and it was proposed as a therapeutic target for metabolic syndromes, including obesity, due to its behavior as a mediator of general adaptive responses of the cell, including proteostasis and inflammation [111,112]. However, the pivotal role of Nrf2 is involved in the regulation of protection against oxidation [113]. Following Nrf2 activation and consequently its translocation to the nucleus, Nrf2 binds to antioxidant response elements (ARE); after binding, it acts on the transcriptional expression of several antioxidant enzymes, including superoxide dismutase (SOD), c-glutamylcysteine synthetase (c-GCS), glutathione S-transferase (GST) and NADPH quinone oxidoreductase-1 (NQO1) [114].

EVOO polyphenols have been reported to interact with Nrf2 and with Nrf2-controlled enzymes. In vivo studies showed that EVOO polyphenols increased, at the mRNA level, the expression of Nrf2 and of its targets paraoxonase-2 (PON2), c-GCS, NQO1, and GST in the heart tissue of senescence-accelerated mouse-prone 8, whose diet included 10% olive oil [115]. These effects have been ascribed to HT. Indeed, a model of metabolic alterations, the high-fat diet (HFD)-fed male mice C57BL/6J, supplemented with HT (5.0 mg/kg), displayed a reduction in oxidative stress by restoring Nrf2 and the activity of the peroxisome proliferator-activated receptor-α (PPAR-α) to normal levels [116]. The same results were obtained when the same model was supplemented with the highest dose of HT (10–50 mg/kg/day), which also resulted in an increase in GST activity in the liver and in the muscle [117]. Finally, spontaneously hypertensive rats fed with OLE (60 mg/kg/day) showed increased levels of Nrf2-dependent phase II enzymes, such as NQO-1 [77]. Anyway, in spite of these and other data, the molecular mechanisms controlled by EVOO polyphenols in terms of antioxidant activity are not still clear; in fact, the reported effects were probably determined by the tissue localization of the enzyme and by the different concentrations of phenols used. Indeed, differently from previous data, in 60-day-old Wistar male rats fed with 7.5 mg/kg/day HT, oxidative stress was increased in heart tissue, probably due to the high concentration used [118]. The latter finding is not surprising; in fact, OLE and HT exert anti-proliferative and pro-apoptotic effects on tumor cells in vitro, inducing an accumulation of hydrogen peroxide mediated by the high doses [119,120].

The activity of EVOO polyphenols on Nrf2 signaling and on the levels of several antioxidant enzymes, such as γ-glutamyl-cysteinyl-ligase (γ-GCL) and SOD, was also reported in in vitro experiments with LPS-treated macrophages [121] and cancer cells [122]. Furthermore, it is widely reported that OLE and HT act on AMPK signaling, and the latter has been considered as an attractive therapeutic target for antioxidant activity. In fact, AMPK signaling plays a fundamental role in the cell defense system against ROS by direct phosphorylation of human FoxO1 (forkhead box O1) at Thr649, with the ensuing increase in FoxO1-dependent transcription of Mn-superoxide dismutase (MN-SOD) and CAT [123].

In conclusion, the data reported in the present and in the previous paragraph convincingly support the idea that EVOO polyphenols, in particular OLE and HT, exert antioxidant activity by interfering with different cellular pathways (Figure 2).

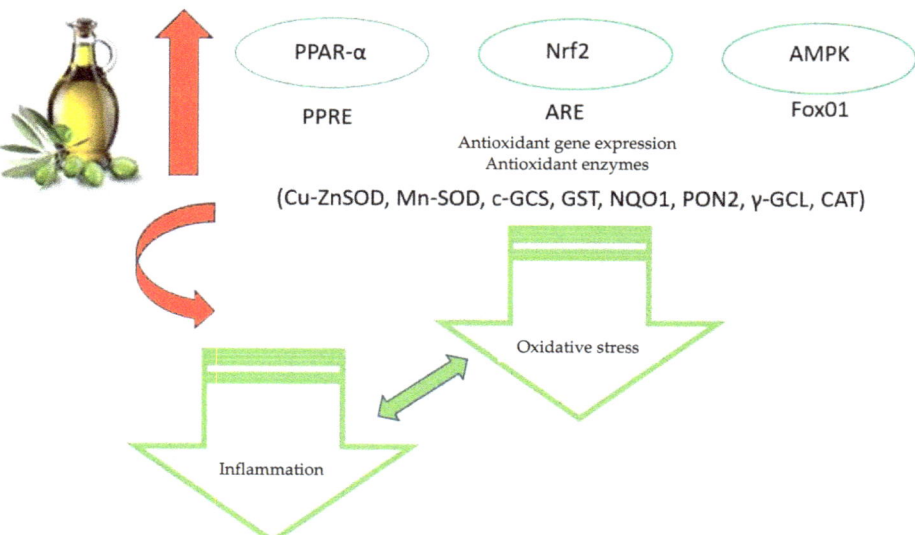

Figure 2. Main antioxidative effects of EVOO polyphenols.

5. Anti-Inflammatory Properties of Olive Polyphenols: Molecular Mechanisms

Inflammation is an essential defense mechanism of the organism by which the immune system recognizes and eliminates harmful agents and infected cells and promotes tissue repair to restore body homeostasis. This process is integrated into many coordinated functions and involves transiently elevated levels of cytokines able to activate both the innate and the adaptive immune systems. The inability to regulate an inflammatory response has multiple detrimental consequences for the organismal homeostasis; when the inflammatory response persists, a shift towards a long-term unresolved and uncontrolled immune response, known as chronic inflammation, involving macrophage- and lymphocyte-accumulated leukocytes does occur, and this results in local or systemic damage to the tissue or organs and in the degradation of normal physiologic function. Chronic inflammation is causally associated with disease onset or progression and increases with age. Indeed, the levels of cytokines, chemokines as well as the expression of genes involved in inflammation are higher in older people or in patients with autoimmune diseases that show a greater propensity to metabolic syndrome, cardiovascular disease and other chronic conditions such as frailty, multimorbidity and a decline in physical and cognitive function. Accordingly, interventions that target inflammatory pathways and restore a deregulated inflammatory response are promising strategies to prevent disease progression.

Convincing evidence highlights that a regular intake of food rich in polyphenols may reduce the risk for the growth of chronic diseases, including obesity, diabetes mellitus and cardiovascular diseases. This healthy effect results largely from the anti-inflammatory power of the polyphenolic compounds that is expressed by various mechanisms such as antioxidant activity (see previous paragraph) and the modulation of signaling pathways and transcriptional events (Figure 3).

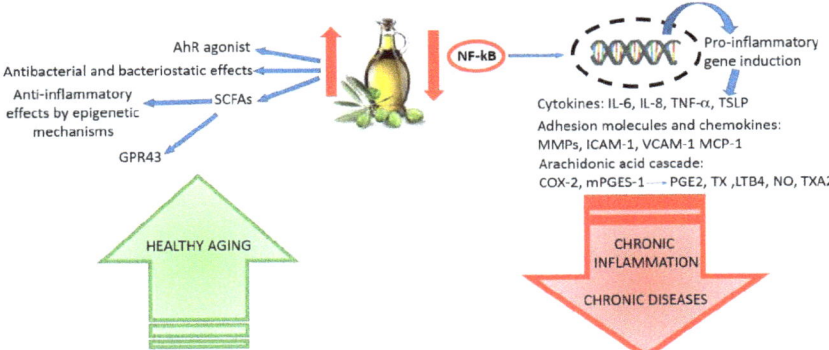

Figure 3. EVOO polyphenols in inflammation inhibition and their healthy effects in aging.

In a rheumatoid arthritis model, the EVOO phenolic extracts showed joint protective properties and reduced proinflammatory mediators by the inhibition of MAPK and NF-κB signaling in activated synovial fibroblasts [124]. In this model, a polyphenolic extract also inhibited IL-1β-induced matrix metalloproteinases, TNF-α and IL-6 production, as well as IL-1β-induced cyclo-oxygenase-2 (COX-2) and microsomal PGE synthase-1 (mPGES-1) [125]. Research on the inflammatory responses in primary human keratinocytes showed that HT and its acetate ester (HTy-Ac), a natural hydroxytyrosyl derivative found in olive oil, interfere with NF-κB signaling by reducing the degradation of IκB (Inhibitor of kB), the nuclear translocation of NF-κB, its recruitment at the promoter, and the ensuing gene transcription. In addition, in this case EVOO polyphenols efficiently attenuated the expression of pro-inflammatory mediators such as thymic stromal lymphopoietin (TSLP) and the expression of several inflammation-related genes, as well as different TSLP isoforms and IL-8, thus restraining harmful processes set off by activated keratinocytes [126]. In endothelial cells, the EVOO phenolic fraction significantly reduced VEGF-induced angiogenic responses and NADPH-oxidase activity dose-dependently, resulting in the inhibition of the expression of Nox2, Nox4, MMP-2 and MMP-9 [127]. Luteolin, one of main phenolic compounds in olive oil, was able to reduce Nox4 and p22phox expression in endothelial cells treated with TNF-α and the TNF-α-induced adhesion of monocytes to human endothelial cells, a key event in the onset of vascular inflammation. The role of luteolin as an inhibitor of this inflammatory event was mediated by suppressing the expression of adhesion molecules, such as MCP-1, ICAM-1 and VCAM-1, and NF-κB signaling. Similar results were also reported with HT, tyrosol, taxifolin and OLE, which were able to inhibit angiogenesis through their inhibition of VEGFR-2 at specific phosphorylation sites [128].

In peripheral blood mononuclear cells and in endothelial cells, HT modulated the inflammatory process through a reduction in the levels of MMP-9, prostaglandin, PGE2 and tromboxanes (TX), by inhibiting COX-2 (but not COX-1). The mechanism suggested for the action of HT, tyrosol and their secoiridoid derivatives (oleacein and oleocanthal) on the inflammatory process is similar to that reported for selective inhibitors of COX-2, such as nonsteroidal anti-inflammatory drugs (NSAIDs) [110,129,130].

Recently, a protective effect, at the intestinal level, of EVOO polyphenols, in terms of the prevention of redox unbalance and of slowdown of the onset and progression of chronic intestinal inflammation, has been described in the human colon adenocarcinoma cell line (Caco-2). In these cells, the phenolic extract allowed the reversion of the oxysterols-driven activation of JNK and p38 and the following phosphorylation of IκB. The inhibition of the NF-kB pathway, iNOS induction and the reduction in IL-6, IL-8 and NO levels were detected after oxysterol stimulation in the presence of the phenolic extract. HT and its metabolites, hydroxytyrosol sulfate, 4-glucuronide and 3′-glucuronide, were able to inhibit the endothelial activation and expression of VCAM-1 and ICAM-1 in the endothelial cells of the human umbilical vein or in the intestinal Caco-2 cells stimulated by LPS or TNF-α or IL-1beta [131–135]. Further evidence has shown that olive oil polyphenols were particularly efficient against LPS-induced inflammation in human macrophages (THP-1 cells) by restoring a normal level of some inflammatory factors such as IL-6, IL-1β and MCP-1 [136].

Oleocanthal, in a dose-dependent manner, induced the inhibition of COX-1 and COX-2 more efficiently than ibuprofen [137]. Tyrosol and hydroxyl-isocroman compounds, a class of ortho-diphenols present in EVOO, displayed an inhibitory effect on NO release and on the arachidonate cascade and the eicosanoid synthesis (PGE2 and LTB4) in cultured macrophages (RAW 264.7) stimulated by phorbol-12-myristate-13-acetate esters [136]. 1-Phenyl-6,7-dihydroxy-isochroman, through the suppression of NF-κB activation and a decrease in COX-2 synthesis, efficiently inhibited the production of TXA2, PGE2, and TNF-α in LPS-primed human monocytes [138]. The data reported above suggest the use of HT or its derivatives as possible innovative drugs to be used in the control of inflammation and of the immune response.

The crucial role of the gut microbiota on the general inflammatory status and cardiovascular, metabolic, and even brain health is becoming more and more convincing via the gut–brain axis. Accumulating data support the beneficial efficacy of EVOO polyphenols on gut microbiota and intestinal immunity. EVOO polyphenols exhibit antibacterial and bacteriostatic effects against pathogenic intestinal microflora, improve the growth of beneficial bacterial strains, and indirectly increase the production of microbially produced short-chain fatty acids (SCFAs), which exhibit anti-inflammatory effects and modulate gene expression through epigenetic mechanisms [139–141]. Moreover, SCFAs are potent activators of GPR43 and play an important role in blood glucose regulation [142].

Olive oil polyphenols, such as HT and other compounds generated from certain bacterial species (e.g., Lactobacillus) favored by EVOO polyphenols, can act as ligands of the aryl hydrocarbon receptor (AhR) that represent a key element in the status of mucosal immunity and in the homeostasis of the gut barrier [143]. Furthermore, as an AhR agonist, HT was shown to favor the induction of angiogenic genes in hypoxic MCF-7 cells and to contribute to slow cancer progression and metastasis [144]. Taken together, these data suggest a significant protective effect by EVOO polyphenols at the intestinal level, supporting the link between diet and the pathogenesis and development of inflammatory bowel diseases [145]. It is worth noting that Lactobacillus and Bifidobacterium are often greatly reduced in patients with AD and in elderly people. These bacterial types, whose populations are increased following EVOO consumption, produce γ-aminobutyric acid (GABA), thus influencing the GABAergic firing pattern in the brain through enteric and vagal systems [146]. In addition, EVOO may protect cognitive performance via its antibacterial activity towards defined pathogenic species of bacteria considered as a key element for AD in the pathogen interaction hypothesis [147].

6. Clinical Trials Highlighting the Antioxidant and Anti-Inflammatory Properties of Olive Polyphenols

Many clinical trials and population studies provide important data on the consistent and efficacious protection resulting from a prolonged olive oil intake against the insurgence of aging-associated pathologies, such as neurodegeneration, cardiovascular diseases, metabolic diseases and cancer. Taking into consideration all the results from these epidemiological studies supporting a causal link between the intake of olive oil polyphenols and effective benefits, in November 2011 the European Food Safety Authority (EFSA) approved two health claims regarding the salutary role of olive oil consumption. The claims recommend the use of olive oil to substitute saturated fats to maintain regular blood cholesterol levels and to protect blood lipids from oxidation. These protective effects can be achieved by the intake of at least 20 g of EVOO or the consumption of 5.0 mg of HT or its derived compounds every day (e.g., oleuropein complex and tyrosol) (http://www.efsa.europa.eu/, accessed on 2012).

One of the most remarkable large dietary intervention randomized trials was the Prevención con Dieta Mediterránea (PREDIMED) trial, carried out in Spain. This trial involved 7447 participants at high cardiovascular risk, or with T2DM or ≥ 3 major risk factors, including smoking, hypertension, elevated LDL-C and low HDL cholesterol levels, overweight or obesity, or with a family history of premature coronary heart disease [148–150]. The results from this trial, at a median of 4.8 years' follow-up, showed that the group following the Mediterranean diet supplemented with EVOO or nuts showed a 30% lower risk of developing cardiovascular pathologies, such as myocardial infarction, stroke, and consequent death, with respect to the group assigned to a low-fat diet.

In a subset of the PREDIMED trial, cognitive performance was also evaluated, with the conclusion that an EVOO-enriched MD significantly improved cognition [151–153]. In another subset of the PREDIMED study, the breast cancer incidence was also investigated in the same cohort. A 68% reduction in the risk of developing cancer was observed in the EVOO group [154]. In addition, results from a subsample (n = 990) of the PREDIMED trial indicated that a continuous intake of VOO containing a high phenolic content, instead of other types of olive oils, was efficient in preserving LDL from oxidation and in increasing the levels of HDL-cholesterol. A controlled, double blind, cross-over, randomized, clinical trial using olive oils with different phenolic concentrations (from 0 mg/L for refined olive oil, ROO, to 629 mg/L for VOO) was conducted in 30 healthy volunteers for 3 weeks, preceded by two-week washout periods. After VOO ingestion, LDL, HT monosulfate and homovanillic acid sulfate, but not tyrosol sulfate, levels were increased, while the concentrations of biomarkers of oxidative stress, including oxidized LDL (oxLDL), conjugated dienes, and hydroxy fatty acids, decreased. ROO ingestion did not affect the levels of LDL phenols and oxidation markers [155,156].

Another randomized, controlled, parallel-arm, clinical trial was carried out to compare the effects of olive oil with high (EVOO) or low (ROO) polyphenol levels in patients undergoing coronary angiography. Forty patients with at least one classic cardiovascular risk factor were randomly divided in two groups and received 25 mL EVOO or ROO daily for 6 weeks. At the end of treatment, the group that received high-polyphenol olive oil had a significant reduction in plasma LDL-cholesterol and plasma CRP. This also resulted in an increased production of inflammatory cytokines, such as IL-10, in LPS-stimulated ex vivo whole blood. Daily uptake of EVOO in subjects under pharmacological treatment could further improve LDL-cholesterol and markers of inflammation [157]. Similar beneficial effects have been demonstrated by "The Three-City Study", carried out in 2009 on 8000 elderly subjects. This first report correlated olive oil consumption with a reduced risk of visual memory decline in a population over 65 years old [35].

The positive impact of EVOO versus low-polyphenol olive oil on markers of CVD risk in a healthy Australian cohort was investigated in a double-blind randomized cross-over study (OLIVAUS). The trial examined markers of CVD risk related to cholesterol transport and metabolism, LDL oxidation, blood pressure (peripheral and central), arterial stiffness, inflammation, and cognitive performances in 50 healthy participants subjected to three weeks of daily administration of EVOO compared to a low-polyphenol olive oil [158].

A cross-over controlled trial (ISRCTN09220811), the EUROLIVE (Effect of Olive Oil Consumption on Oxidative Damage in European Populations) study, was carried out in 25 healthy European men (20–59 years). The participants consumed 25 mL raw olive oil with low or high polyphenol content daily for 3 weeks. The interventions were preceded by a two-week washout period. Then, the effects of olive oil polyphenol intake on plasma LDL concentrations and atherogenicity were evaluated, whereas the effects on lipoprotein lipase (LPL) gene expression were checked in another subset study of EUROLIVE on 18 men. The data obtained from this study showed a decrease in plasma concentrations of apo B-100 and of total and small LDL particles together with the LDL oxidation lag time and LPL gene expression [159]. Another EUROLIVE study confirmed that olive polyphenols increase human HDL functionality, favoring HDL-mediated cholesterol efflux from macrophages [160].

The association between olive oil intake and T2DM incidence in the US population resulted from a 22-year follow-up study involving 59,930 35–65-year-old women from the Nurses' Health Study and 85,157 26–45-year-old women from the NHS II, free of diabetes, CVDs and cancer at baseline. The results suggested that higher olive oil intake was correlated with a moderately reduced risk of T2DM, while the risk increased in women consuming other types of fats and salad dressings [161].

Another short-time study highlighted the effect of EVOO on post-prandial levels of glucose and LDL-cholesterol. Post-prandial glycemic and lipid profiles were investigated in 25 healthy subjects randomly assigned in a cross-over design to a Mediterranean diet supplemented with or without 10 g EVOO/day. The results showed that EVOO improved post-prandial glucose and LDL-cholesterol levels, suggesting an anti-atherosclerotic effect of the MD [162]. Furthermore, the same trial revealed that EVOO consumption resulted in high GLP-1 and gastric inhibitory peptide (GIP) levels in the circulatory system, while in another trial with type 1 diabetes (T1D) patients, an increase in gastric emptying and GPL-1 secretion was observed together with reduced glucose absorption through glucose–lipid competition that can contribute to a lower glycemic response [163]. In addition, an acute intake of EVOO resulted in a significant reduction in the levels of plasma glucose, triglyceride, apolipoprotein B-48, and dipeptidyl peptidase-4 activity and in a significant increase in the peripheral blood levels of insulin and glucagon-like peptide 1 (GLP-1), as revealed by a randomized trial of 30 participants with impaired fasting glucose levels [164].

The MICOIL pilot study was published on 10 November 2020. The trial confirmed that the long-standing benefits against cognitive impairment of polyphenol-enriched olive oil are greater than those granted by "simple" EVOO. The clinical trial divided participants with mild cognitive impairment (MCI) into three randomized groups. Genetic predisposition to AD was taken into account to obtain a homogenous baseline. Each group followed a unique diet: The first group received 50 mL/day of high-polyphenol olive oil, while following an MD. The second group received 50 mL/day of olive oil with moderate phenolic content, along with an MD. The third group only followed a normal MD. Long-term consumption of early harvest high phenolic or moderate phenolic EVOO was associated with an important amelioration of cognitive performance, as opposed to the low phenolic content MD, independent of the presence of genetic predisposition [165]. In 2010, a study on 20 patients with MetS showed that the acute intake of VOO was able to reduce the postprandial inflammatory response and the expression of several pro-inflammatory genes, mainly by decreasing the activation of NF-kB, of the activator protein-1 transcription factor complex AP-1, cytokines, mitogen-activated protein kinases (MAPKs) or arachidonic acid pathways, secondary to the reduction in LPS intestinal absorption following a high-fat meal [166,167].

To describe the exact role of olive oil in the metabolic changes reported above, a network meta-analysis of 30 human intervention studies totalizing 7688 subjects has been performed [168]. Using this approach, it was shown that the effect of olive oil on glycemia and blood lipids cannot be distinguished from the impact of MD adherence. Indeed, the administration of olive polyphenols in the dose suggested by EFSA does not modify glycemia levels, while it ameliorates insulin sensitivity [169]. These data are in accordance with the reported evidence of a direct action of polyphenols on the pancreas [170] and with the improvement of insulin secretion through the anti-inflammatory activity of oleic acid [171]. The only clear effect of the intake of a high-polyphenol olive oil was on HDL-cholesterol levels, on LDL and nucleic acid oxidation and on the plasma antioxidant activity, in agreement with previous meta-analyses [172].

Finally, an MD supplemented with polyphenol-rich EVOO has probiotic effects promoting the growth of bacteria of the Lactobacillus and Bifidobacterium types. These data result from different studies where overweight/obese participants and patients with HIV or with hypercholesterolemia consumed 40–50 g/day of EVOO for 12 weeks [172–174].

7. Conclusions and Future Perspectives

Several data highlight the ability of olive oil polyphenols to counteract aging and to protect against the insurgence of aging-associated pathologies, such as neurodegeneration, cardiovascular and metabolic diseases, and cancer, in part associated with derangement of redox homeostasis and proteostasis. However, recent research supports the idea that the health-promoting properties of olive oil polyphenols go well beyond their anti-amyloid and antioxidant power reported previously, highlighting their multi-target effects.

The claimed benefits of olive oil polyphenols have been supported by positive and encouraging results from many preclinical studies both in vitro and in animal models, as well as by population surveys and clinical trials often involving large numbers of participants. However, to date, there are still some doubts to resolve and therefore definitive results are lacking, even for the bioavailability of these molecules and their effective beneficial dose. In particular, further research is needed to better describe at the molecular and genetic levels the effects of olive polyphenols in several investigated biological systems to provide solid and definitive proof of their positive effects in a number of human pathologies. It must also be considered that the health benefits in humans most likely do not depend on the consumption of a single polyphenol but are the result of a variety of synergistic mechanisms of a combination of several polyphenols or other plant components.

Each factor affecting the bioavailability, bioaccessibility and bioactivity of polyphenols should also be considered. This is crucial because the bioavailability of these molecules is influenced by many factors, including phenolic structure, food processing, the food matrix, and the organism (microbiota composition, efficiency of detoxification mechanisms); furthermore, all these factors can interact with each other, modulating polyphenol bioavailability. Moreover, the latter, and thus the efficacy of these compounds, can be improved by administration in combination with other phytochemicals or drugs or in polyphenol-loaded nanotechnology-based delivery systems.

Finally, it might be more relevant and interesting to investigate the relationship between EVOO polyphenols and the gut microbiota to obtain further dietary indications. In fact, the dietary polyphenols/gut microbiota relation is a bi-directional one. On the one hand, polyphenols can affect the composition of gut microbiota; on the other hand, the microbiota is able to metabolize these molecules into bioactive compounds. Expanding knowledge on the effects of dietary polyphenols on the intestinal microbiota and the relative mechanisms of action and ensuing consequences, in addition to pharmacokinetics and pharmacodynamics of EVOO polyphenols, will be essential to better assess the effective doses and the levels reached by these molecules in different tissues and organs following different routes of introduction.

Author Contributions: M.S., F.C., P.N., M.L. and M.B. wrote and revised the manuscript. All authors have read and agreed to the published version of the manuscript.

Funding: This research was funded by "MONICABUCCIANTINI RICATEN21—Functional food against neurodegenerative disorder.

Acknowledgments: M.L. was supported by Fondazione Umberto Veronesi.

Conflicts of Interest: The authors declare no conflict of interest.

References

1. Mazzocchi, A.; Leone, L.; Agostoni, C.; Pali-Schöll, I. The secrets of the Mediterranean diet. Does [only] olive oil matter? *Nutrients* **2019**, *11*, 2941. [CrossRef]
2. Stefani, M.; Rigacci, S. Beneficial properties of natural phenols: Highlight on protection against pathological conditions associated with amyloid aggregation. *BioFactors* **2014**, *40*, 482–493. [CrossRef] [PubMed]
3. Bach-Faig, A.; Berry, E.M.; Lairon, D.; Reguant, J.; Trichopoulou, A.; Dernini, S.; Medina, F.X.; Battino, M.; Belahsen, R.; Miranda, G.; et al. Mediterranean diet pyramid today. Science and cultural updates. *Public Health Nutr.* **2011**, *14*, 2274–2284. [CrossRef]
4. Williams, R.J.; Spencer, J.P.; Rice-Evans, C. Flavonoids: Antioxidants or signalling molecules? *Free Radic. Biol. Med.* **2004**, *36*, 838–849. [CrossRef]

5. Otręba, M.; Kośmider, L.; Rzepecka-Stojko, A. Polyphenols' cardioprotective potential: Review of rat fibroblasts as well as rat and human cardiomyocyte cell lines research. *Molecules* **2021**, *26*, 774. [CrossRef] [PubMed]
6. Abenavoli, L.; Larussa, T.; Corea, A.; Procopio, A.C.; Boccuto, L.; Dallio, M.; Federico, A.; Luzza, F. Dietary polyphenols and non-alcoholic fatty liver disease. *Nutrients* **2021**, *13*, 494. [CrossRef] [PubMed]
7. Harris, J.; Lang, T.; Thomas, J.P.W.; Sukkar, M.B.; Nabar, N.R.; Kehrl, J.H. Autophagy and inflammasomes. *Mol. Immunol.* **2017**, *86*, 10–15. [CrossRef] [PubMed]
8. Bostancıklıoğlu, M. An update on the interactions between Alzheimer's disease, autophagy and inflammation. *Gene* **2019**, *705*, 157–166. [CrossRef] [PubMed]
9. Liu, W.F.; Wang, Z.Y.; Xia, Y.; Kuang, H.Y.; Liu, S.P.; Li, L.; Tang, C.F.; Yin, D.Z. The balance of apoptosis and autophagy via regulation of the AMPK signal pathway in aging rat striatum during regular aerobic exercise. *Exp. Gerontol.* **2019**, *124*, 110647. [CrossRef] [PubMed]
10. Erdman, V.V.; Nasibullin, T.R.; Tuktarova, I.A.; Somova, R.S.; Mustafina, O.E. Association analysis of polymorphic gene variants in the JAK/STAT signaling pathway with aging and longevity. *Russ. J. Genet.* **2019**, *55*, 728–737. [CrossRef]
11. Yessenkyzy, A.; Saliev, T.; Zhanaliyeva, M.; Masoud, A.R.; Umbayev, B.; Sergazy, S.; Krivykh, E.; Gulyayev, A.; Nurgozhin, T. Polyphenols as caloric-restriction mimetics and autophagy inducers in aging research. *Nutrients* **2020**, *12*, 1344. [CrossRef]
12. Davinelli, S.; de Stefani, D.; de Vivo, I.; Scapagnini, G. Polyphenols as caloric restriction mimetics regulating mitochondrial biogenesis and mitophagy. *Trends Endocrinol. Metab.* **2020**, *31*, 536–550. [CrossRef] [PubMed]
13. Rigacci, S.; Stefani, M. Nutraceutical properties of olive oil polyphenols: An itinerary from cultured cells through animal models to humans. *Int. J. Mol. Sci.* **2016**, *17*, 843. [CrossRef] [PubMed]
14. Leri, M.; Scuto, M.; Ontario, M.L.; Calabrese, V.; Calabrese, E.J.; Bucciantini, M.; Stefani, M. Healthy effects of plant polyphenols: Molecular mechanisms. *Int. J. Mol. Sci.* **2020**, *21*, 1250. [CrossRef]
15. Halliwell, B. Role of free radicals in the neurodegenerative diseases: Therapeutic implications for antioxidant treatment. *Drugs Aging* **2001**, *18*, 685–716. [CrossRef] [PubMed]
16. Fabiani, R.; Vella, N.; Rosignoli, P. Epigenetic modifications induced by olive oil and its phenolic compounds: A systematic review. *Molecules* **2021**, *26*, 273. [CrossRef]
17. Ayissi, V.B.O.; Ebrahimi, A.; Schluesenner, H. Epigenetic effects of natural polyphenols: A focus on SIRT1-mediated mechanisms. *Mol. Nutr. Food Res.* **2014**, *58*, 22–32. [CrossRef]
18. Bartolini, G.; Petruccelli, R. *Classification, Origins, Diffusion and History of the Olive*; Rome Food and Agriculture Organisation in the United Nations: Rome, Italy, 2002.
19. Flemmig, J.; Rusch, D.; Czerwinska, M.E.; Ruwald, H.W.; Arnhold, J. Components of a standardized olive leaf dry extract (Ph. Eur.) promote hypothiocyanate production by lactoperoxidase. *Arch. Biochem. Biophys.* **2014**, *549*, 17–25. [CrossRef] [PubMed]
20. Flemming, J.; Kuchta, K.; Arnhold, J.; Rauwald, H.W. Olea europaea leaf (Ph. Eur.) extract as well as several of its isolated phenolics inhibit the gout-related enzyme xanthine oxidase. *Phytomedicine* **2011**, *18*, 561–566. [CrossRef] [PubMed]
21. Marrano, N.; Spagnuolo, R.; Biondi, G.; Cignarelli, A.; Perrini, S.; Vincenti, L.; Laviola, L.; Giorgino, F.; Natalicchio, A. Effects of extra virgin olive oil polyphenols on beta-cell function and survival. *Plants* **2021**, *10*, 286. [CrossRef]
22. Giacometti, J.; Muhvić, D.; Grubić-Kezele, T.; Nikolić, M.; Šoić-Vranić, T.; Bajek, S. Olive Leaf Polyphenols (OLPs) stimulate GLUT4 expression and translocation in the skeletal muscle of diabetic rats. *Int. J. Mol. Sci.* **2020**, *21*, 8981. [CrossRef]
23. Mehmood, A.; Usman, M.; Patil, P.; Zhao, L.; Wang, C. A review on management of cardiovascular diseases by olive polyphenols. *Food Sci. Nutr.* **2020**, *8*, 4639–4655. [CrossRef] [PubMed]
24. Pintó, X.; Fanlo-Maresma, M.; Corbella, E.; Corbella, X.; Mitjavila, M.T.; Moreno, J.J.; Casas, R.; Estruch, R.; Corella, D.; Bulló, M.; et al. A Mediterranean diet rich in extra-virgin olive oil is associated with a reduced prevalence of nonalcoholic fatty liver disease in older in-dividuals at high cardiovascular risk. *J. Nutr.* **2019**, *149*, 1920–1929. [CrossRef] [PubMed]
25. Mosca, A.; Crudele, A.; Smeriglio, A.; Braghini, M.R.; Panera, N.; Comparcola, D.; Alterio, A.; Sartorelli, M.R.; Tozzi, G.; Raponi, M.; et al. Antioxidant activity of Hydroxytyrosol and Vitamin E reduces systemic inflammation in children with paediatric NAFLD. *Dig. Liver Dis.* **2020**. [CrossRef] [PubMed]
26. Salis, C.; Papageorgiou, L.; Papakonstantinou, E.; Hagidimitriou, M.; Vlachakis, D. live Oil Polyphenols in Neurodegenerative Pathologies. *Adv. Exp. Med. Biol.* **2020**, *1195*, 77–91. [PubMed]
27. Tripoli, E.; Giammanco, M.; Tabacchi, G.; Di Majo, D.; Giammanco, S.; la Guardia, M. The phenolic compounds of olive oil: Structure, biological activity and beneficial effects on human health. *Nutr. Res. Rev.* **2005**, *18*, 98–112. [CrossRef]
28. Casamenti, F.; Stefani, M. Olive polyphenols: New promising agents to combat aging-associated neurodegeneration. *Ext. Rev. Neurother.* **2017**, *17*, 345–358. [CrossRef] [PubMed]
29. Efentakis, P.; Iliodromitis, E.K.; Mikros, E.; Papachristodoulou, A.; Gagres, N.; Skaltsounis, A.-L.; Andreadou, I. Effect of olive tree leaf constituents on myocardial oxidative damage and atherosclerosis. *Planta Med.* **2015**, *81*, 648–654. [CrossRef]
30. Siracusa, R.; Scuto, M.; Fusco, R.; Trovato, A.; Ontario, M.L.; Crea, R.; Di Paola, R.; Cuzzocrea, S.; Calabrese, V. Anti-inflammatory and anti-oxidant activity of Hidrox® in rotenone-induced Parkinson's Disease in mice. *Antioxidants* **2020**, *9*, 824. [CrossRef] [PubMed]
31. Fernández-Prior, Á.; Bermúdez-Oria, A.; Millán-Linares, M.D.C.; Fernández-Bolaños, J.; Espejo-Calvo, J.A.; Rodríguez-Gutiérrez, G. Anti-inflammatory and antioxidant activity of hydroxytyrosol and 3,4-dihydroxyphenylglycol purified from table olive effluents. *Foods* **2021**, *10*, 227. [CrossRef]

32. Cicerale, S.; Lucas, L.; Keast, R. Biological activities of phenolic compounds present in virgin olive oil. *Int. J. Mol. Sci.* **2010**, *11*, 458–479. [CrossRef] [PubMed]
33. Piroddi, M.; Albini, A.; Fabiani, R.; Giovannelli, L.; Luceri, C.; Natella, F.; Rosignoli, P.; Rossi, T.; Taticchi, A.; Servili, M.; et al. Nutrigenomics of extra-virgin olive oil: A review. *Biofactors* **2017**, *43*, 17–41. [CrossRef]
34. Menotti, A.; Puddu, P.E. Coronary heart disease differences across Europe: A contribution from the Seven Countries Study. *J. Cardiovasc. Med.* **2013**, *14*, 767–772. [CrossRef] [PubMed]
35. Berr, C.; Portet, F.; Carriere, I.; Akbaraly, T.N.; Feart, C.; Gourlet, V.; Combe, N.; Barberger-Gateau, P.; Ritchie, K. Olive oil and cognition: Results from the three-city study. *Dement. Geriatr. Cogn. Disord.* **2009**, *28*, 357–364. [CrossRef] [PubMed]
36. Covas, M.I. Bioactive effects of olive oil phenolic compounds in humans: Reduction of heart disease factors and oxidative damage. *Inflammopharmacology* **2008**, *16*, 216–218. [CrossRef]
37. Psaltopoulou, T.; Kosti, R.I.; Haidopoulos, D.; Dimopoulos, M.; Panagiotakos, D.B. Olive oil intake is inversely related to cancer prevalence: A systematic review and a meta-analysis of 13,800 patients and 23,340 controls in 19 observational studies. *Lipids Health Dis.* **2011**, *10*, 127. [CrossRef] [PubMed]
38. Rigacci, S.; Stefani, M. Nutraceuticals and amyloid neurodegenerative diseases: A focus on natural polyphenols. *Exp. Rev. Neurother.* **2014**, *15*, 41–52. [CrossRef]
39. Pandey, K.B.; Rizvi, S.I. Plant polyphenols as dietary antioxidants in human health and disease. *Oxid. Med. Cell. Longev.* **2009**, *2*, 270–278. [CrossRef] [PubMed]
40. Bravo, L. Polyphenols: Chemistry, dietary sources, metabolism and nutritional significance. *Nutr. Rev.* **1998**, *56*, 313–333. [CrossRef] [PubMed]
41. Jimenez-Lopez, C.; Carpena, M.; Lourenço-Lopes, C.; Gallardo-Gomez, M.; Lorenzo, J.M.; Barba, F.J.; Prieto, M.A.; Simal-Gandara, J. Bioactive compounds and quality of extra virgin olive oil. *Foods* **2020**, *9*, 1014. [CrossRef]
42. Servili, M.; Esposto, S.; Fabiani, R.; Urbani, S.; Taticchi, A.; Mariucci, F.; Selvaggini, R.; Montedoro, G.F. Phenolic compounds in olive oil: Antioxidant, health and organoleptic activities according to their chemical structure. *Inflammopharmacology* **2009**, *17*, 76–84. [CrossRef] [PubMed]
43. Gorzynik-Debicka, M.; Przychodzen, P.; Cappello, F.; Kuban-Jankowska, A.; Marino Gammazza, A.; Knap, N.; Wozniak, M.; Gorska-Ponikowska, M. Potential health benefits of olive oil and plant polyphenols. *Int. J. Mol. Sci.* **2018**, *19*, 686. [CrossRef]
44. Dinda, B.; Debnath, S.; Banik, R. Naturally occurring iridoids and secoiridoids. An updated review, part 4. *Chem. Pharm. Bull.* **2011**, *59*, 803–833. [CrossRef]
45. Dinda, B.; Dubnath, S.; Harigaya, Y. Naturally occurring iridoids. A review, part 1. *Chem. Pharm. Bull.* **2007**, *55*, 159–222. [CrossRef] [PubMed]
46. Fabiani, R.; Rosignoli, P.; de Bartolomeo, A.; Fuccelli, R.; Servili, M.; Montedoro, G.F.; Morozzi, G. Oxidative DNA damage is prevented by extracts of olive oil, hydroxytyrosol, and other olive phenolic compounds in human blood mononuclear cells and HL60 cells. *J. Nutr.* **2008**, *138*, 1411–1416. [CrossRef] [PubMed]
47. Tundis, R.; Loizzo, M.; Menichini, F.; Statti, G.; Menichini, F. Biological and pharmacological activities of iridoids: Recent developments. *Mini Rev. Med. Chem.* **2008**, *8*, 399–420. [CrossRef] [PubMed]
48. Ranalli, A.; Marchegiani, D.; Contento, S.; Girardi, F.; Nicolosi, M.P.; Brullo, M.D. Variations of the iridoid oleuropein in Italian olive varieties during growth and maturation. *Eur. J. Lipid Sci. Technol.* **2009**, *111*, 678–687. [CrossRef]
49. Servili, M.; Montedoro, G.F. Contribution of phenolic compounds in virgin olive oil quality. *Eur. J. Lipid Sci. Technol.* **2002**, *104*, 602–613. [CrossRef]
50. Barnes, S.; Prasain, J.; d'Alessandro, T.; Arabshabi, A.; Botting, N.; Lila, M.A.; Jackson, G.; Janle, E.M.; Weaver, C.M. The metabolism and analysis of isoflavones and other dietary polyphenols in foods and biological systems. *Food Funct.* **2012**, *2*, 235–244. [CrossRef]
51. Lee, M.J.; Maliakal, P.; Chen, L.; Meng, X.; Bondoc, F.Y.; Prabhu, S.; Lambert, G.; Mohr, S.; Yang, C.S. Pharmacokinetics of tea catechins after ingestion of green tea and (−)-epigallocatechin-3-gallate by humans: Formation of different metabolites and individual variability. *Cancer Epidemiol. Biomark. Prev.* **2002**, *11*, 1025–1032.
52. Chen, Z.; Zheng, S.; Li, L.; Jiang, H. Metabolism of flavonoids in human: A comprehensive review. *Curr. Drug. Metab.* **2014**, *15*, 48–61. [CrossRef]
53. Manach, C.; Williamson, G.; Morand, C.; Scalbert, A.; Rémésy, C. Bioavailability and bioefficacy of polyphenols in humans. I. Review of 97 bioavailability studies. *Am. J. Clin. Nutr.* **2005**, *81*, 230S–242S. [CrossRef] [PubMed]
54. Wu, B.; Kulkarmi, K.; Basu, S.; Zhang, S.; Hu, M. First-pass metabolism via UDP-lucuronyltransferase: A barrier to oral bioavailability of phenolics. *J. Pharm. Sci.* **2011**, *100*, 3655–3681. [CrossRef]
55. Bazoti, F.N.; Gikas, E.; Tsarbopoulos, A. Simultaneous quantification of oleuropein and its metabolites in rat plasma by liquid chromatography electrospray ionization tandem mass spectrometry. *Biomed. Chromatogr.* **2010**, *24*, 506–515. [CrossRef] [PubMed]
56. Manach, C.; Scalbert, A.; Morand, C.; Remesy, C.; Jimenez, L. Dietary polyphenols: Food sources and bioavailability. *Am. J. Clin. Nutr.* **2004**, *79*, 727–747. [CrossRef] [PubMed]
57. Serra, A.; Rubió, L.; Borràs, X.; Macià, A.; Romero, M.P.; Motilva, M. Distribution of olive oil phenolic compounds in rat tissues after administration of a phenolic extract from olive cake. *J. Mol. Nutr. Food Res.* **2012**, *56*, 486–496. [CrossRef] [PubMed]
58. Vissers, M.N.; Zock, P.L.; Roodenburg, A.J.C.; Leenen, R.; Katan, M.B. Olive oil phenols are absorbed in humans. *J. Nutr.* **2002**, *132*, 409–417. [CrossRef]

59. de Bock, M.; Thorstensen, E.B.; Derraik, J.G.B.; Henderson, H.V.; Hofman, P.L.; Cutfield, W.S. Human absorption and metabolism of oleuropein and hydroxythyrosol ingested as olive (*Olea europaea* L.) leaf extract. *Mol. Nutr. Food Res.* **2013**, *57*, 2079–2085. [CrossRef] [PubMed]
60. Galinano, V.; Villalain, J. Oleuropein aglycone in lipid bilayer membranes. A molecular dynamic study. *Biochim. Biophys. Acta* **2015**, *1848*, 2849–2858. [CrossRef] [PubMed]
61. Camilleri, A.; Zarb, C.; Caruana, M.; Ostermeier, U.; Ghio, S.; Högen, T.; Schmidt, F.; Giese, A.; Vassallo, N. Mitochondrial membrane permeabilisation by amyloid aggregates and protection by polyphenols. *Biochim. Biophys. Acta* **2013**, *1828*, 2532–2543. [CrossRef]
62. Quirantes-Piné, R.; Zurek, G.; Barrajòn-Catalàn, E.; Bäßmann, C.; Micol, V.; Segura-Carretero, A.; Fernàndez-Gutierrez, A. A metabolite-profiling approach to assess the uptake and metabolism of phenolic compounds from olive leaves in SKBR3 cells by HPLC-ESI-QTOF-MS. *J. Pharm. Biomed. Anal.* **2013**, *72*, 121–126. [CrossRef]
63. Mourtzinos, I.; Salta, F.; Yannakopoulou, K.; Chiou, A.; Karathanos, V.T. Encapsulation of olive leaf extract in beta-cyclodextrin. *J. Agric. Food Chem.* **2007**, *55*, 8088–8094. [CrossRef] [PubMed]
64. Mignet, N.; Seguin, J.; Chabot, G.G. Bioavailability of polyphenol liposomes: A challenge ahead. *Pharmaceutics* **2013**, *5*, 457–471. [CrossRef] [PubMed]
65. Soni, M.; Prakash, C.; Dabur, R.; Kumar, V. Protective effect of hydroxytyrosol against oxidative stress mediated by arsenic-induced neurotoxicity in rats. *Appl. Biochem. Biotechnol.* **2018**, *186*, 27–39. [CrossRef] [PubMed]
66. Carrera-González, M.P.; Ramírez-Expósito, M.J.; Mayas, M.D.; Martínez-Martos, J.M. Protective role of oleuropein and its metabolite hydroxytyrosol on cancer. *Trends Food Sci. Technol.* **2013**, *31*, 92–99. [CrossRef]
67. Fernández del Río, L.; Gutiérrez-Casado, E.; Varela-López, A.; Villalba, J.M. Olive oil and the hallmarks of aging. *Molecules* **2016**, *21*, 163. [CrossRef] [PubMed]
68. Serreli, G.; Deiana, M. Extra virgin olive oil polyphenols: Modulation of cellular pathways related to oxidant species and inflammation in aging. *Cells* **2020**, *9*, 478. [CrossRef]
69. Daccache, A.; Lion, C.; Sibille, N.; Gerard, M.; Slomianny, C.; Lippens, G.; Cotelle, P. Oleuropein and derivatives from olives as Tau aggregation inhibitors. *Neurochem. Int.* **2011**, *58*, 700–707. [CrossRef]
70. Sarsour, E.H.; Kumar, M.G.; Kalen, A.L.; Goswami, M.; Buettner, G.R.; Goswami, P.C. MnSOD activity regulates Hydroxytyrosol induced extension of chronological lifespan. *Age* **2012**, *34*, 95–109. [CrossRef] [PubMed]
71. Cañuelo, A.; Gilbert-López, B.; Pacheco-Liñán, P.; Martínez-Lara, E.; Siles, E.; Miranda-Vizuete, A. Tyrosol, a main phenol present in extra virgin olive oil, increases lifespan and stress resistance in *Caenorhabditis elegans*. *Mech. Ageing Dev.* **2012**, *133*, 563–574. [CrossRef]
72. Peng, Y.; Hou, C.; Yang, Z.; Li, C.; Jia, L.; Liu, J.; Tang, Y.; Shi, L.; Li, Y.; Long, J.; et al. Hydroxytyrosol mildly improve cognitive function independent of APP processing in APP/PS1 mice. *Mol. Nutr. Food Res.* **2016**, *60*, 2331–2342. [CrossRef] [PubMed]
73. Sun, W.; Wang, X.; Hou, C.; Yang, L.; Li, H.; Guo, J.; Huo, C.; Wang, M.; Miao, Y.; Liu, J.; et al. Oleuropein improves mitochondrial function to attenuate oxidative stress by activating the Nrf2 pathway in the hypothalamic paraventricular nucleus of spontaneously hypertensive rats. *Neuropharmacology* **2017**, *113*, 556–566. [CrossRef] [PubMed]
74. Wang, W.C.; Xia, Y.M.; Yang, B.; Su, X.N.; Chen, J.K.; Li, W.; Jiang, T. Protective effects of tyrosol against LPS-induced acute lung injury via inhibiting NF-κB and AP-1 activation and activating the HO-1/Nrf2 pathways. *Biol. Pharm. Bull.* **2017**, *40*, 583–593. [CrossRef]
75. Soto-Alarcon, S.A.; Valenzuela, R.; Valenzuela, A.; Videla, L.A. Liver protective effects of extra virgin olive oil: Interaction between its chemical composition and the cell-signaling pathways involved in protection. *Endocr. Metab. Immune Disord. Drug Targets* **2018**, *18*, 75–84. [CrossRef]
76. Ahmed, S.M.; Luo, L.; Namani, A.; Wang, X.J.; Tang, X. Nrf2 signaling pathway: Pivotal roles in inflammation. *Biochim. Biophys. Acta* **2017**, *1863*, 585–597. [CrossRef]
77. Hornedo-Ortega, R.; Cerezo, A.B.; de Pablos, R.M.; Krisa, S.; Richard, T.; García-Parrilla, M.C.; Troncoso, A.M. Phenolic compounds characteristic of the Mediterranean diet in mitigating microglia-mediated neuroinflammation. *Front. Cell. Neurosci.* **2018**, *12*, 373. [CrossRef] [PubMed]
78. Fki, I.; Sayadi, S.; Mahmoudi, A.; Daoued, I.; Marrekchi, R.; Ghorbel, H. Comparative study on beneficial effects of hydroxytyrosol- and oleuropein-rich olive leaf extracts on high-fat diet-induced lipid me-tabolism disturbance and liver injury in rats. *Biomed. Res. Int.* **2020**, 1315202. [CrossRef]
79. Fuccelli, R.; Fabiani, R.; Rosignoli, P. Hydroxytyrosol exerts anti-inflammatory and anti-oxidant activities in a mouse model of systemic inflammation. *Molecules* **2018**, *23*, 3212. [CrossRef] [PubMed]
80. Zhang, Y.J.; Chen, X.; Zhang, L.; Li, J.; Li, S.B.; Zhang, X.; Qin, L.; Sun, F.R.; Li, D.Q.; Ding, G.Z. Protective effects of 3,4-dihydroxyphenylethanol on spinal cord injury-induced oxidative stress and inflammation. *Neuroreport* **2019**, *30*, 1016–1024. [CrossRef]
81. Luccarini, I.; Ed Dami, T.; Grossi, C.; Rigacci, S.; Stefani, M.; Casamenti, F. Oleuropein aglycone counteracts Aβ42 toxicity in the rat brain. *Neurosci. Lett.* **2014**, *558*, 67–72. [CrossRef] [PubMed]
82. Diomede, L.; Rigacci, S.; Romeo, M.; Stefani, M.; Salmona, M. Oleuropein aglycone protects transgenic *C. elegans* strains expressing Aβ42 by reducing plaque load and motor deficit. *PLoS ONE* **2013**, *8*, e58893. [CrossRef]

83. Grossi, C.; Rigacci, S.; Ambrosini, S.; Ed Dami, T.; Luccarini, I.; Traini, C.; Failli, P.; Berti, A.; Casamenti, F.; Stefani, M. The polyphenol oleuropein aglycone protects TgCRND8 mice against Aß plaque pathology. *PLoS ONE* **2013**, *8*, e71702. [CrossRef]
84. Pantano, D.; Luccarini, I.; Nardiello, P.; Servili, M.; Stefani, M.; Casamenti, F. Oleuropein aglycone and polyphenols from olive mill waste water ameliorate cognitive deficits and neuropathology. *Br. J. Clin. Pharmacol.* **2017**, *83*, 54–62. [CrossRef]
85. Luccarini, I.; Grossi, C.; Rigacci, S.; Coppi, E.; Pugliese, A.M.; Pantano, D.; la Marca, G.; Ed Dami, T.; Berti, A.; Stefani, M.; et al. Oleuropein aglycone protects against pyroglutamylated-3 amyloid-ß toxicity: Biochemical, epigenetic and functional correlates. *Neurobiol. Aging* **2015**, *36*, 648–663. [CrossRef] [PubMed]
86. Nardiello, P.; Pantano, D.; Lapucci, A.; Stefani, M.; Casamenti, F. Diet supplementation with hydroxytyrosol ameliorates brain pathology and restores cognitive functions in a mouse model of amyloid-β deposition. *J. Alzheimer's Dis.* **2018**, *63*, 1161–1172. [CrossRef]
87. Adwan, L.; Zawia, N.H. Epigenetics: A novel therapeutic approach for the treatment of Alzheimer's diseas. *Pharmacol. Ther.* **2013**, *139*, 41–50. [CrossRef]
88. Luccarini, I.; Pantano, D.; Nardiello, P.; Cavone, L.; Lapucci, A.; Miceli, C.; Nediani, C.; Berti, A.; Stefani, M.; Casamenti, F. The polyphenol oleuropein aglycone modulates the PARP1-SIRT1 interplay: An in vitro and in vivo study. *J. Alzheimer's Dis.* **2016**, *54*, 737–750. [CrossRef] [PubMed]
89. Rigacci, S.; Miceli, C.; Nediani, C.; Berti, A.; Cascella, R.; Pantano, D.; Nardiello, P.; Luccarini, I.; Casamenti, F.; Stefani, M. Oleuropein aglycone induces autophagy via the AMPK/mTOR signalling pathway: A mechanistic insight. *Oncotarget* **2015**, *6*, 35344–35357. [CrossRef] [PubMed]
90. Wang, M.; Yu, T.; Zhu, C.; Sun, H.; Qiu, Y.; Zhu, X.; Li, J. Resveratrol triggers protective autophagy through the Ceramide/Akt/mTOR pathway in melanoma B16 cells. *Nutr. Cancer* **2014**, *66*, 435–440. [CrossRef] [PubMed]
91. Fu, P.; Hu, Q. 3,4-Dihydroxyphenylethanol alleviates early brain injury by modulating oxidative stress and Akt and nuclear factor-κB pathways in a rat model of subarachnoid hemorrhage. *Exp. Ther. Med.* **2016**, *11*, 1999–2004. [CrossRef] [PubMed]
92. Illesca, P.; Valenzuela, R.; Espinosa, A.; Echeverría, F.; Soto-Alarcon, S.; Ortiz, M.; Videla, L.A. Hydroxytyrosol supplementation ameliorates the metabolic disturbances in white adipose tissue from mice fed a high-fat diet through recovery of transcription factors Nrf2, SREBP-1c, PPAR-γ and NF-κB. *Biomed. Pharmacother.* **2019**, *109*, 2472–2481. [CrossRef] [PubMed]
93. Aparicio-Soto, M.; Sánchez-Hidalgo, M.; Cárdeno, A.; Rosillo, M.T.; Sánchez-Fidalgo, S.; Utrilla, J.; Martín-Lacave, I.; Alarcón-de-la-Lastra, C. Dietary extra virgin olive oil attenuates kidney injury in pristane-induced SLE model via activation of HO-1/Nrf-2 antioxidant pathway and suppression of JAK/STAT, NF-κB and MAPK activation. *J. Nutr. Biochem.* **2016**, *27*, 278–288. [CrossRef] [PubMed]
94. Sun, P.; Zhou, K.; Wang, S.; Li, P.; Chen, S.; Lin, G.; Zhao, Y.; Wang, T. Involvement of MAPK/NF-κB signaling in the activation of the cholinergic anti-inflammatory pathway in experimental colitis by chronic vagus nerve stimulation. *PLoS ONE* **2013**, *8*, e69424. [CrossRef]
95. Arunsundar, M.; Shanmugarajan, T.S.; Ravichandran, V. 3,4-dihydroxyphenylethanol attenuates spatio-cognitive deficits in an Alzheimer's disease mouse model: Modulation of the molecular signals in neuronal survival-apoptotic programs. *Neurotox. Res.* **2015**, *27*, 143–155. [CrossRef] [PubMed]
96. Palazzi, L.; Leri, M.; Cesaro, S.; Stefani, M.; Bucciantini, M.; Polverino de Laureto, P. Insight into the molecular mechanism underlying the inhibition of α-synuclein aggregation by hydroxytyrosol. *Biochem. Pharmacol.* **2020**, *173*, 113722. [CrossRef] [PubMed]
97. Reutzel, M.; Grewal, R.; Silaidos, C.; Zotzel, J.; Marx, S.; Tretzel, J.; Eckert, G.P. Effects of long-term treatment with a blend of highly purified olive secoiridoids on cognition and brain ATP levels in aged NMRI mice. *Oxid. Med. Cell. Longev.* **2018**, *2018*, 4070935. [CrossRef] [PubMed]
98. Zheng, A.; Li, H.; Xu, J.; Cao, K.; Li, H.; Pu, W.; Yang, Z.; Peng, Y.; Long, J.; Liu, J.; et al. Hydroxytyrosol improves mitochondrial function and reduces oxidative stress in the brain of db/db mice: Role of AMP-activated protein kinase activation. *Br. J. Nutr.* **2015**, *113*, 1667–1676. [CrossRef]
99. Qosa, H.; Batarseh, Y.S.; Moyeldin, M.M.; El Sayed, K.A.; Keller, J.N.; Kaddoumi, A. Oleocanthal enhances amyloid-β clearance from the brains of TgSwDI mice and in vitro across a human blood-brain barrier model. *ACS Chem. Neurosci.* **2015**, *6*, 1849–1859. [CrossRef] [PubMed]
100. Abuznait, A.H.; Qosa, H.; Busnena, B.A.; El Sayed, K.A.; Kaddoumi, A. Olive-oil-derived oleocanthal enhances β-amyloid clearance as a potential neuroprotective mechanism against Alzheimer's disease: In vitro and in vivo studies. *ACS Chem. Neurosci.* **2013**, *4*, 973–982. [CrossRef]
101. Halliwell, B. Oxidative stress and cancer: Have we moved forward? *Biochem. J.* **2007**, *401*, 1–11. [CrossRef]
102. Duracková, Z. Some current insights into oxidative stress. *Physiol. Res.* **2010**, *59*, 459–469. [CrossRef]
103. Bjelakovic, G.; Nikolova, D.; Gluud, C. Meta-regression analyses, meta-analyses, and trial sequential analyses of the effects of supplementation with beta-carotene, vitamin A, and vitamin E singly or in different combinations on all-cause mortality: Do we have evidence for lack of harm? *PLoS ONE* **2013**, *8*, e74558. [CrossRef] [PubMed]
104. Jiang, L.; Yang, K.H.; Tian, J.H.; Guan, Q.L.; Yao, N.; Cao, N.; Mi, D.H.; Wu, J.; Ma, B.; Yang, S.H. Efficacy of antioxidant vitamins and selenium supplement in prostate cancer prevention: A meta-analysis of randomized controlled trials. *Nutr. Cancer* **2010**, *62*, 719–727. [CrossRef] [PubMed]

105. Bendini, A.; Cerretani, L.; Carrasco-Pancorbo, A.; Gómez-Caravaca, A.M.; Segura-Carretero, A.; Fernández-Gutiérrez, A.; Lercker, G. Phenolic molecules in virgin olive oils: A survey of their sensory properties, health effects, antioxidant activity and analytical methods: An overview of the last decade. *Molecules* **2007**, *12*, 1679–1719. [CrossRef] [PubMed]
106. Carluccio, M.A.; Massaro, M.; Scoditti, E.; de Caterina, R. Vasculoprotective potential of olive oil components. *Mol. Nutr. Food Res.* **2007**, *51*, 1225–1234. [CrossRef]
107. Cicerale, S.; Lucas, L.J.; Keast, R.S. Antimicrobial, antioxidant and anti-inflammatory phenolic activities in extra virgin olive oil. *Curr. Opin. Biotechnol.* **2012**, *23*, 129–135. [CrossRef]
108. Bulotta, S.; Oliverio, M.; Russo, D.; Procopio, A. Biological activity of oleuropein and its derivatives. In *Natural Products*; Ramawat, K.G., Mérillon, J.M., Eds.; Springer: Berlin/Heidelberg, Germany, 2013; pp. 3605–3638.
109. Visioli, F.; Poli, A.; Gall, C. Antioxidant and other biological activities of phenols from olives and olive oil. *Med. Res. Rev.* **2002**, *22*, 65–75. [CrossRef] [PubMed]
110. Lucas, L.; Russell, A.; Keast, R. Molecular mechanisms of inflammation. Anti-inflammatory benefits of virgin olive oil and the phenolic compound oleocanthal. *Curr. Pharm. Des.* **2011**, *17*, 754–768. [CrossRef] [PubMed]
111. Visioli, F.; Bellomo, G.; Galli, C. Free radical-scavenging properties of olive oil poliphenols. *Biochem. Biophys. Res. Commun.* **1998**, *247*, 60–64. [CrossRef] [PubMed]
112. Kouka, P.; Priftis, A.; Stagos, D.; Angelis, A.; Stathopoulos, P.; Xinos, N.; Skaltsounis, A.L.; Mamoulakis, C.; Tsatsakis, A.M.; Spandidos, D.A.; et al. Assessment of the antioxidant activity of an olive oil total polyphenolic fraction and hydroxytyrosol from a Greek *Olea europea* variety in endothelial cells and myoblasts. *Int. J. Mol. Med.* **2017**, *40*, 703–712. [CrossRef] [PubMed]
113. Tan, B.L.; Norhaizan, M.E.; Liew, W.-P.; Rahman, H.S. Antioxidant and oxidative stress: A mutual interplay in age-related diseases. *Front. Pharmacol.* **2018**, *9*, 1162. [CrossRef]
114. Hayes, J.D.; Dinkova-Kostova, A.T. The Nrf2 regulatory network provides an interface between redox and intermediary metabolism. *Trends Biochem. Sci.* **2014**, *39*, 199–218. [CrossRef] [PubMed]
115. Chapple, S.J.; Siow, R.C.M.; Mann, G.E. Crosstalk between Nrf2 and the proteasome: Therapeutic potential of Nrf2 inducers in vascular disease and aging. *Int. J. Biochem. Cell Biol.* **2012**, *44*, 1315–1320. [CrossRef] [PubMed]
116. Ma, Q. Role of nrf2 in oxidative stress and toxicity. *Annu. Rev. Pharmacol. Toxicol.* **2013**, *53*, 401–426. [CrossRef] [PubMed]
117. Li, B.; Evivie, S.E.; Lu, J.; Jiao, Y.; Wang, C.; Li, Z.; Liu, F.; Huo, G. Lactobacillus helveticus KLDS1.8701 alleviates d-galactose-induced aging by regulating Nrf-2 and gut microbiota in mice. *Food Funct.* **2018**, *9*, 6586–6598. [CrossRef] [PubMed]
118. Bayram, B.; Ozcelik, B.; Grimm, S.; Roeder, T.; Schrader, C.; Ernst, I.M.; Wagner, A.E.; Grune, T.; Frank, J.; Rimbach, G. a diet rich in olive oil phenolics reduces oxidative stress in the heart of SAMP8 mice by induction of Nrf2-dependent gene expression. *Rejuv. Res.* **2012**, *15*, 71–81. [CrossRef]
119. Valenzuela, R.; Illesca, P.; Echeverría, F.; Espinosa, A.; Rincón-Cervera, M.Á.; Ortiz, M.; Hernandez-Rodas, M.C.; Valenzuela, A.; Videla, L.A. Molecular adaptations underlying the beneficial effects of hydroxytyrosol in the pathogenic alterations induced by a high-fat diet in mouse liver: PPAR-α and Nrf2 activation, and NF-κB down-regulation. *Food Funct.* **2017**, *8*, 1526–1537. [CrossRef]
120. Cao, K.; Xu, J.; Zou, X.; Li, Y.; Chen, C.; Zheng, A.; Li, H.; Li, H.; Szeto, I.M.; Shi, Y.; et al. Hydroxytyrosol prevents diet-induced metabolic syndrome and attenuates mitochondrial abnormalities in obese mice. *Free Radic. Biol. Med.* **2014**, *67*, 396–407. [CrossRef]
121. Bigagli, E.; Cinci, L.; Paccosi, S.; Parenti, A.; d'Ambrosio, M.; Luceri, C. Nutritionally relevant concentrations of resveratrol and hydroxytyrosol mitigate oxidative burst of human granulocytes and monocytes and the production of pro-inflammatory mediators in LPS-stimulated RAW 264.7 macrophages. *Int. Immunopharmacol.* **2017**, *43*, 147–155. [CrossRef]
122. Martin, M.A.; Ramos, S.; Granado-Serrano, A.B.; Rodriguez-Ramiro, I.; Trujillo, M.; Bravo, L.; Goya, L. Hydroxytyrosol induces antioxidant/detoxificant enzymes and Nrf2 translocation via extracellular regulated kinases and phosphatidylinositol-3-kinase/protein kinase B pathways in HepG2 cells. *Mol. Nutr. Food Res.* **2010**, *54*, 956–966. [CrossRef] [PubMed]
123. Yun, H.; Park, S.; Kim, M.J.; Yang, W.K.; Im, D.U.; Yang, K.R.; Hong, J.; Choe, W.; Kang, I.; Kim, S.S.; et al. AMP-activated protein kinase mediates the antioxidant effects of resveratrol through regulation of the transcription factor FoxO1. *FEBS J.* **2014**, *281*, 4421–4438. [CrossRef] [PubMed]
124. Rosillo, M.A.; Alarcón-de-la-Lastra, C.; Castejón, M.C.; Montoya, T.; Cejudo-Guillén, M.; Sánchez-Hidalgo, M. Polyphenolic extract from extra virgin olive oil inhibits the inflammatory response in IL-1β-activated synovial fibroblasts. *Br. J. Nutr.* **2019**, *121*, 55–62. [CrossRef]
125. Aparicio-Soto, M.; Redhu, D.; Sánchez-Hidalgo, M.; Fernández-Bolaños, J.G.; Alarcón-de-la-Lastra, C.; Worm, M.; Babina, M. Olive-oil-derived polyphenols effectively attenuate inflammatory responses of human keratinocytes by interfering with the NF-κB pathway. *Nutr. Food Res.* **2019**, *63*, e1900019. [CrossRef]
126. Xia, F.; Wang, C.; Jin, Y.; Liu, Q.; Meng, Q.; Liu, K.; Sun, H. Luteolin protects HUVECs from TNF-α-induced oxidative stress and inflammation via its effects on the Nox4/ROS-NF-κB and MAPK pathways. *J. Atheroscler. Thromb.* **2014**, *21*, 768–783. [CrossRef]
127. Lamy, S.; Ouanouki, A.; Béliveau, R.; Desrosiers, R.R. Olive oil compounds inhibit vascular endothelial growth factor receptor-2 phosphorylation. *Exp. Cell Res.* **2014**, *322*, 89–98. [CrossRef]
128. Lopes de Souza, A.; Marcadenti, A.; Portal, V.L. Effects of olive oil phenolic compounds on inflammation in the prevention and treatment of coronary artery disease. *Nutrients* **2017**, *9*, 1087. [CrossRef] [PubMed]
129. Rosignoli, P.; Fuccelli, R.; Fabiani, R.; Servili, M.; Morozzi, G. Effect of olive oil phenols on the production of inflammatory mediators in freshly isolated human monocytes. *J. Nutr. Biochem.* **2013**, *24*, 1513–1519. [CrossRef] [PubMed]

130. Carluccio, M.A.; Siculella, L.; Ancora, M.A.; Massaro, M.; Scoditti, E.; Storelli, C.; Visioli, F.; Distante, A.; de Caterina, R. Olive oil and red wine antioxidant polyphenols inhibit endothelial activation: Antiatherogenic properties of Mediterranean diet phytochemicals. *Arterioscler. Thromb. Vasc. Biol.* **2003**, *23*, 622–629. [CrossRef] [PubMed]
131. Dell'Agli, M.; Fagnani, R.; Mitro, N.; Scurati, S.; Masciadri, M.; Mussoni, L.; Galli, G.V.; Bosisio, E.; Crestani, M.; de Fabiani, E.; et al. Minor components of olive oil modulate proatherogenic adhesion molecules involved in endothelial activation. *J. Agric. Food Chem.* **2006**, *54*, 3259–3264. [CrossRef]
132. Catalán, Ú.; López de Las Hazas, M.C.; Rubió, L.; Fernández-Castillejo, S.; Pedret, A.; de la Torre, R.; Motilva, M.J.; Solà, R. Protective effect of hydroxytyrosol and its predominant plasmatic human metabolites against endothelial dysfunction in human aortic endothelial cells. *Mol. Nutr. Food Res.* **2015**, *59*, 2523–2536. [CrossRef] [PubMed]
133. Vissers, M.N.; Zock, P.L.; Katan, M.B. Bioavailability and antioxidant effects of olive oil phenols in humans: A review. *Eur. J. Clin. Nutr.* **2004**, *58*, 955–965. [CrossRef]
134. Bordoni, L.; Fedeli, D.; Fiorini, D.; Gabbianelli, R. Extra virgin olive oil and Nigella sativa oil produced in central Italy: A comparison of the nutrigenomic effects of two Mediterranean oils in a low-grade inflammation model. *Antioxidants* **2019**, *9*, 20. [CrossRef] [PubMed]
135. Beauchamp, G.K.; Keast, R.S.; Morel, D.; Lin, J.; Pika, J.; Han, Q.; Lee, C.H.; Smith, A.B.; Breslin, P.A. Phytochemistry: Ibuprofen-like activity in extra-virgin olive oil. *Nature* **2005**, *437*, 45–46. [CrossRef] [PubMed]
136. Moreno, J.J. Effect of olive oil minor components on oxidative stress and arachidonic acid mobilization and metabolism by macrophages RAW 264.7. *Free Radic. Biol. Med.* **2003**, *35*, 1073–1081. [CrossRef]
137. Trefiletti, G.; Togna, A.R.; Latina, V.; Marra, C.; Guiso, M.; Togna, G.I. 1-Phenyl-6,7-dihydroxy-isochromansuppresses lipopolysaccharide-induced pro-inflammatory mediator production in human monocytes. *Br. J. Nutr.* **2011**, *106*, 33–36. [CrossRef]
138. Millman, J.F.; Okamoto, S.; Teruya, T.; Uema, T.; Ikematsu, S.; Shimabukuro, M.; Masuzaki, H. Extra-virgin olive oil and the gut-brain axis: Influence on gut microbiota, mucosal immunity, and cardiometabolic and cognitive health. *Nutr. Rev.* **2021**. [CrossRef] [PubMed]
139. Marcelino, G.; Hiane, P.A.; Freitas, K.C.; Santana, L.F.; Pott, A.; Donadon, J.R.; Guimarães, R.C.A. Effects of olive oil and its minor components on cardiovascular diseases, inflammation, and gut microbiota. *Nutrients* **2019**, *11*, 1826. [CrossRef]
140. Tihana, Ž.; Abdelkebir, R.; Alcantara, C.; Carmen, M.; García-Pérez, J.V.; Meléndez-martínez, A.J.; Re, A.; Lorenzo, J.M.; Barba, F.J. From extraction of valuable compounds to health promoting benefits of olive leaves through bioaccessibility, bioavailability and impact on gut microbiota. *Trends Food Sci. Technol.* **2019**, *83*, 63–77.
141. Gavahian, M.; Khaneghah, A.M.; Lorenzo, J.M.; Munekata, P.E.; Garcia-Mantrana, I.; Collado, M.C.; Meléndez-Martínez, A.J.; Barba, F.J. Health benefits of olive oil and its components: Impacts on gut microbiota antioxidant activities, and prevention of noncommunicable diseases. *Trends Food Sci. Technol.* **2019**, *88*, 220–227. [CrossRef]
142. Koper, J.E.B.; Loonen, L.M.P.; Jerry, M.; Wells, J.M.; Troise, A.D.; Capuano, E.; Fogliano, V. Polyphenols and tryptophan metabolites activate the aryl hydrocarbon receptor in an in vitro model of colonic fermentation. *Mol. Nutr. Food Res.* **2019**, *63*, e1800722. [CrossRef] [PubMed]
143. Calahorra, J.; Martínez-Lara, E.; Granadino-Roldán, J.M.; Martí, J.M.; Cañuelo, A.; Blanco, S.; Oliver, F.J.; Siles, E. Crosstalk between hydroxytyrosol, a major olive oil phenol, and HIF-1 in MCF-7 breast cancer cells. *Sci. Rep.* **2020**, *10*, 6361. [CrossRef] [PubMed]
144. Serra, G.; Incani, A.; Serreli, G.; Porru, L.; Melis, M.P.; Tuberoso, C.I.G.; Rossin, D.; Biasi, F.; Deiana, M. Olive oil polyphenols reduce oxysterols -induced redox imbalance and pro-inflammatory response in intestinal cells. *Redox Biol.* **2018**, *7*, 348–354. [CrossRef] [PubMed]
145. Boonstra, E.; de Kleijn, R.; Colzato, L.S.; Alkemade, A.; Forstmann, B.U.; Nieuwenhuis, S. Neurotransmitters as food supplements: The effects of GABA on brain and behavior. *Front. Psychol.* **2015**, *6*, 1520. [CrossRef] [PubMed]
146. Fulop, T.; Witkowski, J.M.; Bourgade, K.; Khalil, A.; Zerif, E.; Larbi, A.; Hirokawa, K.; Pawelec, G.; Bocti, C.; Lacombe, G.; et al. Can an infection hypothesis explain the beta amyloid hypothesis of Alzheimer's disease? *Front. Aging Neurosci.* **2018**, *10*, 224. [CrossRef]
147. Estruch, R.; Ros, E.; Salas-Salvadó, J.; Covas, M.I.; Corella, D.; Arós, F.; Gómez-Gracia, E.; Ruiz-Gutiérrez, V.; Fiol, M.; Lapetra, J.; et al. Primary prevention of cardiovascular disease with a Mediterranean diet supplemented with extra-virgin olive oil or nuts. *N. Engl. J. Med.* **2018**, *378*, E34. [CrossRef] [PubMed]
148. Guasch-Ferré, M.; Hu, F.B.; Martínez-González, M.A.; Fitó, M.; Bulló, M.; Estruch, R.; Ros, E.; Corella, D.; Recondo, J.; Gómez-Gracia, E.; et al. Olive oil intake and risk of cardiovascular disease and mortality in the PREDIMED Study. *BMC Med.* **2014**, *12*, 78. [CrossRef] [PubMed]
149. Guo, X.; Tresserra-Rimbau, A.; Estruch, R.; Martínez-González, M.A.; Medina-Remón, A.; Castañer, O.; Corella, D.; Salas-Salvadó, J.; Lamuela-Raventós, R.M. Effects of polyphenol, measured by a biomarker of total polyphenols in urine, on cardiovascular risk factors after a long-term follow-up in the PREDIMED Study. *Oxid. Med. Cell Longev.* **2016**, *2016*, 2572606. [CrossRef] [PubMed]
150. Martínez-Lapiscina, E.H.; Clavero, P.; Toledo, E.; Estruch, R.; Salas-Salvadó, J.; San Julián, B.; Sanchez-Tainta, A.; Ros, E.; Valls-Pedret, C.; Martinez-Gonzalez, M.Á. Mediterranean diet improves cognition: The PREDIMED-NAVARRA randomised trial. *J. Neurol. Neurosurg. Psychiatry* **2013**, *84*, 1318–1325. [CrossRef]

151. Martínez-Lapiscina, E.H.; Galbete, C.; Corella, D.; Toledo, E.; Buil-Cosiales, P.; Salas-Salvado, J.; Ros, E.; Martinez-Gonzalez, M.A. Genotype patterns at CLU, CR1, PICALM and APOE, cognition and Mediterranean diet: The PREDIMED-NAVARRA trial. *Genes Nutr.* **2014**, *9*, 393. [CrossRef] [PubMed]
152. Valls-Pedret, C.; Lamuela-Raventós, R.M.; Medina-Remón, A.; Quintana, M.; Corella, D.; Pintó, X.; Martínez-González, M.Á.; Estruch, R.; Ros, E. Polyphenol-rich foods in the Mediterranean diet are associated with better cognitive function in elderly subjects at high cardiovascular risk. *J. Alzheimer's Dis.* **2012**, *29*, 773–782. [CrossRef]
153. Toledo, E.; Salas-Salvadó, J.; Donat-Vargas, C.; Buil-Cosiales, P.; Estruch, R.; Ros, E.; Corella, D.; Fitó, M.; Hu, F.B.; Arós, F.; et al. Mediterranean diet and invasive breast cancer risk among women at high cardiovascular risk in the PREDIMED Trial: A randomized clinical trial. *JAMA Intern. Med.* **2015**, *175*, 1752–1760. [CrossRef]
154. de la Torre-Carbot, K.; Chávez-Servín, J.L.; Jaúregui, O.; Castellote, A.I.; Lamuela-Raventós, R.M.; Nurmi, T.; Poulsen, H.E.; Gaddi, A.V.; Kaikkonen, J.; Zunft, H.F.; et al. Elevated circulating LDL phenol levels in men who consumed virgin rather than refined olive oil are associated with less oxidation of plasma LDL. *J. Nutr.* **2010**, *140*, 501–508. [CrossRef]
155. Marrugat, J.; Covas, M.I.; Fitó, M.; Schröder, H.; Miró-Casas, E.; Gimeno, E.; López-Sabater, M.C.; de la Torre, R.; Farré, M. Effects of differing phenolic content in dietary olive oils on lipids and LDL oxidation—A randomized controlled trial. *Eur. J. Nutr.* **2004**, *43*, 140–147. [CrossRef] [PubMed]
156. Khandouzi, N.; Zahedmehr, A.; Nasrollahzadeh, J. Effect of polyphenol-rich extra-virgin olive oil on lipid profile and inflammatory biomarkers in patients undergoing coronary angiography: A randomised, controlled, clinical trial. *Int. J. Food Sci. Nutr.* **2021**, *72*, 548–558. [CrossRef]
157. Marx, W.; George, E.S.; Mayr, H.L.; Thomas, C.J.; Sarapis, K.; Moschonis, G.; Kennedy, G.; Pipingas, A.; Willcox, J.C.; Prendergast, L.A.; et al. Effect of high polyphenol extra virgin olive oil on markers of cardiovascular disease risk in healthy Australian adults (OLIVAUS): A protocol for a double-blind randomised, controlled, cross-over study. *Nutr. Diet.* **2020**, *77*, 523–528. [CrossRef]
158. Hernáez, Á.; Remaley, A.T.; Farràs, M.; Fernández-Castillejo, S.; Subirana, I.; Schröder, H.; Fernández-Mampel, M.; Muñoz-Aguayo, D.; Sampson, M.; Solà, R.; et al. Olive oil polyphenols decrease LDL concentrations and LDL atherogenicity in men in a randomized controlled trial. *J. Nutr.* **2015**, *145*, 1692–1697. [CrossRef] [PubMed]
159. Hernáez, Á.; Fernàndez-Castillejo, S.; Farràs, M.; Catalán, Ú.; Subirana, I.; Montes, R.; Solà, R.; Muñoz-Aguayo, D.; Gelabert-Gorgues, A.; Díaz-Gil, Ó.; et al. Olive oil polyphenols enhance high-density lipoprotein function in humans. A randomized controlled trial. *Arterioscler. Thromb. Vasc. Biol.* **2014**, *34*, 2115–2119. [CrossRef] [PubMed]
160. Guasch-Ferré, M.; Hruby, A.; Salas-Salvadò, J.; Martinez-Gonzàlez, M.A.; Sun, Q.; Willett, W.C.; Hu, F.B. Olive oil consumption and risk of type 2 diabetes in US women. *Am. J. Clin. Nutr.* **2015**, *102*, 479–486. [CrossRef] [PubMed]
161. Violi, F.; Loffredo, L.; Pignatelli, P.; Angelico, F.; Bartimoccia, S.; Nocella, C.; Cangemi, R.; Petruccioli, A.; Monticolo, R.; Pastori, D.; et al. Extra virgin olive oil use is associated with improved post-prandial blood glucose and LDL-cholesterol in healthy subjects. *Nutr. Diabetes* **2015**, *5*, e172. [CrossRef] [PubMed]
162. Bozzetto, L.; Alderisio, A.; Clemente, G.; Giorgini, M. Gastrointestinal effects of extra-virgin olive oil associated with lower postprandial glycemia in type 1 diabetes. *Clin. Nutr.* **2019**, *38*, 2645–2651. [CrossRef]
163. Carnevale, R.; Loffredo, L.; del Ben, M.; Angelico, F.; Nocella, C.; Petruccioli, A.; Bartimoccia, S.; Monticolo, R.; Cava, E.; Violi, F. Extra virgin olive oil improves post-prandial glycemic and lipid profile in patients with impaired fasting glucose. *Clin. Nutr.* **2017**, *36*, 782–787. [CrossRef] [PubMed]
164. Tsolaki, M.; Lazarou, E.; Kozori, M.; Petridou, N.; Tabakis, I.; Lazarou, I.; Karakota, M.; Saoulidis, I.; Melliou, E.; Magiatis, P. A Randomized clinical trial of Greek high phenolic early harvest extra virgin olive oil in mild cognitive impairment: The MICOIL pilot study. *J. Alzheimer's Dis.* **2020**, *78*, 801–817. [CrossRef]
165. Camargo, A.; Ruano, J.; Fernandez, J.M.; Parnell, L.D.; Jimenez, A.; Santos-Gonzalez, M.; Marin, C.; Perez-Martinez, P.; Uceda, M.; Lopez-Miranda, J.; et al. Gene expression changes in mononuclear cells in patients with metabolic syndrome after acute intake of phenol-rich virgin olive oil. *BMC Genom.* **2010**, *11*, 253. [CrossRef] [PubMed]
166. Perez-Herrera, A.; Delgado-Lista, J.; Torres-Sanchez, L.A.; Rangel-Zuñiga, O.A.; Camargo, A.; Moreno-Navarrete, J.M.; Garcia-Olid, B.; Quintana-Navarro, G.M.; Alcala-Diaz, J.F.; Muñoz-Lopez, C.; et al. The postprandial inflammatory response after ingestion of heated oils in obese persons is reduced by the presence of phenol compounds. *Mol. Nutr. Food Res.* **2012**, *56*, 510–514. [CrossRef] [PubMed]
167. Tsartsou, E.; Proutsos, N.; Castanas, E.; Kampa, M. Network meta-analysis of metabolic effects of olive-oil in humans shows the importance of olive oil consumption with moderate polyphenol levels as part of the Mediterranean diet. *Front. Nutr.* **2019**, *12*, 6. [CrossRef]
168. Peroulis, N.; Androutsopoulos, V.P.; Notas, G.; Koinaki, S.; Giakoumaki, E.; Spyros, A.; Manolopoulou, E.; Kargaki, S.; Tzardi, M.; Moustou, E.; et al. Significant metabolic improvement by a water extract of olives: Animal and human evidence. *Eur. J. Nutr.* **2019**, *58*, 2545–2560. [CrossRef] [PubMed]
169. Lee, H.; Im, S.W.; Jung, C.H.; Jang, Y.J.; Ha, T.Y.; Ahn, J. Tyrosol, an olive oil polyphenol, inhibits ER stress-induced apoptosis in pancreatic beta-cell through JNK signaling. *Biochem. Biophys. Res. Commun.* **2016**, *469*, 748–752. [CrossRef] [PubMed]
170. Vassiliou, E.K.; Gonzalez, A.; Garcia, C.; Tadros, J.H.; Chakraborty, G.; Toney, J.H. Oleic acid and peanut oil high in oleic acid reverse the inhibitory effect of insulin production of the inflammatory cytokine TNF-alpha both in vitro and in vivo systems. *Lipids Health Dis.* **2009**, *8*, 25. [CrossRef]

171. Schwingshackl, L.; Christoph, M.; Hoffmann, G. Effects of olive oil on markers of inflammation and endothelial function-a systematic review and meta-analysis. *Nutrients* **2015**, *7*, 7651–7675. [CrossRef]
172. Luisi, M.L.E.; Lucarini, L.; Biffi, B.; Rafanelli, E.; Pietramellara, G.; Durante, M.; Vidali, S.; Provensi, G.; Madiai, S.; Gheri, C.F.; et al. Effect of Mediterranean diet enriched in high quality extra virgin olive oil on oxidative stress, inflammation and gut microbiota in obese and normal weight adult subjects. *Front. Pharmacol.* **2019**, *10*, 1366. [CrossRef] [PubMed]
173. Olalla, J.; García de Lomas, J.M.; Chueca, N.; Pérez-Stachowski, X.; de Salazar, A.; del Arco, A.; Plaza-Díaz, J.; de la Torre, J.; Prada, J.L.; García-Alegría, J.; et al. Effect of daily consumption of extra virgin olive oil on the lipid profile and microbiota of HIV-infected patients over 50 years of age. *Medicine* **2019**, *98*, e17528. [CrossRef] [PubMed]
174. Martín-Peláez, S.; Mosele, J.I.; Pizarro, N.; Farràs, M.; de la Torre, R.; Subirana, I.; Pérez-Cano, F.J.; Castañer, O.; Solà, R.; Fernandez-Castillejo, S.; et al. Effect of virgin olive oil and thyme phenolic compounds on blood lipid profile: Implications of human gut microbiota. *Eur. J. Nutr.* **2017**, *56*, 119–131. [CrossRef] [PubMed]

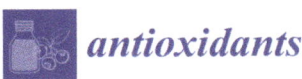

Review

Therapeutic Potential of Polyphenols in Amyotrophic Lateral Sclerosis and Frontotemporal Dementia

Valentina Novak [1], Boris Rogelj [1,2] and Vera Župunski [1,*]

[1] Chair of Biochemistry, Faculty of Chemistry and Chemical Technology, University of Ljubljana, SI-1000 Ljubljana, Slovenia; vn4556@student.uni-lj.si (V.N.); boris.rogelj@ijs.si (B.R.)
[2] Department of Biotechnology, Jozef Stefan Institute, SI-1000 Ljubljana, Slovenia
* Correspondence: vera.zupunski@fkkt.uni-lj.si

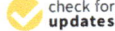

Abstract: Amyotrophic lateral sclerosis (ALS) and frontotemporal dementia (FTD) are severe neurodegenerative disorders that belong to a common disease spectrum. The molecular and cellular aetiology of the spectrum is a highly complex encompassing dysfunction in many processes, including mitochondrial dysfunction and oxidative stress. There is a paucity of treatment options aside from therapies with subtle effects on the post diagnostic lifespan and symptom management. This presents great interest and necessity for the discovery and development of new compounds and therapies with beneficial effects on the disease. Polyphenols are secondary metabolites found in plant-based foods and are well known for their antioxidant activity. Recent research suggests that they also have a diverse array of neuroprotective functions that could lead to better treatments for neurodegenerative diseases. We present an overview of the effects of various polyphenols in cell line and animal models of ALS/FTD. Furthermore, possible mechanisms behind actions of the most researched compounds (resveratrol, curcumin and green tea catechins) are discussed.

Keywords: ALS; FTD; polyphenols; neurodegeneration; resveratrol; curcumin; catechin; EGCG

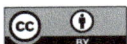

1. Introduction

With the ageing population, the treatment and management of neurodegenerative diseases is a major and increasing challenge for health care systems and societies around the world [1]. Amyotrophic lateral sclerosis (ALS) is a neurodegenerative disease that affects motor neurons, resulting in deterioration of motor function, and frontotemporal dementia (FTD) is a neurodegenerative disorder characterised by changes in personality, behaviour, and language. The development of both diseases is a progressive and ultimately fatal multistep process with a complex genetic and molecular background. Despite extensive research efforts, only two treatment options with limited effects on survival and motor function are currently approved for ALS. The vast majority of compounds researched as possible ALS therapies until today were found to be ineffective in clinical trials, highlighting the need for further research [2]. Currently, only symptomatic treatments with limited effects are available for FTD [3].

Polyphenols are natural compounds whose neuroprotective effects have been demonstrated in various models of neurodegenerative diseases such as Alzheimer's and Parkinson's disease. These compounds are being explored for possible dietary intervention and supplementation as preventive measures against neurodegenerative diseases, and also as possible candidates for therapies to slow disease progression and alleviate symptoms [4]. Due to the lack of disease-changing treatments for ALS/FTD and the growing interest in natural compounds as therapeutic agents, this article reviews an intriguing topic of potential use of polyphenols in the development of treatments for ALS/FTD symptoms.

1.1. Amyotrophic Lateral Sclerosis and Frontotemporal Dementia

ALS is a neurodegenerative disease characterised by progressive loss of both upper and lower motor neurons. Initial signs of the disease may include weakness of the limbs (in spinal-onset ALS) or difficulties with speech and swallowing (in bulbar-onset ALS) [5]. Disease progression eventually leads to paralysis and death from respiratory failure, on average 24 to 50 months after onset [6–10]. The worldwide incidence of ALS is 1.75 with a reported mean age at diagnosis between 51 and 69 years [11,12]. ALS cases can be divided into the familial form of the disease (fALS, 5–15% of patients), where there is a clear family history, and the predominant sporadic form (sALS) [13]. Frontotemporal dementia (FTD) is a type of dementia primarily associated with alterations in the frontal and temporal lobes. Symptoms manifest as changes in behaviour, personality, language, and motor skills [14,15]. The incidence of FTD is 1.6 and the mean age of onset is 65 years [16]. FTD can be divided into one behavioural (bvFTD) and two language variants (or primary progressive aphasias (PPA)) [14]. Mean survival time for most forms of FTD is approximately 8 years [17]. Up to 40% of FTD patients have a family history of the disease [18,19].

Clinical, genetic, pathological and biochemical data show that there is an overlap between ALS and FTD. First observations that ALS and FTD might be connected were made in the early 1990s [20,21]. Data show that about half of ALS patients have cognitive impairment and 15% meet the criteria for FTD [22,23]. Similarly, about 30% of patients with FTD develop signs of motor dysfunction and 10–15% have ALS [24,25]. The discovery of common genetic causes and biological mechanisms further confirmed that ALS and FTD are closely associated (Figure 1) [5,26].

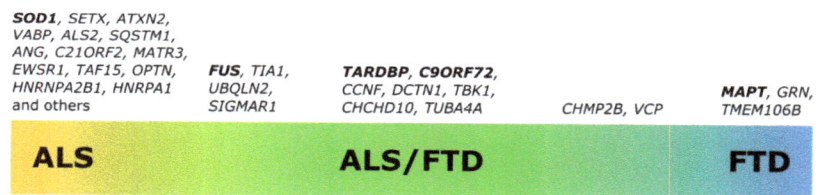

Figure 1. Genes involved in pathologies along the ALS-FTD spectrum. The most common genetic causes of the disease are highlighted in bold.

ALS and FTD pathologies are multistep processes that affect many aspects of cellular activity. The most prominent pathological hallmark of both ALS and FTD are changes in protein homeostasis, including protein misfolding and aggregation, altered localisation, and defects in autophagic and proteasomal degradation. The combination of these mechanisms leads to the formation of toxic cytoplasmic inclusions in motor neurons and surrounding cells. Proteins that predominantly form these structures are two RNA-binding proteins, TAR DNA binding protein (TDP-43, protein product of *TARDBP*), and fused in sarcoma (FUS), microtubule-associated protein tau (gene *MAPT*), and superoxide dismutase 1 (SOD1) [27,28]. The correlation between pathology and genetics is complex [29–31]. Pathologically, 97% of ALS cases have pathognomonic TDP-43 aggregates, while only 1% of those are associated with mutations in TDP-43 and in the rest TDP-43 is not mutated. A total of 1% of ALS shows FUS aggregates, all of which are associated with mutations in FUS. Mutations in FUS or TDP-43 are extremely rare in FTD; however, 50% of FTD have TDP-43 aggregates and 10% of FTD have FUS aggregates. A total of 40% of FTD is tau aggregates. Impairments in protein turnover and clearance are also observed. Mutations in genes associated with different stages of autophagy are also causative for ALS/FTD, from autophagy regulating activities of C9ORF72 to impaired functions of autophagic receptors SQSTM1 and optineurin [32–37].

In healthy cells, TDP-43 and FUS are predominantly nuclear RNA/DNA-binding proteins with functions in RNA splicing, transcription, microRNA biogenesis, and mRNA transport [38–47]. Both play important parts in ribonucleoprotein coacervates that form membrane-less organelles such as stress granules in the cytoplasm and paraspeckles in the nucleus [48,49]. In ALS/FTD, FUS or TDP-43 mislocalise to the cytoplasm and form aggregates that are most likely toxic, although loss of function from the nucleus may also be the key disease-causing factor. This mislocalisation is instigated by a number of disruptions, including dysfunctions in proteostasis, nucleocytoplasmic shuttling, and the cellular stress response [50–52]. Upon stress, TDP-43, FUS, and some other ALS-associated RNA-binding proteins separate into stress granules, which may be the first step in the formation of insoluble aggregates [53,54]. Another common factor in the disruption of RNA metabolism is G4C2 repeat expansions in the C9ORF72 gene, which are the most common cause of familiar forms of ALS/FTD [55–57]. The repeats form stable nucleic acid secondary structures known as G-quadruplexes, hairpin loops, and i-motifs, that sequester RNA-binding proteins and form nuclear foci similar to paraspeckles, or can be translated into toxic dipeptide repeats via repeat-associated non-ATG translation [58–65].

Mitochondria play a central role in neurons, primarily fulfilling high needs for energy. ALS/FTD-associated changes include defects in oxidative phosphorylation and calcium homeostasis, elevated production of ROS, structural impairments, and reduced clearance of damaged mitochondria [66]. Changes in mitochondrial morphology are observed in cells overexpressing mutant SOD1, FUS, or TDP-43 [67–70]. The increased localisation of mutant SOD1 in the mitochondrial intermembrane space causes mitochondrial dysfunction and toxicity to neurons [71–73]. Overall, mitochondrial changes result in decreased electron transport chain activity and reduced ATP production [66]. Moreover, oxidative stress has been proposed to be crucial in ALS pathogenesis and has been well documented in patient samples [74–76].

1.2. Currently Used Therapies for ALS/FTD

Treatments currently in clinical trials for ALS/FTD were comprehensively reviewed by Liscic et al. [26]. Therapeutic targets include a reduction in glutamate excitotoxicity and protein aggregation, upregulation of certain heat shock proteins, and activation of troponin in skeletal muscle. Interesting novel strategies for ALS/FTD treatment may also come from stem cell therapy, non-invasive brain stimulation, and the growing knowledge of the influence of the gut microbiota on the development of neurological diseases [26]. Currently, only two drugs are approved for the treatment of ALS. Riluzole was approved for clinical use in 1995 and trials observed reduced one year mortality and slower deterioration of muscle function [26,77,78]. The mechanisms behind the beneficial effects of riluzole are not entirely clear. Different neuroprotective actions have been proposed, such as inhibition of glutamate excitotoxicity, blockade of Ca^{2+}- or Na^+-ion channels, and modulation of GABA pathways [79]. In recent years, some countries have also approved the use of edaravone (also known as MCI-186 or Radicava) for the treatment of ALS [26]. Its actions could benefit a subgroup of patients with early onset and rapidly progressive disease [80]. Edaravone is thought to act as an antioxidant and free radical scavenger, but the mechanisms are not well understood [81]. There are currently no approved direct treatments for FTD, other than symptom management [82].

2. Therapeutic Potentials of Polyphenols in ALS/FTD

Many potential therapeutic compounds have antioxidant and anti-inflammatory properties. Polyphenols (Figure 2) are a diverse group of naturally occurring compounds with a characteristic chemical structure that has one or more phenolic rings. They are found in plant foods such as fruits, vegetables, and whole grains [83,84]. In plants, polyphenols are categorised as secondary metabolites and have functions in normal growth as well as in the plant defense system [85]. They are synthesised in the shikimate and phenylpropanoid pathways [86]. Many different polyphenols have been described to have neuroprotective effects in mammalian cell and animal models of ALS/FTD [87]. In this review, the focus will be on resveratrol, epigallocatechin gallate (EGCG), and curcumin (Figure 2). We will also explore the effects of some other flavonoids and phenolic acids in the context of ALS/FTD.

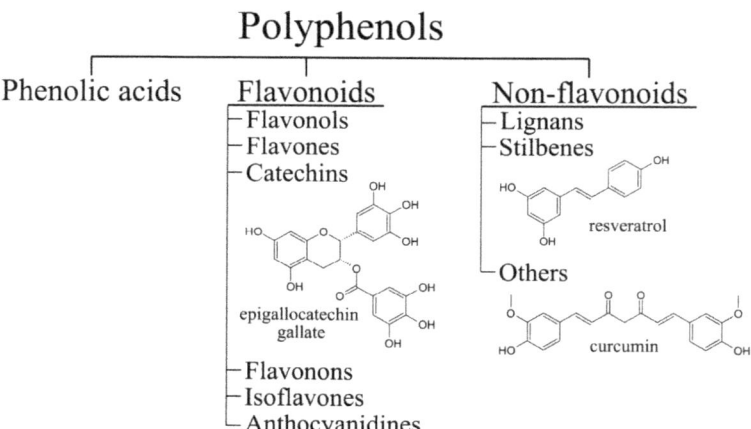

Figure 2. Classification of polyphenols with structural formulas of epigallocatechin gallate (EGCG), resveratrol and curcumin.

2.1. Resveratrol

Resveratrol (3,5,4'-trihydroxystilbene) is a polyphenol found in grapes, red wine, berries, and peanuts [88]. Both cis- and trans- isomers occur naturally, with trans-form being the focus in terms of potential neuroprotective activity [89]. Effects of resveratrol in ALS were first demonstrated in neuronal cell lines expressing the SOD1^{G93A} mutant [90–92]. Resveratrol treatment halved the cell death observed as a consequence of SOD1-mediated toxicity [90]. Treatments of mouse motor neuron cells NSC34 expressing SOD1^{G93A} showed a minor dose-dependent improvement in cell viability and a simultaneous reduction in the concentration of cytosolic ROS [91]. Administration of resveratrol protected rat cortical motor neurons from the toxic effects of cerebrospinal fluid (CSF) from ALS patients [93]. Further studies in mice ALS models expressing mutant SOD1^{G93A} showed conflicting results, which are probably a consequence of different protocols on dosing and route of administration. Chronic oral administration of resveratrol at 25 mg/kg/day did not improve motor abilities and life span of ALS mice [94]. On the other hand, intraperitoneal injections of 20 mg/kg/twice a week improved survival and delayed the onset of ALS [95]. A similar positive effect on survival and motor function was observed with a higher dose (160 mg/kg/day) administered orally [96]. The neuroprotective effects of resveratrol in ALS mice have been further demonstrated in coadministration with other potential therapeutics [97,98]. Resveratrol has also been researched in models of tauopathies, a hallmark of FTD, but the overall effects on tau aggregation are inconclusive [99].

The predominant mechanism behind the neuroprotective effect of resveratrol is the activation of SIRT1, a NAD$^+$-dependent protein deacetylase [90,92,95,96,100]. Structural studies suggested a mechanism in which resveratrol acts as an adaptor for the interaction between the peptide substrate and SIRT1 [101]. Many downstream mechanisms of SIRT1 targets have been proposed as possible mediators of the beneficial effects. SIRT1 deacetylates p53 [90,96], a known tumor suppressor protein involved in mechanisms of motor neuron cell death [102]. Resveratrol treatment upregulates factors involved in mitochondrial biogenesis, which could improve altered energy metabolism observed in ALS [92,96]. SIRT1 also targets HSF1 (heat shock factor 1) that activates several heat shock proteins. Their activity as chaperones possibly mitigates formation of toxic protein aggregates [95]. Normalisation of autophagic flux was also observed in resveratrol-treated ALS mice, but it is not clear whether SIRT1 is involved [96]. Independent of SIRT1, resveratrol can also activate AMPK (AMP-activated protein kinase) [96,103] that has downstream targets involved in neuroprotective mechanisms [104]. Moreover, a molecular mechanistic study on

SOD1^{G93A} showed a stabilising effect of resveratrol that could impede the aggregation of mutant protein [105]. A similar inhibitory effect was observed in aggregation studies of wt SOD1 [106].

2.2. Curcumin

Curcumin (diferuloylmethane) is the predominant curcuminoid found in turmeric (*Curcuma longa*), which is widely used in traditional Indian medicine. The potential benefits of curcumin are being explored in many neurodegenerative diseases. In models of Alzheimer's and Parkinson's disease, curcumin can reduce oxidative stress, affect toxic protein aggregation, and protect against apoptosis [107,108].

Regarding ALS, curcumin was shown to impede aggregation of reduced wt SOD1 in vitro by binding its aggregation prone regions. Curcumin-bound SOD1 aggregates were smaller, unstructured, and less cytotoxic [109]. A similar effect of inhibiting beta-sheet formation and aggregation was observed with tau, a protein involved in FTD [110]. In contrast, the binding of curcumin to tau aggregates was not observed in post-mortem brain tissue sections from FTD patients [111].

Curcumin presents a challenge for in vivo use due to its poor absorption, fast metabolism, and rapid elimination. Several strategies can be utilised to overcome the low oral bioavailability of curcumin [112]. The protective effect of an analogue, dimethoxy curcumin, was demonstrated in a neuronal cell line expressing TDP-43 mutants Q331K or M337V. Dimethoxy curcumin restored mitochondrial damage by improving transmembrane potential, increasing electron transfer chain complex I activity, and upregulating UCP2 (uncoupling protein 2) [113]. The same compound also improved abnormally high excitability of cells expressing mutant TDP-43 [114]. Furthermore, an improved curcumin analogue, monocarbonyl dimethoxycurcumin C, prevented aggregation of mutant TDP-43 and reduced oxidative stress, possibly due to increased expression of heme oxygenase-1 [115].

Another approach to improve the bioavailability of curcumin is delivery using nanoparticles. The potential for ALS treatment was demonstrated with curcumin-loaded inulin-D-alfa-tocopherol succinate micelles, which were effectively delivered into mesenchymal stromal cells [116]. Furthermore, the efficiency of a turmeric supplement in nanomicelles was tested in a clinical trial involving 54 ALS patients treated primarily with riluzole. Nanocurcumin improved the survival probability of the patients, but did not significantly improve their motor function [117].

2.3. Catechins

Green tea, produced from the leaves and buds of *Camellia sinensis*, is rich in polyphenols catechins, predominantly (−)epigallocatechin gallate (EGCG), but also (−)-epigallocatechin (EGC), (−)-epicatechin gallate (ECG), (−)-epicatechin (EC), and (+)-catechin [118]. In ALS models, EGCG has been shown to protect motor neuron cells from oxidative stress and mitochondrial damage [119]. Presymptomatic oral supplementation of EGCG at doses of at least 2.9 mg EGCG/kg body weight in SOD1^{G93A} mice significantly delayed symptom onset, improved motor function, and increased lifespan [120,121].

EGCG likely acts by upregulating a prosurvival signaling pathway PI3K/Akt. Among other pathways, PI3K/Akt regulates the activity of GSK-3. Increased GSK-3 levels are associated with the formation of neurofibrillary tangles and neuronal death. In addition, GSK-3 induces apoptosis through downstream signaling, including mitochondrial damage and caspase-3 activation. It was shown that Akt phosphorylates GSK-3, resulting in less mitochondrial damage [119]. Observations in ALS mice further confirm an increase in PI3K/Akt and a decrease in death signals such as caspase-3, cytosolic cytochrome c, and cleaved PARP (poly (ADP-ribose) polymerase) [120]. EGCG also has antioxidant and anti-inflammatory effects on microglia and astrocytes [121]. In addition, it can decrease lipid peroxidation, but has no effect on iron metabolism despite its presumed chelating abilities [122]. A molecular docking study showed the potential of EGCG to reduce mutant SOD1 aggregates [123]. In vitro studies confirmed an inhibitory effect on apo-SOD1 aggregation [124]. It has also been shown that the addition of EGCG induces oligomerisation of TDP-43 and inhibits its degradation into toxic aggregation-prone fragments [125]. In FTD, inhibition of tau filament formation was observed for ECG, but not for EC [126].

2.4. Other Flavonoids

In addition to green tea catechins, several other flavonoids have been tested in ALS/FTD models. Presymptomatic administration of 2 mg/kg body weight of an anthocyanin-enriched strawberry extract with callistephin (pelargonidin 3-glucoside) as the predominant component delayed ALS onset, preserved grip strength, and prolonged survival in SOD1^{G93A} mice [127]. Oral supplementation of fisetin (3,3,4,7-tetrahydroxyflavone) improved motor functions, delayed disease onset, and increased survival in SOD1^{G93A} mice (at a dosage of 9 mg/kg) and SOD1^{G85R} *Drosophila melanogaster*. The predominant mechanism behind the activity of fisetin in motor neuron cell lines expressing SOD1^{G93A} appears to be the activation of the ERK pathway involved in the regulation of cell survival. Moreover, fisetin decreased both wt and mutant SOD1 levels in cells, possibly by activating autophagy [128].

A computational study confirmed the binding of kaempferol (3,4',5,7-tetrahydroxyflavone) and kaempferide to mutant SOD1^{G85R} [129]. Both compounds were experimentally shown to have antioxidant properties and could reduce the formation of SOD1^{G85R} aggregates in N2a mouse neuroblastoma cells. Kaempferol could act via increased phosphorylation of AMPK and downstream induction of autophagy [130]. The antioxidant effect of quercetin (3,3',4',5,7-pentahyroxyflavone) was first observed in lymphoblast cell lines from ALS patients [131]. In vitro tests showed that quercetin glycosides, namely quercitrin and quercetin 3-beta-d-glucoside, inhibit misfolding and aggregation of SOD1^{A4V} mutant [132]. A similar effect on aggregation was observed with quercetin and baicalein [133]. Furthermore, preventive administration of quercetin in rats reduced oxidative stress, defective mitochondria, and brain cell death caused by aluminium exposure [134].

SOD1^{G93A} mice treated with 5 mg/kg 7,8-dihydroxyflavone exhibited significantly improved motor performance and increased numbers of spinal motor neurons compared with untreated animals [135]. Interestingly, it was observed that treatment with 16 mg/kg genistein (4',5,7-trihydroxyisoflavone) had a protective effect on disease progression in male SOD1^{G93A} mice [136]. In contrast, in further studies, a delay in symptoms and higher survival of motor neurons was observed in both sexes, possibly due to anti-inflammatory effects and restored autophagy [137]. Twice-daily administration of 700 mg luteolin (3',4',5,7-tetrahydroxyflavone) in combination with palmitoylethanolamide showed some improvement of symptoms in patients with FTD [138].

2.5. Phenolic Acids and Derivatives

Phenolic acids are found in fruits, coffee, tea, and grains. Their diverse neuroprotective effects make them interesting candidates for better ALS therapies. It has been reported that protocatechuic acid administration at 100 mg/kg in SOD1^{G93A} mice prolongs survival, improves motor function, and reduces gliosis [139]. Caffeic acid phenethyl ester (CAPE) showed a dose-dependent improvement in survival and a simultaneous reduction in cytosolic ROS in the NCS34 cell line expressing SOD1^{G93A}. CAPE decreased the activation of the oxidative stress-associated transcription factor NF-κB and activated the antioxidant response element (ARE) [91]. Further studies in SOD1^{G93A} mice confirmed that daily administration of 10 mg/kg CAPE after disease onset slowed symptom progression and prolonged survival. A reduction in glial activation and phospho-p38 levels was observed as a result [140]. Gallic acid and wedelolactone improved locomotor function and motor learning abilities in an aluminium or quinolinic acid-induced rat model of sALS. The effects may be due to a reduction in inflammatory cytokines, normalisation of L-glutamate levels, and decreased activation of caspase-3 [141,142]. Rosmarinic acid, the main compound in rosemary (*Rosmarinus officinalis*) extract, reduced weight loss, improved motor performance, and prolonged survival of SOD1^{G93A} mice [143,144]. The effects of treatment with higher doses were compared with the established ALS therapeutic agent riluzole, but were not found to be more effective [144].

2.6. Overview of Potential Therapeutic Effects of Polyphenols in ALS and FTD

We have summarised the therapeutic implications of polyphenols, including their proposed mechanisms in animal and cell line models of ALS and FTD (Table 1). The predominant mechanism behind the neuroprotective role of resveratrol is the activation of SIRT1. Its downstream targets may impact processes such as neuronal survival, mitochondrial biogenesis, and prevention of protein aggregate formation, all of which contribute to the observed delay in symptoms and increased viability in ALS models [90,92,95,96]. Curcumin derivatives show neuroprotective value through several mechanisms, such as restoring mitochondrial functions, normalising cell excitability, and preventing the formation of toxic protein aggregates [113–115]. Green tea catechin EGCG has been observed to upregulate a prosurvival signaling pathway PI3K/Akt and decrease signals leading to cell death, such as activation of caspase-3, which is associated with apoptosis [119,120]. Both resulted in the delayed onset of ALS and increased survival in mice models treated with EGCG [120,121]. Fisetin acts by activating the ERK pathway, which modulates cell survival and upregulates HO-1, both of which contribute to the cellular response against oxidative stress [128]. Another mechanism exerted by some polyphenols is the downregulation of the NF-κB pathway that, overall, has an anti-inflammatory effect [91].

Table 1. Therapeutic implications of different polyphenols in ALS and FTD models.

Compound	Animal/Cell Line	Mechanism of Action	Outcome	Ref.
resveratrol	rat cortical primary neurons expressing SOD1^{G93A}	activation of SIRT1	reduced cell death	[90]
	NCS34 cell line expressing SOD1^{G93A}	antioxidant activity	reduction in ROS, increased viability	[91]
	VSC4.1 cell line expressing hSOD1^{G93A}	activation of SIRT1, mitochondrial biogenesis	increased viability, reduced apoptosis	[92]
	rat cortical neurons with ALS-patient CSF	possibly reduction in cytosolic Ca^{2+} concentration	increased viability	[93]
	mice expressing SOD1^{G93A}	activation of SIRT1, heat shock protein response	delayed onset, increased survival	[95]
	mice expressing SOD1^{G93A}	activation of SIRT1, mitochondrial biogenesis, normalised autophagic flux	delayed onset, improved motor function, increased survival	[96]
	bone marrow-mesenchymal stem cells of ALS patients	activation of SIRT1 and AMPK	increased differentiation rate	[103]
dimethoxy curcumin	NSC34 cell line expressing TDP-43^{Q331K}, TDP-43^{M337V}	decreased expression of UCP2, improved mitochondrial transmembrane potential and morphology	improved mitochondrial function	[113]
	NSC34 cell line expressing TDP-43^{Q331K}	not determined	lowered excitability, no observed change in survival	[114]
monocarbonyl dimethoxycurcumin	NSC34 cell line expressing TDP-43^{Q331K}	upregulation of HO-1	reduced oxidative stress and toxicity	[115]
epigallocatechin gallate	VSC4.1 cell line expressing SOD1^{G93A}	protection from oxidative stress, increase in survival signals through PI3K	increased viability, reduced apoptosis	[119]
	mice expressing SOD1^{G93A}	increase in survival signals through PI3K	delayed onset, increased lifespan	[120]
	mice expressing SOD1^{G93A}	reduced activation of NF-κB and caspase-3	delayed onset, increased lifespan	[121]
	rat spinal cord culture with THA (induced glutamate excitotoxicity)	decrease of lipid peroxidation	increased viability	[122]

Table 1. Cont.

Compound	Animal/Cell Line	Mechanism of Action	Outcome	Ref.
anthocyanin enriched strawberry extract	mice expressing SOD1^{G93A}	preservation of neuromuscular junctions, reduction in reactive astrocytes	delayed onset, increased survival	[127]
fisetin	NCS34 cell line expressing SOD1^{G93A}	antioxidant activity, activation of ERK pathway	increased viability	[128]
	Drosophila melanogaster expressing SOD1^{G85R}	antioxidant activity, activation of ERK pathway	increased survival, improved motor function	[128]
	mice expressing SOD1^{G93A}	antioxidant activity	delayed onset, increased survival, improved motor function	[128]
kaempferol	N2a cells expressing SOD1^{G85R}	reduction in mutant SOD1 aggregates, induction of autophagy (AMPK)	increased viability	[130]
quercetin	lymphoblast cell lines from ALS patients	reduction in ROS	not determined	[131]
	rats, aluminium-induced neurodegeneration	reduced oxidative stress, improved mitochondrial function	increased neuronal viability, inhibition of apoptosis	[134]
7,8-dihydroxyflavone	mice expressing SOD1^{G93A}	not determined, possibly as TrkB agonist	improved motor function, higher motor neuron count and density	[135]
genistein	mice expressing SOD1^{G93A}	not determined	delayed onset and increased survival in males	[136]
	mice expressing SOD1^{G93A}	anti-inflammatory, autophagy promotion	delayed onset and improved motor performance, increased survival in both sexes	[137]
protocatechuic acid	mice expressing SOD1^{G93A}	anti-inflammatory, preservation of neuromuscular junctions	increased survival, improved motor performance	[139]
caffeic acid phenethyl ester	NCS34 cell line expressing SOD1^{G93A}	reduced activation of NF-κB, activation of antioxidant response element	increased viability, reduction in ROS	[91]
	mice expressing SOD1^{G93A}	anti-inflammatory, anti-cell death signals	slower progression, increased survival	[140]
gallic acid	rats, aluminium- or quinolinic acid-induced neurodegeneration	antioxidant and anti-inflammatory activity, prevention of apoptosis, reduction in glutamate	improved motor function	[141, 142]
rosmarinic acid	mice expressing SOD1^{G93A}	not determined	increased survival, improved motor function, reduced weight loss	[143]
	mice expressing SOD1^{G93A}	antioxidant activity	increased survival, improved motor function	[144]
nordihydroguaiaretic acid	mice expressing SOD1^{G93A}	TNFα antagonist	increased survival, reduced weight loss	[145]

The importance of the gut–brain axis in ALS/FTD has been recognised. On the one hand, polyphenols may serve as prebiotics and alter the gut microbiota, affecting disease pathogenesis [146], (for a detailed review, see [147]). On the other hand, certain polyphenols such as EGCG are degraded by some gut microbiota, which reduces their bioavailability [148,149]. However, some metabolites do target the brain and have beneficial effects on neurons [118,150].

3. Conclusions

Polyphenols offer new possibilities for the development of therapies for ALS/FTD. However, more research is needed in this field, including strategies for effective targeting and delivery to the site of action. When evaluating the therapeutic potential of polyphenols, we must also consider their uptake in the gut, degradation by the microbiota, and the delivery to the brain. Therefore, it is important whether polyphenols are consumed or administered intravenously and how well they can cross the blood–brain barrier [151,152]. Another hurdle for potential ALS/FTD medication is translating findings from animal models into successful clinical trials. Additional aspect of potential variability in successful treatment lies in the use of purified polyphenols or plant extracts that may act synergistically. Most of the findings reviewed here come from various successful preclinical stages and have yet to be tested in humans. Nevertheless, polyphenols have the potential to improve the treatment of ALS/FTD, either through the development of new drugs or as dietary supplements.

Funding: This work was funded by Slovenian Research Agency grants (P4-0127, P1-0207, J3-9263, J3-8201, J7-9399 and N3-0141) and CRP-ICGEB research grant (CRP/SVN19-03).

Conflicts of Interest: The authors declare no conflict of interest.

References

1. Shah, H.; Albanese, E.; Duggan, C.; Rudan, I.; Langa, K.M.; Carrillo, M.C.; Chan, K.Y.; Joanette, Y.; Prince, M.; Rossor, M.; et al. Research priorities to reduce the global burden of dementia by 2025. *Lancet Neurol.* **2016**, *15*, 1285–1294. [CrossRef]
2. Petrov, D.; Mansfield, C.; Moussy, A.; Hermine, O. ALS clinical trials review: 20 years of failure. Are we any closer to registering a new treatment? *Front. Aging Neurosci.* **2017**, *9*, 1–11. [CrossRef]
3. Panza, F.; Lozupone, M.; Seripa, D.; Daniele, A.; Watling, M.; Giannelli, G.; Imbimbo, B.P. Development of disease-modifying drugs for frontotemporal dementia spectrum disorders. *Nat. Rev. Neurol.* **2020**, *16*, 213–228. [CrossRef]
4. Silva, R.F.M.; Pogačnik, L. Polyphenols from food and natural products: Neuroprotection and safety. *Antioxidants* **2020**, *9*, 61. [CrossRef] [PubMed]
5. Hardiman, O.; Al-Chalabi, A.; Chio, A.; Corr, E.M.; Logroscino, G.; Robberecht, W.; Shaw, P.J.; Simmons, Z.; Van Den Berg, L.H. Amyotrophic lateral sclerosis. *Nat. Rev. Dis. Prim.* **2017**, *3*, 17071. [CrossRef] [PubMed]
6. Longinetti, E.; Regodón Wallin, A.; Samuelsson, K.; Press, R.; Zachau, A.; Ronnevi, L.O.; Kierkegaard, M.; Andersen, P.M.; Hillert, J.; Fang, F.; et al. The Swedish motor neuron disease quality registry. *Amyotroph. Lateral Scler. Front. Degener.* **2018**, *19*, 528–537. [CrossRef]
7. Jun, K.Y.; Park, J.; Oh, K.W.; Kim, E.M.; Bae, J.S.; Kim, I.; Kim, S.H. Epidemiology of ALS in Korea using nationwide big data. *J. Neurol. Neurosurg. Psychiatry* **2019**, *90*, 395–403. [CrossRef]
8. Benjaminsen, E.; Alstadhaug, K.B.; Gulsvik, M.; Baloch, F.K.; Odeh, F. Amyotrophic lateral sclerosis in Nordland county, Norway, 2000–2015: Prevalence, incidence, and clinical features. *Amyotroph. Lateral Scler. Front. Degener.* **2018**, *19*, 522–527. [CrossRef]
9. Ryan, M.; Zaldívar Vaillant, T.; McLaughlin, R.L.; Doherty, M.A.; Rooney, J.; Heverin, M.; Gutierrez, J.; Lara-Fernández, G.E.; Pita Rodríguez, M.; Hackembruch, J.; et al. Comparison of the clinical and genetic features of amyotrophic lateral sclerosis across Cuban, Uruguayan and Irish clinic-based populations. *J. Neurol. Neurosurg. Psychiatry* **2019**, *90*, 659–665. [CrossRef] [PubMed]
10. Qadri, S.; Langefeld, C.D.; Milligan, C.; Caress, J.B.; Cartwright, M.S. Racial differences in intervention rates in individuals with ALS: A case-control study. *Neurology* **2019**, *92*, E1969–E1974. [CrossRef]
11. Marin, B.; Boumé diene, F.; Logroscino, G.; Couratier, P.; Babron, M.C.; Leutenegger, A.L.; Copetti, M.; Preux, P.M.; Beghi, E. Variation in world wide incidence of amyotrophic lateral sclerosis: A meta-analysis. *Int. J. Epidemiol.* **2017**, *46*, 57–74. [CrossRef]
12. Longinetti, E.; Fang, F. Epidemiology of amyotrophic lateral sclerosis: An update of recent literature. *Curr. Opin. Neurol.* **2019**, *32*, 771–776. [CrossRef]
13. van Es, M.A.; Hardiman, O.; Chio, A.; Al-Chalabi, A.; Pasterkamp, R.J.; Veldink, J.H.; van den Berg, L.H. Amyotrophic lateral sclerosis. *Lancet* **2017**, *390*, 2084–2098. [CrossRef]
14. Greaves, C.V.; Rohrer, J.D. An update on genetic frontotemporal dementia. *J. Neurol.* **2019**, *266*, 2075–2086. [CrossRef]
15. Couratier, P.; Corcia, P.; Lautrette, G.; Nicol, M.; Marin, B. ALS and frontotemporal dementia belong to a common disease spectrum. *Rev. Neurol. (Paris)* **2017**, *173*, 273–279. [CrossRef] [PubMed]
16. Coyle-Gilchrist, I.T.S.; Dick, K.M.; Patterson, K.; Rodríquez, P.V.; Wehmann, E.; Wilcox, A.; Lansdall, C.J.; Dawson, K.E.; Wiggins, J.; Mead, S.; et al. Prevalence, characteristics, and survival of frontotemporal lobar degeneration syndromes. *Neurology* **2016**, *86*, 1736–1743. [CrossRef] [PubMed]
17. Kansal, K.; Mareddy, M.; Sloane, K.L.; Minc, A.A.; Rabins, P.V.; McGready, J.B.; Onyike, C.U. Survival in Frontotemporal Dementia Phenotypes: A Meta-Analysis. *Dement. Geriatr. Cogn. Disord.* **2016**, *41*, 109–122. [CrossRef] [PubMed]

18. Goldman, J.S.; Farmer, J.M.; Wood, E.M.; Johnson, J.K.; Boxer, A.; Neuhaus, J.; Lomen-Hoerth, C.; Wilhelmsen, K.C.; Lee, V.M.Y.; Grossman, M.; et al. Comparison of family histories in FTLD subtypes and related tauopathies. *Neurology* **2005**, *65*, 1817–1819. [CrossRef]
19. Rohrer, J.D.; Guerreiro, R.; Vandrovcova, J.; Uphill, J.; Reiman, D.; Beck, J.; Isaacs, A.M.; Authier, A.; Ferrari, R.; Fox, N.C.; et al. The heritability and genetics of frontotemporal lobar degeneration. *Neurology* **2009**, *73*, 1451–1456. [CrossRef]
20. Neary, D.; Snowden, J.S.; Mann, D.M.A.; Northern, B.; Goulding, P.J.; Macdermott, N. Frontal lobe dementia and motor neuron disease. *J. Neurol. Neurosurg. Psychiatry* **1990**, *53*, 23–32. [CrossRef]
21. Mitsuyama, Y. Presenile dementia with motor neuron disease. *Dement. Geriatr. Cogn. Disord.* **1993**, *4*, 137–142. [CrossRef]
22. Ringholz, G.M.; Appel, S.H.; Bradshaw, M.; Cooke, N.A.; Mosnik, D.M.; Schulz, P.E. Prevalence and patterns of cognitive impairment in sporadic ALS. *Neurology* **2005**, *65*, 586–590. [CrossRef]
23. Wheaton, M.W.; Salamone, A.R.; Mosnik, D.M.; McDonald, R.O.; Appel, S.H.; Schmolck, H.I.; Ringholz, G.M.; Schulz, P.E. Cognitive impairment in familial ALS. *Neurology* **2007**, *69*, 1411–1417. [CrossRef] [PubMed]
24. Burrell, J.R.; Kiernan, M.C.; Vucic, S.; Hodges, J.R. Motor Neuron dysfunction in frontotemporal dementia. *Brain* **2011**, *134*, 2582–2594. [CrossRef] [PubMed]
25. Van Langenhove, T.; Piguet, O.; Burrell, J.R.; Leyton, C.; Foxe, D.; Abela, M.; Bartley, L.; Kim, W.S.; Jary, E.; Huang, Y.; et al. Predicting development of amyotrophic lateral sclerosis in frontotemporal dementia. *J. Alzheimer Dis.* **2017**, *58*, 163–170. [CrossRef]
26. Liscic, R.M.; Alberici, A.; Cairns, N.J.; Romano, M.; Buratti, E. From basic research to the clinic: Innovative therapies for ALS and FTD in the pipeline. *Mol. Neurodegener.* **2020**, *15*, 1–17. [CrossRef]
27. Gao, F.; Almeida, S.; Lopez-Gonzalez, R. Dysregulated molecular pathways in amyotrophic lateral sclerosis–frontotemporal dementia spectrum disorder. *EMBO J.* **2017**, *36*, 2931–2950. [CrossRef]
28. Ling, S.C.; Polymenidou, M.; Cleveland, D.W. Converging mechanisms in ALS and FTD: Disrupted RNA and protein homeostasis. *Neuron* **2013**, *79*, 416–438. [CrossRef] [PubMed]
29. Bampton, A.; Gittings, L.M.; Fratta, P.; Lashley, T.; Gatt, A. The role of hnRNPs in frontotemporal dementia and amyotrophic lateral sclerosis. *Acta Neuropathol.* **2020**, *140*, 599–623. [CrossRef]
30. Vance, C.; Rogelj, B.; Hortobágyi, T.; De Vos, K.J.; Nishimura, A.L.; Sreedharan, J.; Hu, X.; Smith, B.; Ruddy, D.; Wright, P.; et al. Mutations in FUS, an RNA processing protein, cause familial amyotrophic lateral sclerosis type 6. *Science* **2009**, *323*, 1208–1211. [CrossRef] [PubMed]
31. Sreedharan, J.; Blair, I.P.; Tripathi, V.B.; Hu, X.; Vance, C.; Rogelj, B.; Ackerley, S.; Durnall, J.C.; Williams, K.L.; Buratti, E.; et al. TDP-43 mutations in familial and sporadic amyotrophic lateral sclerosis. *Science* **2008**, *319*, 1668–1672. [CrossRef]
32. Webster, C.P.; Smith, E.F.; Bauer, C.S.; Moller, A.; Hautbergue, G.M.; Ferraiuolo, L.; Myszczynska, M.A.; Higginbottom, A.; Walsh, M.J.; Whitworth, A.J.; et al. The C9orf72 protein interacts with Rab1a and the ULK 1 complex to regulate initiation of autophagy. *EMBO J.* **2016**, *35*, 1656–1676. [CrossRef]
33. Goode, A.; Butler, K.; Long, J.; Cavey, J.; Scott, D.; Shaw, B.; Sollenberger, J.; Gell, C.; Johansen, T.; Oldham, N.J.; et al. Defective recognition of LC3B by mutant SQSTM1/p62 implicates impairment of autophagy as a pathogenic mechanism in ALS-FTLD. *Autophagy* **2016**, *12*, 1094–1104. [CrossRef] [PubMed]
34. Wong, Y.C.; Holzbaur, E.L.F. Optineurin is an autophagy receptor for damaged mitochondria in parkin-mediated mitophagy that is disrupted by an ALS-linked mutation. *Proc. Natl. Acad. Sci. USA* **2014**, *111*, E4439–E4448. [CrossRef]
35. Hortobágyi, T.; Troakes, C.; Nishimura, A.L.; Vance, C.; van Swieten, J.C.; Seelaar, H.; King, A.; Al-Sarraj, S.; Rogelj, B.; Shaw, C.E. Optineurin inclusions occur in a minority of TDP-43 positive ALS and FTLD-TDP cases and are rarely observed in other neurodegenerative disorders. *Acta Neuropathol.* **2011**, *121*, 519–527. [CrossRef] [PubMed]
36. Markovinovic, A.; Cimbro, R.; Ljutic, T.; Kriz, J.; Rogelj, B.; Munitic, I. Optineurin in amyotrophic lateral sclerosis: Multifunctional adaptor protein at the crossroads of different neuroprotective mechanisms. *Prog. Neurobiol.* **2017**, *154*, 1–20. [CrossRef] [PubMed]
37. Chua, J.P.; De Calbiac, H.; Kabashi, E.; Barmada, S.J. Autophagy and ALS: Mechanistic insights and therapeutic implications. *Autophagy* **2021**, 1–29. [CrossRef]
38. Buratti, E.; Baralle, F.E. Characterization and functional implications of the RNA binding properties of nuclear factor TDP-43, a novel splicing regulator of CFTR exon 9. *J. Biol. Chem.* **2001**, *276*, 36337–36343. [CrossRef]
39. Fallini, C.; Bassell, G.J.; Rossoll, W. The ALS disease protein TDP-43 is actively transported in motor neuron axons and regulates axon outgrowth. *Hum. Mol. Genet.* **2012**, *21*, 3703–3718. [CrossRef] [PubMed]
40. Butti, Z.; Patten, S.A. RNA dysregulation in amyotrophic lateral sclerosis. *Front. Genet.* **2019**, *10*, 1–18. [CrossRef]
41. Tollervey, J.R.; Curk, T.; Rogelj, B.; Briese, M.; Cereda, M.; Kayikci, M.; König, J.; Hortobágyi, T.; Nishimura, A.L.; Zupunski, V.; et al. Characterizing the RNA targets and position-dependent splicing regulation by TDP-43. *Nat. Neurosci.* **2011**, *14*, 452–458. [CrossRef]
42. Rogelj, B.; Easton, L.E.; Bogu, G.K.; Stanton, L.W.; Rot, G.; Curk, T.; Zupan, B.; Sugimoto, Y.; Modic, M.; Haberman, N.; et al. Widespread binding of FUS along nascent RNA regulates alternative splicing in the brain. *Sci. Rep.* **2012**, *2*, 603. [CrossRef] [PubMed]
43. Wang, X.; Arai, S.; Song, X.; Reichart, D.; Du, K.; Pascual, G.; Tempst, P.; Rosenfeld, M.G.; Glass, C.K.; Kurokawa, R. Induced ncRNAs allosterically modify RNA-binding proteins in cis to inhibit transcription. *Nature* **2008**, *454*, 126–130. [CrossRef] [PubMed]

44. Tan, A.Y.; Riley, T.R.; Coady, T.; Bussemaker, H.J.; Manley, J.L. TLS/FUS (translocated in liposarcoma/fused in sarcoma) regulates target gene transcription via single-stranded DNA response elements. *Proc. Natl. Acad. Sci. USA* **2012**, *109*, 6030–6035. [CrossRef] [PubMed]
45. Hoell, J.I.; Larsson, E.; Runge, S.; Nusbaum, J.D.; Duggimpudi, S.; Farazi, T.A.; Hafner, M.; Borkhardt, A.; Sander, C.; Tuschl, T. RNA targets of wild-type and mutant FET family proteins. *Nat. Struct. Mol. Biol.* **2011**, *18*, 1428–1431. [CrossRef] [PubMed]
46. Ishigaki, S.; Masuda, A.; Fujioka, Y.; Iguchi, Y.; Katsuno, M.; Shibata, A.; Urano, F.; Sobue, G.; Ohno, K. Position-dependent FUS-RNA interactions regulate alternative splicing events and transcriptions. *Sci. Rep.* **2012**, *2*, 1–8. [CrossRef] [PubMed]
47. Wang, W.Y.; Pan, L.; Su, S.C.; Quinn, E.J.; Sasaki, M.; Jimenez, J.C.; MacKenzie, I.R.A.; Huang, E.J.; Tsai, L.H. Interaction of FUS and HDAC1 regulates DNA damage response and repair in neurons. *Nat. Neurosci.* **2013**, *16*, 1383–1391. [CrossRef]
48. Webber, C.J.; Lei, S.E.; Wolozin, B. The pathophysiology of neurodegenerative disease: Disturbing the balance between phase separation and irreversible aggregation. *Prog. Mol. Biol. Transl. Sci.* **2020**, *174*, 187–223. [CrossRef]
49. Modic, M.; Grosch, M.; Rot, G.; Schirge, S.; Lepko, T.; Yamazaki, T.; Lee, F.C.Y.; Rusha, E.; Shaposhnikov, D.; Palo, M.; et al. Cross-Regulation between TDP-43 and Paraspeckles Promotes Pluripotency-Differentiation Transition. *Mol. Cell* **2019**, *74*, 951–965.e13. [CrossRef]
50. Prpar Mihevc, S.; Darovic, S.; Kovanda, A.; Bajc Česnik, A.; Županjski, V.; Rogelj, B. Nuclear trafficking in amyotrophic lateral sclerosis and frontotemporal lobar degeneration. *Brain* **2017**, *140*, 13–26. [CrossRef]
51. Pasha, T.; Zatorska, A.; Sharipov, D.; Rogelj, B.; Hortobágyi, T.; Hirth, F. Karyopherin abnormalities in neurodegenerative proteinopathies. *Brain* **2021**. [CrossRef] [PubMed]
52. Cicardi, M.E.; Marrone, L.; Azzouz, M.; Trotti, D. Proteostatic imbalance and protein spreading in amyotrophic lateral sclerosis. *EMBO J.* **2021**, *40*, e106389. [CrossRef]
53. Vance, C.; Scotter, E.L.; Nishimura, A.L.; Troakes, C.; Mitchell, J.C.; Kathe, C.; Urwin, H.; Manser, C.; Miller, C.C.; Hortobágyi, T.; et al. ALS mutant FUS disrupts nuclear localization and sequesters wild-type FUS within cytoplasmic stress granules. *Hum. Mol. Genet.* **2013**, *22*, 2676–2688. [CrossRef] [PubMed]
54. Portz, B.; Lee, B.L.; Shorter, J. FUS and TDP-43 Phases in Health and Disease. *Trends Biochem. Sci.* **2021**, *46*, 550–563. [CrossRef] [PubMed]
55. Renton, A.E.; Majounie, E.; Waite, A.; Simón-Sánchez, J.; Rollinson, S.; Gibbs, J.R.; Schymick, J.C.; Laaksovirta, H.; van Swieten, J.C.; Myllykangas, L.; et al. A hexanucleotide repeat expansion in C9ORF72 is the cause of chromosome 9p21-linked ALS-FTD. *Neuron* **2011**, *72*, 257–268. [CrossRef]
56. DeJesus-Hernandez, M.; Mackenzie, I.R.; Boeve, B.F.; Boxer, A.L.; Baker, M.; Rutherford, N.J.; Nicholson, A.M.; Finch, N.A.; Flynn, H.; Adamson, J.; et al. Expanded GGGGCC hexanucleotide repeat in noncoding region of C9ORF72 causes chromosome 9p-linked FTD and ALS. *Neuron* **2011**, *72*, 245–256. [CrossRef]
57. Smith, B.N.; Newhouse, S.; Shatunov, A.; Vance, C.; Topp, S.; Johnson, L.; Miller, J.; Lee, Y.; Troakes, C.; Scott, K.M.; et al. The C9ORF72 expansion mutation is a common cause of ALS+/−FTD in Europe and has a single founder. *Eur. J. Hum. Genet.* **2013**, *21*, 102–108. [CrossRef]
58. Malnar, M.; Rogelj, B. SFPQ regulates the accumulation of RNA foci and dipeptide repeat proteins from the expanded repeat mutation in C9orf72. *J. Cell Sci.* **2021**, *134*. [CrossRef]
59. Božič, T.; Zalar, M.; Rogelj, B.; Plavec, J.; Šket, P. Structural Diversity of Sense and Antisense RNA Hexanucleotide Repeats Associated with ALS and FTLD. *Molecules* **2020**, *25*, 525. [CrossRef]
60. Bajc Česnik, A.; Darovic, S.; Prpar Mihevc, S.; Štalekar, M.; Malnar, M.; Motaln, H.; Lee, Y.-B.; Mazej, J.; Pohleven, J.; Grosch, M.; et al. Nuclear RNA foci from C9ORF72 expansion mutation form paraspeckle-like bodies. *J. Cell Sci.* **2019**, *132*. [CrossRef]
61. Solomon, D.A.; Stepto, A.; Au, W.H.; Adachi, Y.; Diaper, D.C.; Hall, R.; Rekhi, A.; Boudi, A.; Tziortzouda, P.; Lee, Y.-B.; et al. A feedback loop between dipeptide-repeat protein, TDP-43 and karyopherin-α mediates C9orf72-related neurodegeneration. *Brain* **2018**, *141*, 2908–2924. [CrossRef]
62. Lee, Y.-B.; Baskaran, P.; Gomez-Deza, J.; Chen, H.-J.; Nishimura, A.L.; Smith, B.N.; Troakes, C.; Adachi, Y.; Stepto, A.; Petrucelli, L.; et al. C9orf72 poly GA RAN-translated protein plays a key role in amyotrophic lateral sclerosis via aggregation and toxicity. *Hum. Mol. Genet.* **2017**, *26*, 4765–4777. [CrossRef]
63. Kovanda, A.; Zalar, M.; Šket, P.; Plavec, J.; Rogelj, B. Anti-sense DNA d(GGCCCC)n expansions in C9ORF72 form i-motifs and protonated hairpins. *Sci. Rep.* **2015**, *5*, 17944. [CrossRef]
64. Šket, P.; Pohleven, J.; Kovanda, A.; Štalekar, M.; Županski, V.; Zalar, M.; Plavec, J.; Rogelj, B. Characterization of DNA G-quadruplex species forming from C9ORF72 G4C2-expanded repeats associated with amyotrophic lateral sclerosis and frontotemporal lobar degeneration. *Neurobiol. Aging* **2015**, *36*, 1091–1096. [CrossRef]
65. Vatovec, S.; Kovanda, A.; Rogelj, B. Unconventional features of C9ORF72 expanded repeat in amyotrophic lateral sclerosis and frontotemporal lobar degeneration. *Neurobiol. Aging* **2014**, *35*, 2421.e1–2421.e12. [CrossRef]
66. Smith, E.F.; Shaw, P.J.; De Vos, K.J. The role of mitochondria in amyotrophic lateral sclerosis. *Neurosci. Lett.* **2019**, *710*, 132933. [CrossRef]
67. Wang, W.; Li, L.; Lin, W.L.; Dickson, D.W.; Petrucelli, L.; Zhang, T.; Wang, X. The ALS disease-associated mutant TDP-43 impairs mitochondrial dynamics and function in motor neurons. *Hum. Mol. Genet.* **2013**, *22*, 4706–4719. [CrossRef] [PubMed]

68. Magrané, J.; Cortez, C.; Gan, W.-B.; Manfredi, G. Abnormal mitochondrial transport and morphology are common pathological denominators in SOD1 and TDP43 ALS mouse models. *Hum. Mol. Genet.* **2014**, *23*, 1413–1424. [CrossRef] [PubMed]
69. Higgins, C.M.J.; Jung, C.; Xu, Z. ALS-associated mutant SODIG93A causes mitochondrial vacuolation by expansion of the intermembrane space by involvement of SODI aggregation and peroxisomes. *BMC Neurosci.* **2003**, *4*, 1–14. [CrossRef] [PubMed]
70. Deng, J.; Yang, M.; Chen, Y.; Chen, X.; Liu, J.; Sun, S.; Cheng, H.; Li, Y.; Bigio, E.H.; Mesulam, M.; et al. FUS interacts with HSP60 to promote mitochondrial damage. *PLoS Genet.* **2015**, *11*, e1005357. [CrossRef] [PubMed]
71. Magrané, J.; Hervias, I.; Henning, M.S.; Damiano, M.; Kawamata, H.; Manfredi, G. Mutant SOD1 in neuronal mitochondria causes toxicity and mitochondrial dynamics abnormalities. *Hum. Mol. Genet.* **2009**, *18*, 4552–4564. [CrossRef]
72. Cozzolino, M.; Pesaresi, M.G.; Amori, I.; Crosio, C.; Ferri, A.; Nencini, M.; Carrì, M.T. Oligomerization of mutant SOD1 in mitochondria of motoneuronal cells drives mitochondrial damage and cell toxicity. *Antioxid. Redox Signal.* **2009**, *11*, 1547–1558. [CrossRef] [PubMed]
73. Igoudjil, A.; Magrané, J.; Fischer, L.R.; Kim, H.J.; Hervias, I.; Dumont, M.; Cortez, C.; Glass, J.D.; Starkov, A.A.; Manfredi, G. In vivo pathogenic role of mutant SOD1 localized in the mitochondrial intermembrane space. *J. Neurosci.* **2011**, *31*, 15826–15837. [CrossRef]
74. Bogdanov, M.; Brown, R.H.; Matson, W.; Smart, R.; Hayden, D.; O'Donnell, H.; Flint Beal, M.; Cudkowicz, M. Increased oxidative damage to DNA in ALS patients. *Free Radic. Biol. Med.* **2000**, *29*, 652–658. [CrossRef]
75. Simpson, E.P.; Henry, Y.K.; Henkel, J.S.; Smith, R.G.; Appel, S.H. Increased lipid peroxidation in sera of ALS patients: A potential biomarker of disease burden. *Neurology* **2004**, *62*, 1758–1765. [CrossRef]
76. Mitsumoto, H.; Santella, R.; Liu, X.; Bogdanov, M.; Zipprich, J.; Wu, H.C.; Mahata, J.; Kilty, M.; Bednarz, K.; Bell, D.; et al. Oxidative stress biomarkers in sporadic ALS. *Amyotroph. Lateral Scler.* **2008**, *9*, 177–183. [CrossRef]
77. Bensimon, G.; Lacomblez, L.; Meininger, V. A controlled trial of riluzole in amyotrophic lateral sclerosis. *N. Engl. J. Med.* **1994**, *330*, 585–591. [CrossRef] [PubMed]
78. Lacomblez, L.; Bensimon, G.; Leigh, P.N.; Guillet, P.; Meininger, V. Dose-ranging study of riluzole in amyotrophic lateral sclerosis. *Lancet* **1996**, *347*, 1425–1431. [CrossRef]
79. Cheah, B.C.; Vucic, S.; Krishnan, A.; Kiernan, M.C. Riluzole, neuroprotection and amyotrophic lateral sclerosis. *Curr. Med. Chem.* **2010**, *17*, 1942–1959. [CrossRef]
80. Abe, K.; Aoki, M.; Tsuji, S.; Itoyama, Y.; Sobue, G.; Togo, M.; Hamada, C.; Tanaka, M.; Akimoto, M.; Nakamura, K.; et al. Safety and efficacy of edaravone in well defined patients with amyotrophic lateral sclerosis: A randomised, double-blind, placebo-controlled trial. *Lancet Neurol.* **2017**, *16*, 505–512. [CrossRef]
81. Jaiswal, M.K. Riluzole and edaravone: A tale of two amyotrophic lateral sclerosis drugs. *Med. Res. Rev.* **2019**, *39*, 733–748. [CrossRef]
82. Hodges, J.R.; Piguet, O. Progress and challenges in frontotemporal dementia research: A 20-year review. *J. Alzheimer Dis.* **2018**, *62*, 1467–1480. [CrossRef] [PubMed]
83. Swallah, M.S.; Sun, H.; Affoh, R.; Fu, H.; Yu, H. Antioxidant Potential Overviews of Secondary Metabolites (Polyphenols) in Fruits. *Int. J. Food Sci.* **2020**, *2020*, 1–8. [CrossRef] [PubMed]
84. Rambaran, T.F. Nanopolyphenols: A review of their encapsulation and anti-diabetic effects. *SN Appl. Sci.* **2020**, *2*, 1–26. [CrossRef]
85. Yang, B.; Dong, Y.; Wang, F.; Zhang, Y. Nanoformulations to enhance the bioavailability and physiological functions of polyphenols. *Molecules* **2020**, *25*, 4613. [CrossRef] [PubMed]
86. Tsao, R. Chemistry and biochemistry of dietary polyphenols. *Nutrients* **2010**, *2*, 1231–1246. [CrossRef]
87. Solanki, I.; Parihar, P.; Mansuri, M.L.; Parihar, M.S. Flavonoid-based therapies in the early management of neurodegenerative diseases. *Adv. Nutr.* **2015**, *6*, 64–72. [CrossRef]
88. Tian, B.; Liu, J. Resveratrol: A review of plant sources, synthesis, stability, modification and food application. *J. Sci. Food Agric.* **2020**, *100*, 1392–1404. [CrossRef]
89. Tellone, E.; Galtieri, A.; Russo, A.; Giardina, B.; Ficarra, S. Resveratrol: A focus on several neurodegenerative diseases. *Oxid. Med. Cell. Longev.* **2015**, *2015*. [CrossRef]
90. Kim, D.; Nguyen, M.D.; Dobbin, M.M.; Fischer, A.; Sananbenesi, F.; Rodgers, J.T.; Delalle, I.; Baur, J.A.; Sui, G.; Armour, S.M.; et al. SIRT1 deacetylase protects against neurodegeneration in models for Alzheimer's disease and amyotrophic lateral sclerosis. *EMBO J.* **2007**, *26*, 3169–3179. [CrossRef]
91. Barber, S.C.; Higginbottom, A.; Mead, R.J.; Barber, S.; Shaw, P.J. An in vitro screening cascade to identify neuroprotective antioxidants in ALS. *Free Radic. Biol. Med.* **2009**, *46*, 1127–1138. [CrossRef]
92. Wang, J.; Zhang, Y.; Tang, L.; Zhang, N.; Fan, D. Protective effects of resveratrol through the up-regulation of SIRT1 expression in the mutant hSOD1-G93A-bearing motor neuron-like cell culture model of amyotrophic lateral sclerosis. *Neurosci. Lett.* **2011**, *503*, 250–255. [CrossRef] [PubMed]
93. Yáñez, M.; Galán, L.; Matías-Guiu, J.; Vela, A.; Guerrero, A.; García, A.G. CSF from amyotrophic lateral sclerosis patients produces glutamate independent death of rat motor brain cortical neurons: Protection by resveratrol but not riluzole. *Brain Res.* **2011**, *1423*, 77–86. [CrossRef] [PubMed]
94. Markert, C.D.; Kim, E.; Gifondorwa, D.J.; Childers, M.K.; Milligan, C.E. A single-dose resveratrol treatment in a mouse model of amyotrophic lateral sclerosis. *J. Med. Food* **2010**, *13*, 1081–1085. [CrossRef] [PubMed]

95. Han, S.; Choi, J.R.; Soon Shin, K.; Kang, S.J. Resveratrol upregulated heat shock proteins and extended the survival of G93A-SOD1 mice. *Brain Res.* **2012**, *1483*, 112–117. [CrossRef]
96. Mancuso, R.; del Valle, J.; Modol, L.; Martinez, A.; Granado-Serrano, A.B.; Ramirez-Núñez, O.; Pallás, M.; Portero-Otin, M.; Osta, R.; Navarro, X. Resveratrol improves motoneuron function and extends survival in SOD1G93A ALS Mice. *Neurotherapeutics* **2014**, *11*, 419–432. [CrossRef]
97. Mancuso, R.; Del Valle, J.; Morell, M.; Pallás, M.; Osta, R.; Navarro, X. Lack of synergistic effect of resveratrol and sigma-1 receptor agonist (PRE-084) in SOD1G93A ALS mice: Overlapping effects or limited therapeutic opportunity? *Orphanet J. Rare Dis.* **2014**, *9*, 1–11. [CrossRef]
98. Schiaffino, L.; Bonafede, R.; Scambi, I.; Parrella, E.; Pizzi, M.; Mariotti, R. Acetylation state of RelA modulated by epigenetic drugs prolongs survival and induces a neuroprotective effect on ALS murine model. *Sci. Rep.* **2018**, *8*, 1–13. [CrossRef]
99. Yu, K.C.; Kwan, P.; Cheung, S.K.K.; Ho, A.; Baum, L. Effects of resveratrol and morin on insoluble tau in tau transgenic mice. *Transl. Neurosci.* **2018**, *9*, 54–60. [CrossRef]
100. Laudati, G.; Mascolo, L.; Guida, N.; Sirabella, R.; Pizzorusso, V.; Bruzzaniti, S.; Serani, A.; Di Renzo, G.; Canzoniero, L.M.T.; Formisano, L. Resveratrol treatment reduces the vulnerability of SH-SY5Y cells and cortical neurons overexpressing SOD1-G93A to Thimerosal toxicity through SIRT1/DREAM/PDYN pathway. *Neurotoxicology* **2019**, *71*, 6–15. [CrossRef]
101. Cao, D.; Wang, M.; Qiu, X.; Liu, D.; Jiang, H.; Yang, N.; Xu, R.M. Structural basis for allosteric, substratedependent stimulation of SIRT1 activity by resveratrol. *Genes Dev.* **2015**, *29*, 1316–1325. [CrossRef] [PubMed]
102. Ranganathan, S.; Bowser, R. p53 and cell cycle proteins participate in spinal motor neuron cell death in ALS. *Open Pathol. J.* **2010**, *4*, 11–22. [CrossRef] [PubMed]
103. Yun, Y.C.; Jeong, S.G.; Kim, S.H.; Cho, G.W. Reduced sirtuin 1/adenosine monophosphate-activated protein kinase in amyotrophic lateral sclerosis patient-derived mesenchymal stem cells can be restored by resveratrol. *J. Tissue Eng. Regen. Med.* **2019**, *13*, 110–115. [CrossRef] [PubMed]
104. Dasgupta, B.; Milbrandt, J. Resveratrol stimulates AMP kinase activity in neurons. *Proc. Natl. Acad. Sci. USA* **2007**, *104*, 7217–7222. [CrossRef]
105. Srinivasan, E.; Rajasekaran, R. Quantum chemical and molecular mechanics studies on the assessment of interactions between resveratrol and mutant SOD1 (G93A) protein. *J. Comput. Aided Mol. Des.* **2018**, *32*, 1347–1361. [CrossRef]
106. Zhuang, X.; Li, X.; Zhao, B.; Liu, Z.; Song, F.; Lu, J. Native mass spectrometry based method for studying the interactions between superoxide dismutase 1 and stilbenoids. *ACS Chem. Neurosci.* **2020**, *11*, 184–190. [CrossRef]
107. Adami, R.; Bottai, D. Curcumin and neurological diseases. *Nutr. Neurosci.* **2020**, 1–21. [CrossRef]
108. Soo, S.K.; Rudich, P.D.; Traa, A.; Harris-Gauthier, N.; Shields, H.J.; Van Raamsdonk, J.M. Compounds that extend longevity are protective in neurodegenerative diseases and provide a novel treatment strategy for these devastating disorders. *Mech. Ageing Dev.* **2020**, *190*, 111297. [CrossRef]
109. Bhatia, N.K.; Srivastava, A.; Katyal, N.; Jain, N.; Khan, M.A.I.; Kundu, B.; Deep, S. Curcumin binds to the pre-fibrillar aggregates of Cu/Zn superoxide dismutase (SOD1) and alters its amyloidogenic pathway resulting in reduced cytotoxicity. *Biochim. Biophys. Acta Proteins Proteom.* **2015**, *1854*, 426–436. [CrossRef]
110. Rane, J.S.; Bhaumik, P.; Panda, D. Curcumin inhibits tau aggregation and disintegrates preformed tau filaments in vitro. *J. Alzheimer's Dis.* **2017**, *60*, 999–1014. [CrossRef]
111. den Haan, J.; Morrema, T.H.J.; Rozemuller, A.J.; Bouwman, F.H.; Hoozemans, J.J.M. Different curcumin forms selectively bind fibrillar amyloid beta in post mortem Alzheimer's disease brains: Implications for in-vivo diagnostics. *Acta Neuropathol. Commun.* **2018**, *6*, 75. [CrossRef]
112. Ma, Z.; Wang, N.; He, H.; Tang, X. Pharmaceutical strategies of improving oral systemic bioavailability of curcumin for clinical application. *J. Control. Release* **2019**, *316*, 359–380. [CrossRef]
113. Lu, J.; Duan, W.; Guo, Y.; Jiang, H.; Li, Z.; Huang, J.; Hong, K.; Li, C. Mitochondrial dysfunction in human TDP-43 transfected NSC34 cell lines and the protective effect of dimethoxy curcumin. *Brain Res. Bull.* **2012**, *89*, 185–190. [CrossRef] [PubMed]
114. Dong, H.; Xu, L.; Wu, L.; Wang, X.; Duan, W.; Li, H.; Li, C. Curcumin abolishes mutant TDP-43 induced excitability in a motoneuron-like cellular model of ALS. *Neuroscience* **2014**, *272*, 141–153. [CrossRef] [PubMed]
115. Duan, W.; Guo, Y.; Xiao, J.; Chen, X.; Li, Z.; Han, H.; Li, C. Neuroprotection by monocarbonyl dimethoxycurcumin C: Ameliorating the toxicity of mutant TDP-43 via HO-1. *Mol. Neurobiol.* **2014**, *49*, 368–379. [CrossRef] [PubMed]
116. Tripodo, G.; Chlapanidas, T.; Perteghella, S.; Vigani, B.; Mandracchia, D.; Trapani, A.; Galuzzi, M.; Tosca, M.C.; Antonioli, B.; Gaetani, P.; et al. Mesenchymal stromal cells loading curcumin-INVITE-micelles: A drug delivery system for neurodegenerative diseases. *Colloids Surf. B Biointerfaces* **2015**, *125*, 300–308. [CrossRef]
117. Ahmadi, M.; Agah, E.; Nafissi, S.; Jaafari, M.R.; Harirchian, M.H.; Sarraf, P.; Faghihi-Kashani, S.; Hosseini, S.J.; Ghoreishi, A.; Aghamollaii, V.; et al. Safety and efficacy of nanocurcumin as add-on therapy to riluzole in patients with amyotrophic lateral sclerosis: A pilot randomized clinical trial. *Neurotherapeutics* **2018**, *15*, 430–438. [CrossRef]
118. Pervin, M.; Unno, K.; Takagaki, A.; Isemura, M.; Nakamura, Y. Function of green tea catechins in the brain: Epigallocatechin gallate and its metabolites. *Int. J. Mol. Sci.* **2019**, *20*, 3630. [CrossRef]
119. Koh, S.H.; Kwon, H.; Kim, K.S.; Kim, J.; Kim, M.H.; Yu, H.J.; Kim, M.; Lee, K.W.; Do, B.R.; Jung, H.K.; et al. Epigallocatechin gallate prevents oxidative-stress-induced death of mutant Cu/Zn-superoxide dismutase (G93A) motoneuron cells by alteration of cell survival and death signals. *Toxicology* **2004**, *202*, 213–225. [CrossRef]

120. Koh, S.H.; Lee, S.M.; Kim, H.Y.; Lee, K.Y.; Lee, Y.J.; Kim, H.T.; Kim, J.; Kim, M.H.; Hwang, M.S.; Song, C.; et al. The effect of epigallocatechin gallate on suppressing disease progression of ALS model mice. *Neurosci. Lett.* **2006**, *395*, 103–107. [CrossRef]
121. Xu, Z.; Chen, S.; Li, X.; Luo, G.; Li, L.; Le, W. Neuroprotective effects of (-)-epigallocatechin-3-gallate in a transgenic mouse model of amyotrophic lateral sclerosis. *Neurochem. Res.* **2006**, *31*, 1263–1269. [CrossRef]
122. Che, F.; Wang, G.; Yu, J.; Wang, X.; Lu, Y.; Fu, Q.; Su, Q.; Jiang, J.; Du, Y. Effects of epigallocatechin-3-gallate on iron metabolismin spinal cord motor neurons. *Mol. Med. Rep.* **2017**, *16*, 3010–3014. [CrossRef]
123. Srinivasan, E.; Rajasekaran, R. Probing the inhibitory activity of epigallocatechin-gallate on toxic aggregates of mutant (L84F) SOD1 protein through geometry based sampling and steered molecular dynamics. *J. Mol. Graph. Model.* **2017**, *74*, 288–295. [CrossRef] [PubMed]
124. Zhao, B.; Zhuang, X.; Pi, Z.; Liu, S.; Liu, Z.; Song, F. Determining the effect of catechins on SOD1 conformation and aggregation by ion mobility mass spectrometry combined with optical spectroscopy. *J. Am. Soc. Mass Spectrom.* **2018**, *29*, 734–741. [CrossRef] [PubMed]
125. Wang, I.F.; Chang, H.Y.; Hou, S.C.; Liou, G.G.; Der Way, T.; James Shen, C.K. The self-interaction of native TDP-43 C terminus inhibits its degradation and contributes to early proteinopathies. *Nat. Commun.* **2012**, *3*. [CrossRef] [PubMed]
126. Taniguchi, S.; Suzuki, N.; Masuda, M.; Hisanaga, S.I.; Iwatsubo, T.; Goedert, M.; Hasegawa, M. Inhibition of heparin-induced tau filament formation by phenothiazines, polyphenols, and porphyrins. *J. Biol. Chem.* **2005**, *280*, 7614–7623. [CrossRef]
127. Winter, A.N.; Ross, E.K.; Wilkins, H.M.; Stankiewicz, T.R.; Wallace, T.; Miller, K.; Linseman, D.A. An anthocyanin-enriched extract from strawberries delays disease onset and extends survival in the hSOD1G93A mouse model of amyotrophic lateral sclerosis. *Nutr. Neurosci.* **2018**, *21*, 414–426. [CrossRef] [PubMed]
128. Wang, T.H.; Wang, S.Y.; Wang, X.D.; Jiang, H.Q.; Yang, Y.Q.; Wang, Y.; Cheng, J.L.; Zhang, C.T.; Liang, W.W.; Feng, H.L. Fisetin exerts antioxidant and neuroprotective effects in multiple mutant hSOD1 models of amyotrophic lateral sclerosis by activating ERK. *Neuroscience* **2018**, *379*, 152–166. [CrossRef] [PubMed]
129. Srinivasan, E.; Rajasekaran, R. Comparative binding of kaempferol and kaempferide on inhibiting the aggregate formation of mutant (G85R) SOD1 protein in familial amyotrophic lateral sclerosis: A quantum chemical and molecular mechanics study. *BioFactors* **2018**, *44*, 431–442. [CrossRef] [PubMed]
130. Ueda, T.; Inden, M.; Shirai, K.; Sekine, S.I.; Masaki, Y.; Kurita, H.; Ichihara, K.; Inuzuka, T.; Hozumi, I. The effects of Brazilian green propolis that contains flavonols against mutant copper-zinc superoxide dismutase-mediated toxicity. *Sci. Rep.* **2017**, *7*, 1–11. [CrossRef]
131. Said Ahmed, M.; Hung, W.Y.; Zu, J.S.; Hockberger, P.; Siddique, T. Increased reactive oxygen species in familial amyotrophic lateral sclerosis with mutations in SOD1. *J. Neurol. Sci.* **2000**, *176*, 88–94. [CrossRef]
132. Ip, P.; Sharda, P.R.; Cunningham, A.; Chakrabartty, S.; Pande, V.; Chakrabartty, A. Quercitrin and quercetin 3-β-d-glucoside as chemical chaperones for the A4V SOD1 ALS-causing mutant. *Protein Eng. Des. Sel.* **2017**, *30*, 431–440. [CrossRef]
133. Bhatia, N.K.; Modi, P.; Sharma, S.; Deep, S. Quercetin and baicalein act as potent antiamyloidogenic and fibril destabilizing agents for SOD1 fibrils. *ACS Chem. Neurosci.* **2020**, *11*, 1129–1138. [CrossRef] [PubMed]
134. Sharma, D.R.; Wani, W.Y.; Sunkaria, A.; Kandimalla, R.J.; Sharma, R.K.; Verma, D.; Bal, A.; Gill, K.D. Quercetin attenuates neuronal death against aluminum-induced neurodegeneration in the rat hippocampus. *Neuroscience* **2016**, *324*, 163–176. [CrossRef]
135. Korkmaz, O.T.; Aytan, N.; Carreras, I.; Choi, J.K.; Kowall, N.W.; Jenkins, B.G.; Dedeoglu, A. 7,8-Dihydroxyflavone improves motor performance and enhances lower motor neuronal survival in a mouse model of amyotrophic lateral sclerosis. *Neurosci. Lett.* **2014**, *566*, 286–291. [CrossRef] [PubMed]
136. Trieu, V.N.; Uckun, F.M. Genistein is neuroprotective in murine models of familial amyotrophic lateral sclerosis and stroke. *Biochem. Biophys. Res. Commun.* **1999**, *258*, 685–688. [CrossRef] [PubMed]
137. Zhao, Z.; Fu, J.; Li, S.; Li, Z. Neuroprotective effects of genistein in a SOD1-G93A transgenic mouse model of amyotrophic lateral sclerosis. *J. Neuroimmune Pharmacol.* **2019**, *14*, 688–696. [CrossRef]
138. Assogna, M.; Casula, E.P.; Borghi, I.; Bonnì, S.; Samà, D.; Motta, C.; Di Lorenzo, F.; D'Acunto, A.; Porrazzini, F.; Minei, M.; et al. Effects of palmitoylethanolamide combined with luteoline on frontal lobe functions, high frequency oscillations, and GABAergic transmission in patients with frontotemporal dementia. *J. Alzheimer Dis.* **2020**, *76*, 1297–1308. [CrossRef]
139. Koza, L.A.; Winter, A.N.; Holsopple, J.; Baybayon-Grandgeorge, A.N.; Pena, C.; Olson, J.R.; Mazzarino, R.C.; Patterson, D.; Linseman, D.A. Protocatechuic acid extends survival, improves motor function, diminishes gliosis, and sustains neuromuscular junctions in the hSOD1G93A mouse model of amyotrophic lateral sclerosis. *Nutrients* **2020**, *12*, 1824. [CrossRef]
140. Fontanilla, C.V.; Wei, X.; Zhao, L.; Johnstone, B.; Pascuzzi, R.M.; Farlow, M.R.; Du, Y. Caffeic acid phenethyl ester extends survival of a mouse model of amyotrophic lateral sclerosis. *Neuroscience* **2012**, *205*, 185–193. [CrossRef]
141. Maya, S.; Prakash, T.; Goli, D. Evaluation of neuroprotective effects of wedelolactone and gallic acid on aluminium-induced neurodegeneration: Relevance to sporadic amyotrophic lateral sclerosis. *Eur. J. Pharmacol.* **2018**, *835*, 41–51. [CrossRef] [PubMed]
142. Maya, S.; Prakash, T.; Goli, D. Effect of wedelolactone and gallic acid on quinolinic acid-induced neurotoxicity and impaired motor function: Significance to sporadic amyotrophic lateral sclerosis. *Neurotoxicology* **2018**, *68*, 1–12. [CrossRef]
143. Shimojo, Y.; Kosaka, K.; Noda, Y.; Shimizu, T.; Shirasawa, T. Effect of rosmarinic acid in motor dysfunction and life span in a mouse model of familial amyotrophic lateral sclerosis. *J. Neurosci. Res.* **2010**, *88*, 896–904. [CrossRef]
144. Seo, J.-S.; Choi, J.; Leem, Y.-H.; Han, P.-L. Rosmarinic acid alleviates neurological symptoms in the G93A-SOD1 transgenic mouse model of amyotrophic lateral sclerosis. *Exp. Neurobiol.* **2015**, *24*, 341–350. [CrossRef]

145. West, M.; Mhatre, M.; Ceballos, A.; Floyd, R.A.; Grammas, P.; Gabbita, S.P.; Hamdheydari, L.; Mai, T.; Mou, S.; Pye, Q.N.; et al. The arachidonic acid 5-lipoxygenase inhibitor nordihydroguaiaretic acid inhibits tumor necrosis factor α activation of microglia and extends survival of G93A-SOD1 transgenic mice. *J. Neurochem.* **2004**, *91*, 133–143. [CrossRef]
146. Blacher, E.; Bashiardes, S.; Shapiro, H.; Rothschild, D.; Mor, U.; Dori-Bachash, M.; Kleimeyer, C.; Moresi, C.; Harnik, Y.; Zur, M.; et al. Potential Roles of Gut Microbiome and Metabolites in Modulating ALS in Mice. *Nature* **2019**, *572*, 474–480. [CrossRef]
147. Casani-Cubel, J.; Benlloch, M.; Sanchis-Sanchis, C.E.; Marin, R.; Lajara-Romance, J.M.; de la Rubia Orti, J.E. The impact of microbiota on the pathogenesis of amyotrophic lateral sclerosis and the possible benefits of polyphenols. An overview. *Metabolites* **2021**, *11*, 120. [CrossRef] [PubMed]
148. Unno, T.; Takeo, T. Absorption of (−)-epigallocatechin gallate into the circulation system of rats. *Biosci. Biotechnol. Biochem.* **1995**, *59*, 1558–1559. [CrossRef] [PubMed]
149. Liu, A.B.; Tao, S.; Lee, M.-J.; Hu, Q.; Meng, X.; Lin, Y.; Yang, C.S. Effects of gut microbiota and time of treatment on tissue levels of green tea polyphenols in mice. *BioFactors* **2018**, *44*, 348–360. [CrossRef] [PubMed]
150. Gasperotti, M.; Passamonti, S.; Tramer, F.; Masuero, D.; Guella, G.; Mattivi, F.; Vrhovsek, U. Fate of microbial metabolites of dietary polyphenols in rats: Is the brain their target destination? *ACS Chem. Neurosci.* **2015**, *6*, 1341–1352. [CrossRef] [PubMed]
151. Pogačnik, L.; Pirc, K.; Palmela, I.; Skrt, M.; Kim, K.S.; Brites, D.; Brito, M.A.; Ulrih, N.P.; Silva, R.F.M. Potential for brain accessibility and analysis of stability of selected flavonoids in relation to neuroprotection in vitro. *Brain Res.* **2016**, *1651*, 17–26. [CrossRef] [PubMed]
152. Pervin, M.; Unno, K.; Nakagawa, A.; Takahashi, Y.; Iguchi, K.; Yamamoto, H.; Hoshino, M.; Hara, A.; Takagaki, A.; Nanjo, F.; et al. Blood brain barrier permeability of (−)-epigallocatechin gallate, its proliferation-enhancing activity of human neuroblastoma SH-SY5Y cells, and its preventive effect on age-related cognitive dysfunction in mice. *Biochem. Biophys. Rep.* **2017**, *9*, 180–186. [CrossRef] [PubMed]

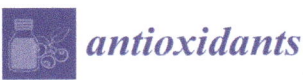

Article

Differential Effects of Polyphenols on Insulin Proteolysis by the Insulin-Degrading Enzyme

Qiuchen Zheng [†], Micheal T. Kebede [†], Bethany Lee [†], Claire A. Krasinski, Saadman Islam, Liliana A. Wurfl, Merc M. Kemeh, Valerie A. Ivancic, Charles E. Jakobsche, Donald E. Spratt and Noel D. Lazo *

Gustaf H. Carlson School of Chemistry and Biochemistry, Clark University, Worcester, MA 01610, USA; qzheng@clarku.edu (Q.Z.); mkebede@clarku.edu (M.T.K.); blee@clarku.edu (B.L.); ckrasinski@clarku.edu (C.A.K.); sislam@clarku.edu (S.I.); lwurfl@clarku.edu (L.A.W.); mkemeh@clarku.edu (M.M.K.); vivancic@clarku.edu (V.A.I.); cjakobsche@clarku.edu (C.E.J.); dspratt@clarku.edu (D.E.S.)
* Correspondence: nlazo@clarku.edu
† These authors contributed equally to this work.

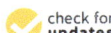

Citation: Zheng, Q.; Kebede, M.T.; Lee, B.; Krasinski, C.A.; Islam, S.; Wurfl, L.A.; Kemeh, M.M.; Ivancic, V.A.; Jakobsche, C.E.; Spratt, D.E.; et al. Differential Effects of Polyphenols on Insulin Proteolysis by the Insulin-Degrading Enzyme. *Antioxidants* **2021**, *10*, 1342. https:// doi.org/10.3390/antiox10091342

Academic Editors: Rui F. M. Silva and Lea Pogačnik

Received: 26 July 2021
Accepted: 23 August 2021
Published: 25 August 2021

Publisher's Note: MDPI stays neutral with regard to jurisdictional claims in published maps and institutional affiliations.

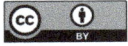

Copyright: © 2021 by the authors. Licensee MDPI, Basel, Switzerland. This article is an open access article distributed under the terms and conditions of the Creative Commons Attribution (CC BY) license (https:// creativecommons.org/licenses/by/ 4.0/).

Abstract: The insulin-degrading enzyme (IDE) possesses a strong ability to degrade insulin and Aβ42 that has been linked to the neurodegeneration in Alzheimer's disease (AD). Given this, an attractive IDE-centric strategy for the development of therapeutics for AD is to boost IDE's activity for the clearance of Aβ42 without offsetting insulin proteostasis. Recently, we showed that resveratrol enhances IDE's activity toward Aβ42. In this work, we used a combination of chromatographic and spectroscopic techniques to investigate the effects of resveratrol on IDE's activity toward insulin. For comparison, we also studied epigallocatechin-3-gallate (EGCG). Our results show that the two polyphenols affect the IDE-dependent degradation of insulin in different ways: EGCG inhibits IDE while resveratrol has no effect. These findings suggest that polyphenols provide a path for developing therapeutic strategies that can selectively target IDE substrate specificity.

Keywords: polyphenols; resveratrol; epigallocatechin-3-gallate; insulin-degrading enzyme

1. Introduction

Insulin-degrading enzyme (IDE), aka insulysin, is a ubiquitous zinc-dependent protease belonging to the M16 family of metalloendopeptidases [1]. Members of this family form a catalytic chamber, also referred to as crypt, the volume of which in IDE (~15,700 Å^3 [2]) limits the length of substrates to less than 70 amino acids [3]. Biophysical studies using X-ray crystallography [2,4,5] and cryogenic electron microscopy [6] have revealed mechanisms by which IDE encloses and degrades a diverse group of metabolically important and pathologically relevant substrates including insulin, a key hormone for glucose metabolism, amyloid-β(1-42) (Aβ42), which self-assembles to form the proximate neurotoxic assemblies in Alzheimer's disease (AD) [7], and islet amyloid polypeptide (IAPP), which self-assembles to form pancreatic amyloid in type 2 diabetes (T2D) [8]. IDE consists of two bowl-shaped halves, IDE-N and IDE-C, held together by an unstructured linker (Figure 1a). The flexibility of the linker allows IDE to exist in two major conformational states during its catalytic cycle: an open conformational state, which facilitates substrate entry and anchoring to IDE's exosite; and a closed conformational state, which expedites substrate degradation. IDE bears the HXXEH catalytic motif arranged so that the two histidine residues (His108 and His112) coordinate Zn^{2+} and the catalytic role of Glu111 in the hydrolysis of peptide bonds is facilitated (Figure 1b).

Given IDE's ability to degrade insulin, IAPP and Aβ42, it is no surprise that there has been strong academic and pharmaceutical interest in developing small molecules that modulate IDE's activity [9–12]. Several small-molecule and peptidic IDE inhibitors have been developed and investigated for their effects on insulin levels in cells or mice. Ii1 [13] and P12-3A [14] inhibited degradation of extracellular insulin in cells and fibroblasts, respectively. BDM44768 [15], B35 [16], and 6bk [17] elevated plasma insulin levels in mice. Despite these advances, significant challenges remain, as noted in a recent review by Leissring et al. [12]. First and foremost, inhibiting IDE may lead to increased levels of IAPP and Aβ, increasing the risk for T2D and AD, respectively (Figure 2).

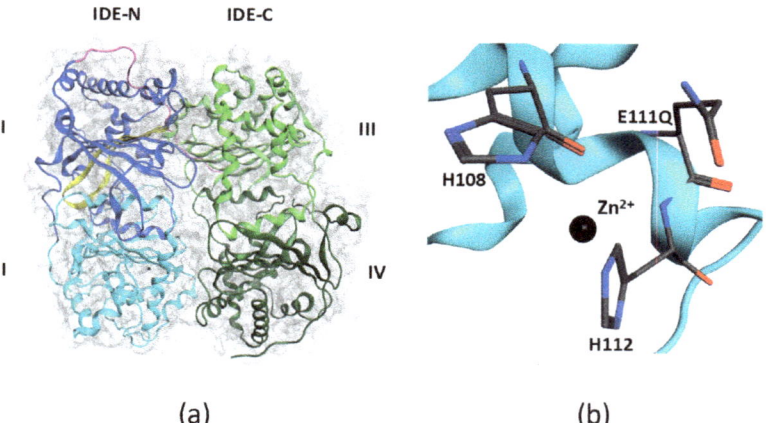

Figure 1. X-ray structure of insulin-degrading enzyme in its closed conformational state (PDB: 4PES). (**a**) IDE is composed of an N-terminal half (IDE-N) containing domains I and II, and a C-terminal half (IDE-C) containing domains III and IV. The two halves are joined by an unstructured linker (magenta). Domain I contains the HXXEH zinc-binding and catalytic motif. Domain II contains the exosite (yellow) in an anti-parallel β-sheet conformation. (**b**) The HXXEH motif includes H108 and H112 that coordinate Zn^{2+} and the catalytically important glutamate (E111) residue. When E111 is mutated to a glutamine as in 4PES, the enzyme becomes inactive.

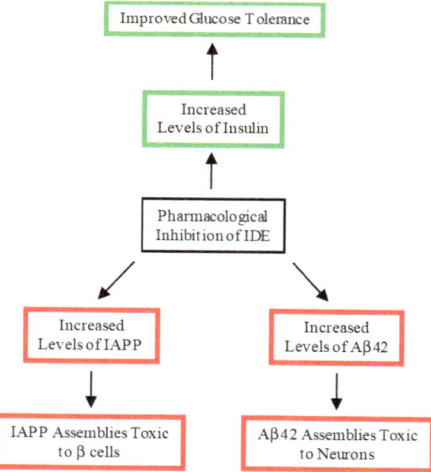

Figure 2. Beneficial and deleterious consequences of the pharmacological inhibition of IDE. A beneficial consequence of the inhibition of IDE is increased levels of insulin, leading to an improvement in glucose tolerance. Deleterious consequences include increased levels of Aβ42 and IAPP, leading to the formation of cytotoxic assemblies in the brain and pancreas, respectively.

An attractive alternative to the development of small-molecule inhibitors of IDE is a nutritional strategy that implicates polyphenols. Polyphenols are naturally occurring compounds that possess antioxidant [18–20], anti-inflammatory [19–21], and anti-amyloidogenic [22] properties. As such, polyphenols have been hypothesized to prevent T2D [23] and AD [24]. Recently, we showed that IDE's activity toward Aβ42 is sustained in the presence of resveratrol (Figure 3a) [25]. The effect of resveratrol on the IDE-dependent degradation of insulin, the enzyme's most physiologically important substrate, however, remains unknown. In this work, we used a combination of chromatographic and spectroscopy-based kinetic analysis to investigate the effects of resveratrol on IDE's activity toward insulin. For comparison, similar experiments were conducted in the presence of epigallocatechin-3-gallate (EGCG, Figure 3b), which is approximately two times larger than resveratrol, and is similar in size to BDM44768 [15]. Our results show that EGCG inhibits the IDE-dependent degradation of insulin, whereas resveratrol has no effect, presumably because of its smaller size. The implications of these results in the development of IDE-centric therapeutic strategies for T2D and AD are discussed.

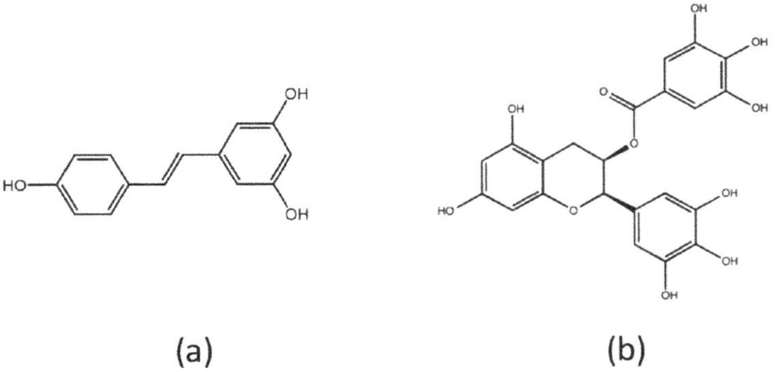

Figure 3. Chemical structures of polyphenols used in this study. (**a**) Resveratrol ($C_{14}H_{12}O_3$) is found in red wine and red grapes. (**b**) Epigallocatechin-3-gallate ($C_{22}H_{18}O_{11}$) is found in green tea.

2. Materials and Methods

2.1. Insulin-Degrading Enzyme Expression and Purification

The bacterial expression vector encoding IDE fused to GST was kindly provided by Dr. Malcolm A. Leissring of the University of California at Irvine. GST-IDE was overexpressed in *E. coli* BL21-CodonPlus RIL cells (EMD Biosciences Inc., San Diego, CA, USA), and purified as previously described [25–27]. Cleavage of the GST tag was accomplished using GST PreScission protease and further purification of IDE was accomplished by standard gel filtration [25–27]. UV absorbance at 280 nm was used to determine the concentration of IDE using an extinction coefficient of $\varepsilon_{280nm} = 113{,}570$ M^{-1} cm^{-1} [28].

2.2. Preparation of Stock Solutions

Recombinant human insulin (99% pure), EGCG (>98% pure), and resveratrol (>99% pure) were purchased from Sigma-Aldrich (St. Louis, MO, USA). Stock solutions of insulin and EGCG were prepared in 50 mM Tris buffer (pH 7.4). Stock solutions of resveratrol were prepared in 100% ethanol. The concentrations of the stock solutions were detected by UV absorbance at the following wavelengths: 276 nm for insulin ($\varepsilon_{276nm} = 6190$ M^{-1} cm^{-1}) [29]; 275 nm for EGCG ($\varepsilon_{275nm} = 11{,}500$ M^{-1} cm^{-1}) [30]; and 306 nm for resveratrol ($\varepsilon_{306nm} = 15{,}400$ M^{-1} cm^{-1}) [31]. All stock solutions were freshly prepared, and used immediately after preparation.

2.3. Circular Dichroism Spectroscopy

2.3.1. Monitoring the Loss of Insulin's Helical Circular Dichroic Signals with Digestion Time

We used circular dichroism spectroscopy to detect the changes in insulin's secondary structure as its proteolysis proceeds. All far UV circular dichroic (CD) spectra were recorded at 37 °C using a JASCO J-815 spectropolarimeter equipped with a Peltier temperature control unit. Each sample was prepared with a volume of 200 µL. The substrate-to-enzyme molar ratio of insulin-to-IDE was 100:1 (20 µM insulin: 0.2 µM IDE) for limited proteolysis [26], and the molar ratio of insulin-to-polyphenol was set as 1:2 (20 µM insulin: 40 µM EGCG or resveratrol), similar to the molar ratio of Aβ42-to-resveratrol we previously used [25]. We determined that by setting the insulin concentration at 20 µM, CD spectra of good signal-to-noise ratios were recorded in the far UV range (i.e., from 260 to 198 nm). All samples were incubated in quartz cuvettes with a path length of 1 mm. Each CD spectrum was recorded from 260 to 198 nm using an averaging time of 1 s and four accumulations. All samples were kept at 37 °C in between recording of spectra. The Savitzsky–Golay method with convolution width equal to 7 was applied to smoothen all CD spectra.

2.3.2. Kinetic Parameters from Insulin's Helical Circular Dichroic Ellipticity at 222 nm

Steady-state kinetic parameters for the IDE-dependent degradation of insulin were determined using insulin's helical circular dichroic ellipticity at 222 nm ($[\theta_{obs(222nm)}]$), as described in detail elsewhere [26]. Briefly, seven substrate solutions with concentrations of 15, 20, 25, 30, 50, 80, and 110 µM were prepared in 50 mM Tris buffer (pH 7.4). EGCG or resveratrol was added at a concentration of 20 or 40 µM. Proteolysis was initiated with the addition of IDE at a concentration of 1 µM. After mixing, the solution was transferred into a 1-mm path length quartz cuvette and loaded into the sample holder of our circular dichroism spectrometer that was pre-warmed to 37 °C. After a brief equilibration period, $[\theta_{obs(222nm)}]$ was recorded for 5 min. The real-time $[\theta_{obs(222nm)}]$ data were then used to calculate the amount of digested insulin ([DI]) using the equation below:

$$[DI]_t = [I]_0 \times \left(1 - \frac{[\theta_{obs(222nm)}]_t}{[\theta_{obs(222nm)}]_0}\right) \quad (1)$$

where $[DI]_t$ is the amount of digested insulin at real-time t; $[I]_0$ is the initial amount of undigested insulin; and $[\theta_{obs(222nm)}]_t$ and $[\theta_{obs(222nm)}]_0$ are the observed ellipticity at real-time t and observed initial ellipticity at time = 0, respectively. Plots of [DI] against time were used to determine the initial rates (V_0) of insulin proteolysis by IDE. Michaelis–Menten (V_0 plotted against [S], Lineweaver–Burk ($1/V_0$ plotted against $1/[S]$), and Hanes–Woolf ([S]/V_0 plotted against [S]) plots were then constructed from which the kinetic constants K_M, V_{max}, k_{cat} and k_{cat}/K_M were determined.

2.4. Reversed Phase High Performance Liquid Chromatography

Proteolysis samples were prepared for RP HPLC analysis by setting the substrate-to-enzyme molar ratio to 100:1, and the polyphenol-to-insulin molar ratio to 2:1. These included: (1) insulin + EGCG + IDE (20 µM insulin + 40 µM EGCG + 0.2 µM IDE); and (2) insulin + RES + IDE (20 µM insulin + 40 µM RES + 0.2 µM IDE). Control samples that only contain insulin + IDE (20 µM insulin + 0.2 µM IDE) were also prepared. All reactions were started by the addition of IDE followed by incubation at 37 °C. Aliquots (200 µL) of each digests were removed at the desired time points and quenched by acidification to low pH with 15 µL of 5% (v/v) trifluoroacetic acid in water.

The IDE-dependent proteolysis of insulin was monitored using a Varian Pro Star 210 HPLC system, equipped with a ProStar 325 Variable Wavelength UV–Visible Detector. RP HPLC fractionation of insulin digests was carried out at room temperature using an analytical Agilent AdvanceBio mAb C4 column. Solvents A and B were 0.1% (v/v) formic acid in H₂O and 0.1% (v/v) formic acid in acetonitrile, respectively. Aliquots (20 µL) of solutions containing insulin digests were injected into the HPLC manually and eluted with a 20-min linear gradient of 0–100% B at a flow rate of 1 mL/min. The elution of analytes was monitored by UV absorbance at 214 and 254 nm.

3. Results and Discussion

Insulin's CD spectrum indicates a predominantly α-helical structure as indicated by the following features [32]: (1) a positive $\pi \to \pi^*$ band at 195 nm, polarized $\perp$ to the helix axis; (2) a negative $\pi \to \pi^*$ band at 208 nm, polarized $\parallel$ to the helix axis; and (3) a negative $n \to \pi^*$ band at 222 nm, also polarized $\parallel$ to the helix axis. Recently, we showed that the CD spectrum of insulin is sensitive to the extent of IDE-dependent degradation [26]. In particular, we noted that as proteolysis occurs, the intensities of insulin's helical CD signals decrease with an increase in digestion time. The complete degradation of insulin by IDE is indicated by a CD spectrum with a single minimum near 198 nm, consistent with the dominant presence of unstructured or random coil peptides [26].

Figure 4 presents the CD spectra of insulin IDE digests in the absence of polyphenols and in the presence of EGCG or resveratrol. The time-dependent spectra recorded in the absence of polyphenols (Figure 4a) were similar to those we reported recently [26]. The intensities of the signals at 222 and 208 nm decreased with time, indicating the progressive loss of α-helical insulin. Similar results were obtained in the digestions that contained resveratrol (Figure 4b), which suggest that the polyphenol has no effect on the IDE-dependent degradation of insulin. In sharp contrast, insulin's CD helical signals persisted in the presence of EGCG (Figure 4c), indicating inhibition of the proteolysis of insulin by IDE. We noted, however, that the intensities of the helical signals, particularly at 222 and 198 nm, decreased, suggesting that the inhibition is partial and not complete.

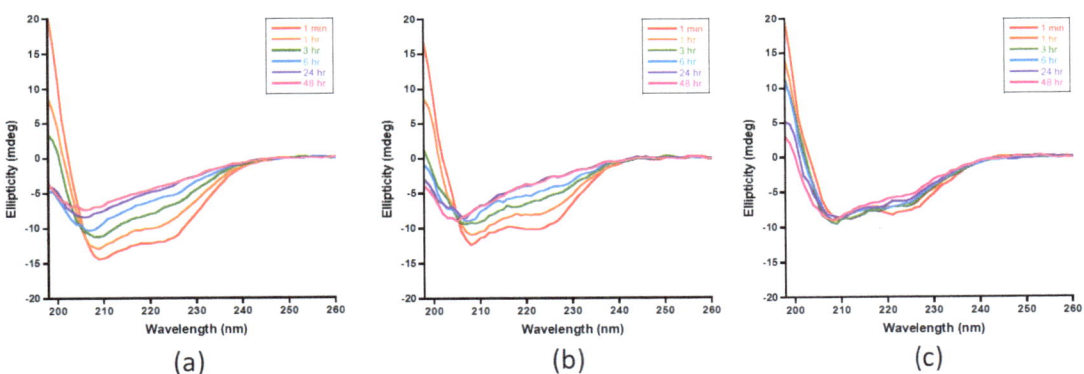

Figure 4. CD spectra of IDE-dependent degradation of insulin in the absence and presence of polyphenols at 37 °C. (**a**) Spectra recorded for insulin digests that do not contain polyphenols (control samples) show the progressive loss on insulin's helical CD signals at 222, 208, and 198 nm, consistent with the loss of α-helical structure. (**b**) Spectra recorded for insulin digests in the presence of resveratrol were similar to the spectra recorded for the control samples, indicating that the polyphenol had no effect on IDE's activity toward insulin. (**c**) Spectra recorded for insulin digests in the presence of EGCG showed that the helical signals of insulin persist, indicating that EGCG inhibits insulin proteolysis by IDE. The insulin concentration in all samples was set at 20 µM in 50 mM Tris buffer (pH 7.4). The substrate-to-enzyme molar ratio and the polyphenol-to-insulin molar ratio were set to 100:1 and 2:1, respectively. All samples were kept at 37 °C in between spectral acquisition.

We also used reversed phase HPLC to monitor the proteolytic activity of IDE toward insulin over the same incubation periods used in the digestions that yielded the CD spectra shown in Figure 4. Representative chromatograms of control samples are shown in Figure 5a. As the digestion time increased, the intensity of the insulin peak decreased and peaks at shorter retention times appeared due to the production of insulin fragments. Digestion is complete within 24 h. Figure 5b presents chromatograms of the digests in the presence of resveratrol. With the exception of the peak for resveratrol, the chromatograms were similar to those of the control samples. Insulin degradation was also complete within 24 h. Figure 5c shows the chromatograms of the digests in the presence of EGCG. In contrast to the corresponding chromatograms in Figure 5a,b, the chromatograms of the 24- and 48-h digests showed the presence of the insulin peak indicating inhibition of IDE-dependent degradation. The intensity of the insulin peak, however, decreased with time, suggesting that the inhibition of IDE was not complete. The intensity of the peak for EGCG decreased with incubation time, presumably because it epimerizes to gallocatechin-3-gallate and/or dimerizes to form digallate dimers [22,33]. Our cumulative CD (Figure 4) and RP HPLC (Figure 5) results clearly demonstrate that resveratrol has no effect on IDE's activity toward insulin. EGCG, on the other hand, partially inhibits IDE.

Next, the steady-state kinetic parameters for the IDE-dependent degradation of insulin in the absence and presence of polyphenols were determined using insulin's helical CD ellipticity at 222 nm ($[\theta_{obs(222nm)}]$). Because our analysis was limited to 5 min of digestion time, complications due to the epimerization and oxidation of EGCG were circumvented. Figures S1a and S2a present representative real-time ellipticity data obtained from proteolysis experiments in the presence of resveratrol and EGCG, respectively. As digestion proceeded, $[\theta_{obs(222nm)}]$ became less negative indicating loss of helicity. We calculated the amount of digested insulin $[DI]_t$ using Equation (1) and these were plotted against digestion time (Figures S1b and S2b). Linear regression analysis yielded V_0, the initial velocity (or initial rate) of insulin proteolysis. Figure 6a,b present the resulting Michaelis–Menten plots for the digestions carried out in the presence of resveratrol and EGCG, respectively, at polyphenol concentrations of 0 (control), 20, and 40 µM. Lineweaver–Burk and Hanes–Woolf plots for the digestions in the presence of resveratrol and EGCG are shown in Figures S3 and S4, respectively. The Michaelis–Menten (Figure 6a), Lineweaver–Burk (Figure S3), and Hanes–Woolf (Figure S3) plots for resveratrol are invariant to concentration, indicating that the polyphenol has no effect on IDE's activity. In sharp contrast, the corresponding plots for EGCG clearly indicate that IDE's activity decreased as the concentration of the polyphenol increased (Figure 6b and Figure S4). Table 1 summarizes the kinetic constants obtained from the Michaelis–Menten plots. Similar values were obtained from the Lineweaver–Burk (Table S1) and Hanes–Woolf (Table S2) plots. IDE's catalytic efficiency, as given by k_{cat}/K_M, was not affected by resveratrol. In sharp contrast, k_{cat}/K_M decreased by 54 and 67% relative to the control in the presence of 20 and 40 µM of EGCG, respectively. The Lineweaver–Burk plots (Figure S4a) show straight lines with different slopes and a common intercept that is not on the $1/V_0$ axis, suggesting mixed inhibition by EGCG. Mixed inhibitors bind at a site separate from the enzyme's active site, but may bind to either the enzyme or enzyme-substrate complex [34]. A schematic representation of the mixed inhibition by IDE is shown in Scheme 1.

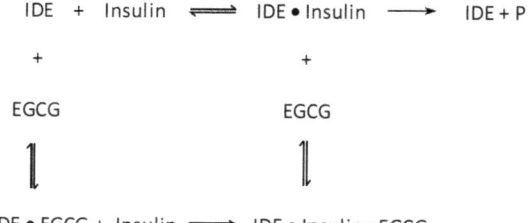

Scheme 1. Schematic representation of the mixed inhibition of IDE-dependent degradation of insulin by EGCG. EGCG binds to either IDE or IDE•insulin complex, leading to a decrease in catalytic activity.

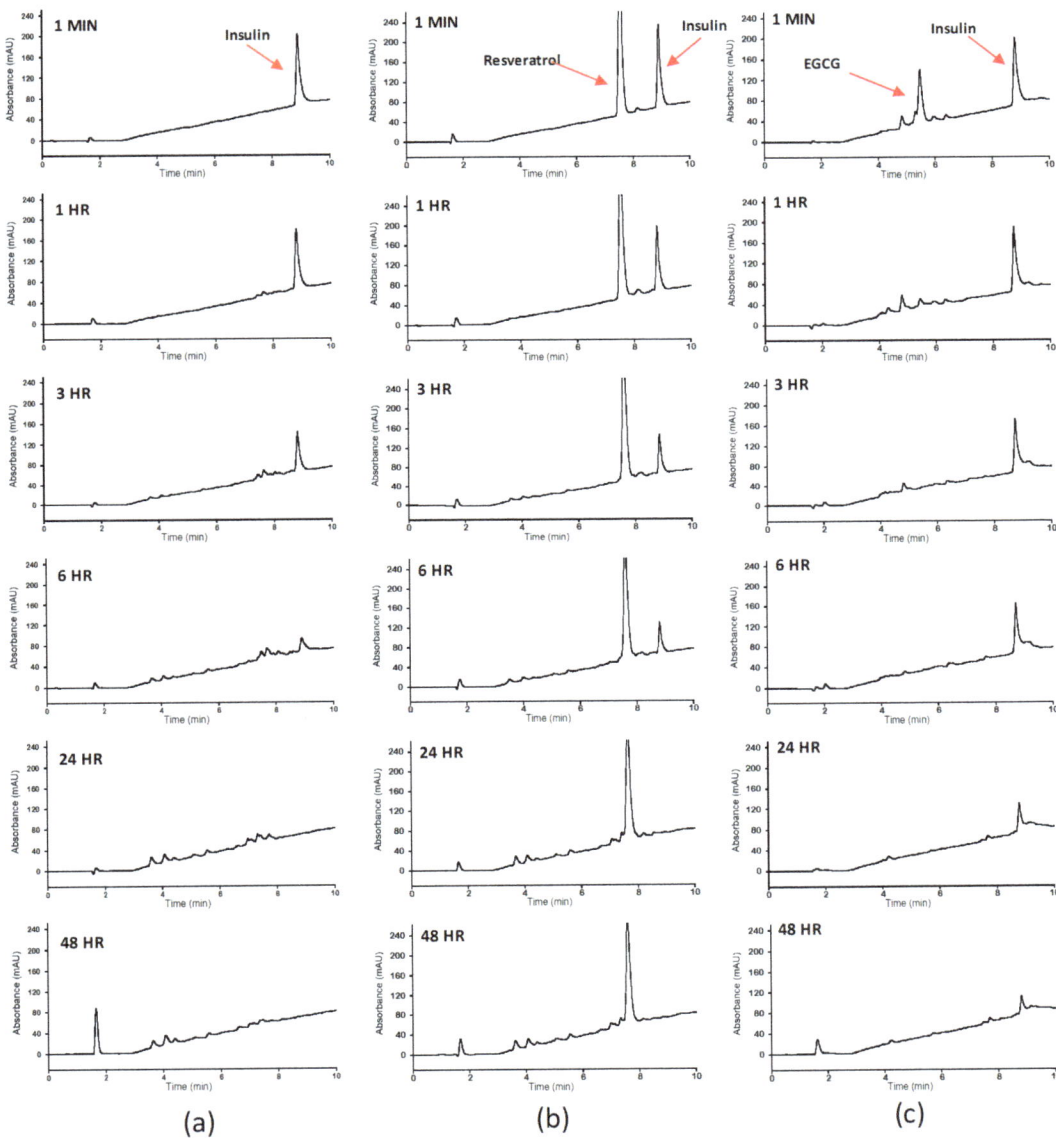

Figure 5. RP HPLC analysis of IDE-dependent degradation of insulin in the absence and presence of polyphenols at 37 °C. (**a**) Chromatograms of insulin digests in the absence of polyphenols (control samples) show the progressive loss of the insulin peak over the digestion period. This loss is accompanied by new peaks at shorter retention times due to the formation of insulin fragments. The chromatogram recorded for the 24-hr digest shows the absence of the insulin peak, indicating complete degradation of insulin. (**b**) Chromatograms of insulin digests in the presence of resveratrol are similar to the chromatograms in (**a**) with the exception of the peak for the polyphenol at a retention time of 7.5 min. Digestion of insulin is complete within 24 h. (**c**) Chromatograms of insulin digests in the presence of EGCG show that the digestion of insulin was not complete, even after 48 h of digestion. The intensity of the insulin peak, however, decreased with digestion time, suggesting that the inhibition by EGCG was partial and not complete. The intensity of the peak for EGCG decreased with incubation time presumably because of epimerization and/or dimerization.

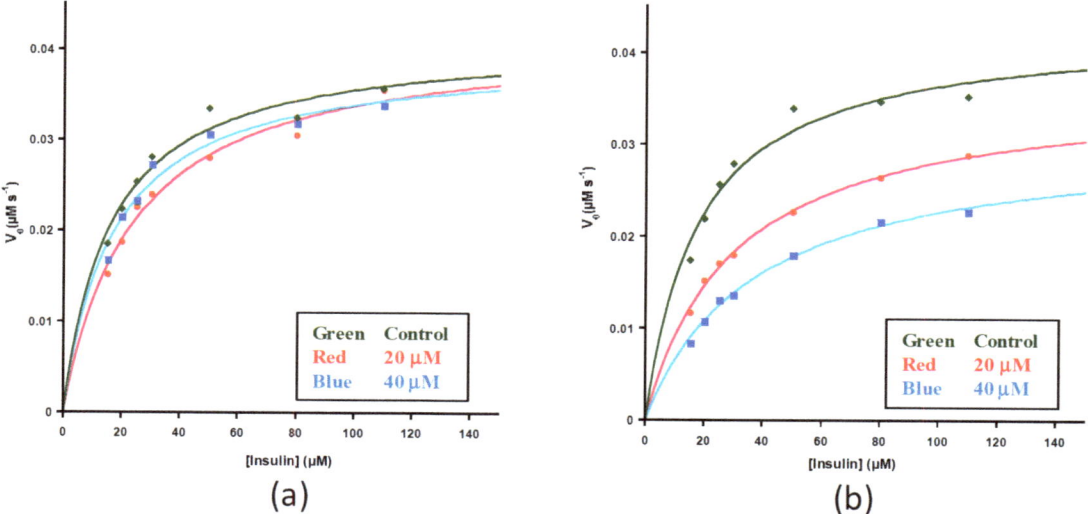

Figure 6. Kinetics of IDE-dependent degradation of insulin in the absence and presence of polyphenols at 37 °C. (**a**) Michaelis–Menten plots for insulin digests in the absence and presence of resveratrol were similar to one another, indicating that the polyphenol has no effect on IDE's activity toward insulin. (**b**) Corresponding plots for the digestions in the absence and presence of EGCG clearly show that IDE's activity decreased as the concentration of EGCG increased. Plots for polyphenol concentrations of 0, 20, and 40 µM are shown in green, red, and blue, respectively. Each data point represents the mean from three trials. The solid lines are fits to the Michaelis–Menten equation.

Table 1. Steady-state kinetic parameters for the IDE-dependent proteolysis of insulin determined from Michaelis–Menten plots.

Polyphenol	K_M (M)	k_{cat} (s^{-1})	k_{cat}/K_M (M^{-1}S^{-1})
None	$1.8 \pm 0.2 \times 10^{-5}$	0.043 ± 0.0006	$2.4 \pm 0.3 \times 10^3$
None/Ethanol *	$1.6 \pm 0.2 \times 10^{-5}$	0.041 ± 0.001	$2.6 \pm 0.3 \times 10^3$
Resveratrol (20 µM)	$2.6 \pm 1.2 \times 10^{-5}$	0.043 ± 0.003	$1.8 \pm 0.6 \times 10^3$
Resveratrol (40 µM)	$1.7 \pm 0.3 \times 10^{-5}$	0.040 ± 0.004	$2.3 \pm 0.1 \times 10^3$
EGCG (20 µM)	$3.2 \pm 1.2 \times 10^{-5}$	0.037 ± 0.002	$1.3 \pm 0.4 \times 10^3$
EGCG (40 µM)	$3.7 \pm 0.9 \times 10^{-5}$	0.031 ± 0.0008	$0.83 \pm 0.2 \times 10^3$

* Control experiments to test the effect of ethanol that was used to dissolve resveratrol.

In vivo studies on animals have identified beneficial effects of EGCG including decreased adipose mass [35], reduction in body weight [36], and improvement in glucose homeostasis [35–37]. The effects of EGCG on glucose metabolism associated with T2D have been reported to be mediated in several ways including decreased gluconeogenesis [38], increased insulin sensitivity [39], and increased glucose uptake in skeletal muscle [40], which is an important regulator of glucose homeostasis [41]. The direct molecular targets of EGCG in vivo are not known. This work shows that EGCG directly targets IDE, and in doing so, the IDE-dependent degradation of insulin is inhibited, providing molecular basis for the improvement in glucose homeostasis observed in the in vivo studies.

How might our resveratrol results be used in the development of therapeutic and/or preventive strategies for AD? Recently, we showed that resveratrol sustains IDE activity toward Aβ42 monomer [25]. This conclusion, together with this work's finding that resveratrol does not affect IDE's activity toward insulin, has an important implication. Given that insulin and Aβ42 are IDE's most physiologically important and most pathologically significant substrates in the brain, respectively, resveratrol is an IDE substrate-selective activator. Resveratrol's selectivity toward Aβ42 and its ability to cross the blood–brain barrier [24,42,43] suggest that this polyphenol can potentially act as an ideal naturally-occurring molecule for an IDE-centric therapeutic for AD.

Supplementary Materials: The following are available online at https://www.mdpi.com/article/10.3390/antiox10091342/s1, Figure S1: Early-stage kinetics of IDE-dependent degradation of insulin in the absence and presence of resveratrol using insulin's observed ellipticity at 222 nm [$\theta_{obs(222nm)}$], Figure S2: Early-stage kinetics of IDE-dependent degradation of insulin in the absence and presence of EGCG using observed ellipticity at 222 nm [$\theta_{obs(222nm)}$], Figure S3: Kinetics of IDE-dependent degradation of insulin in the absence and presence of resveratrol at 37 °C, Figure S4: Kinetics of IDE-dependent degradation of insulin in the absence and presence of EGCG at 37 °C, Table S1: Steady-state kinetic parameters of the IDE-dependent proteolysis of insulin determined from Lineweaver–Burk plots, Table S2: Steady-state kinetic parameters of IDE-dependent proteolysis of insulin determined from Hanes–Woolf plots.

Author Contributions: Conceptualization and overall direction of the project, N.D.L.; Circular dichroism and kinetic studies, Q.Z., B.L., S.I., L.A.W., C.A.K., V.A.I., M.M.K., RP HPLC, M.T.K. and C.E.J.; IDE production, B.L., V.A.I., C.A.K. and D.E.S.; Writing—original draft preparation, Q.Z., M.T.K. and N.D.L.; Writing—review and editing, all authors. All authors have read and agreed to the published version of the manuscript.

Funding: This research was funded by the National Institute on Aging through R15AG055043 to N.D.L.

Institutional Review Board Statement: Not applicable.

Informed Consent Statement: Not applicable.

Data Availability Statement: Data is contained within the article.

Acknowledgments: The authors thank Malcolm A. Leissring of the University of California at Irvine for providing the bacterial expression vector encoding IDE fused to GST.

Conflicts of Interest: The authors declare no conflict of interest. The funders had no role in the design of the study; in the collection, analyses, or interpretation of data; in the writing of the manuscript, or in the decision to publish the results.

References

1. Barrett, A.J.; Rawlings, N.D.; Woessner, J.F. *Handbook of Proteolytic Enzymes*; Academic Press: Cambridge, MA, USA, 2012.
2. Manolopoulou, M.; Guo, Q.; Malito, E.; Schilling, A.B.; Tang, W.J. Molecular basis of catalytic chamber-assisted unfolding and cleavage of human insulin by human insulin-degrading enzyme. *J. Biol. Chem.* **2009**, *284*, 14177–14188. [CrossRef]
3. Malito, E.; Hulse, R.E.; Tang, W.J. Amyloid β-degrading cryptidases: insulin degrading enzyme, presequence peptidase, and neprilysin. *Cell. Mol. Life Sci.* **2008**, *65*, 2574–2585. [CrossRef]
4. Shen, Y.; Joachimiak, A.; Rosner, M.R.; Tang, W.J. Structures of human insulin-degrading enzyme reveal a new substrate recognition mechanism. *Nature* **2006**, *443*, 870–874. [CrossRef]
5. McCord, L.A.; Liang, W.G.; Dowdell, E.; Kalas, V.; Hoey, R.J.; Koide, A.; Koide, S.; Tang, W.J. Conformational states and recognition of amyloidogenic peptides of human insulin-degrading enzyme. *Proc. Natl. Acad. Sci. USA* **2013**, *110*, 13827–13832. [CrossRef] [PubMed]
6. Zhang, Z.; Liang, W.G.; Bailey, L.J.; Tan, Y.Z.; Wei, H.; Wang, A.; Farcasanu, M.; Woods, V.A.; McCord, L.A.; Lee, D.; et al. Ensemble cryoEM elucidates the mechanism of insulin capture and degradation by human insulin degrading enzyme. *Elife* **2018**, *7*, e33572. [CrossRef]
7. Selkoe, D.J.; Hardy, J. The amyloid hypothesis of Alzheimer's disease at 25 years. *EMBO Mol. Med.* **2016**, *8*, 595–608. [CrossRef] [PubMed]
8. Milardi, D.; Gazit, E.; Radford, S.E.; Xu, Y.; Gallardo, R.U.; Caflisch, A.; Westermark, G.T.; Westermark, P.; Rosa, C.; Ramamoorthy, A. Proteostasis of Islet Amyloid Polypeptide: A Molecular Perspective of Risk Factors and Protective Strategies for Type II Diabetes. *Chem. Rev.* **2021**, *121*, 1845–1893. [CrossRef]
9. Tang, W.J. Targeting Insulin-Degrading Enzyme to Treat Type 2 Diabetes Mellitus. *Trends Endocrinol. Metab.* **2016**, *27*, 24–34. [CrossRef]
10. Kurochkin, I.V.; Guarnera, E.; Berezovsky, I.N. Insulin-Degrading Enzyme in the Fight against Alzheimer's Disease. *Trends Pharmacol. Sci.* **2018**, *39*, 49–58. [CrossRef]

11. Gonzalez-Casimiro, C.M.; Merino, B.; Casanueva-Alvarez, E.; Postigo-Casado, T.; Camara-Torres, P.; Fernandez-Diaz, C.M.; Leissring, M.A.; Cozar-Castellano, I.; Perdomo, G. Modulation of Insulin Sensitivity by Insulin-Degrading Enzyme. *Biomedicines* 2021, 9, 86. [CrossRef]
12. Leissring, M.A.; Gonzalez-Casimiro, C.M.; Merino, B.; Suire, C.N.; Perdomo, G. Targeting Insulin-Degrading Enzyme in Insulin Clearance. *Int. J. Mol. Sci.* 2021, 22, 2235. [CrossRef]
13. Abdul-Hay, S.O.; Lane, A.L.; Caulfield, T.R.; Claussin, C.; Bertrand, J.; Masson, A.; Choudhry, S.; Fauq, A.H.; Maharvi, G.M.; Leissring, M.A. Optimization of peptide hydroxamate inhibitors of insulin-degrading enzyme reveals marked substrate-selectivity. *J. Med. Chem.* 2013, 56, 2246–2255. [CrossRef]
14. Suire, C.N.; Nainar, S.; Fazio, M.; Kreutzer, A.G.; Paymozd-Yazdi, T.; Topper, C.L.; Thompson, C.R.; Leissring, M.A. Peptidic inhibitors of insulin-degrading enzyme with potential for dermatological applications discovered via phage display. *PLoS ONE* 2018, 13, e0193101. [CrossRef]
15. Deprez-Poulain, R.; Hennuyer, N.; Bosc, D.; Liang, W.G.; Enee, E.; Marechal, X.; Charton, J.; Totobenazara, J.; Berte, G.; Jahklal, J.; et al. Catalytic site inhibition of insulin-degrading enzyme by a small molecule induces glucose intolerance in mice. *Nat Commun.* 2015, 6, 8250. [CrossRef]
16. Yang, D.; Qin, W.; Shi, X.; Zhu, B.; Xie, M.; Zhao, H.; Teng, B.; Wu, Y.; Zhao, R.; Yin, F.; et al. Stabilized β-Hairpin Peptide Inhibits Insulin Degrading Enzyme. *J. Med. Chem.* 2018, 61, 8174–8185. [CrossRef]
17. Maianti, J.P.; McFedries, A.; Foda, Z.H.; Kleiner, R.E.; Du, X.Q.; Leissring, M.A.; Tang, W.J.; Charron, M.J.; Seeliger, M.A.; Saghatelian, A.; et al. Anti-diabetic activity of insulin-degrading enzyme inhibitors mediated by multiple hormones. *Nature* 2014, 511, 94–98. [CrossRef]
18. Baroni, L.; Sarni, A.R.; Zuliani, C. Plant Foods Rich in Antioxidants and Human Cognition: A Systematic Review. *Antioxidants* 2021, 10, 714. [CrossRef] [PubMed]
19. Bucciantini, M.; Leri, M.; Nardiello, P.; Casamenti, F.; Stefani, M. Olive Polyphenols: Antioxidant and Anti-Inflammatory Properties. *Antioxidants* 2021, 10, 1044. [CrossRef] [PubMed]
20. Silva, R.F.M.; Pogacnik, L. Polyphenols from Food and Natural Products: Neuroprotection and Safety. *Antioxidants* 2020, 9, 61. [CrossRef] [PubMed]
21. Kim, H.; Castellon-Chicas, M.J.; Arbizu, S.; Talcott, S.T.; Drury, N.L.; Smith, S.; Mertens-Talcott, S.U. Mango (*Mangifera indica* L.) Polyphenols: Anti-Inflammatory Intestinal Microbial Health Benefits, and Associated Mechanisms of Actions. *Molecules* 2021, 26, 2732. [CrossRef]
22. Zheng, Q.; Kebede, M.T.; Kemeh, M.M.; Islam, S.; Lee, B.; Bleck, S.D.; Wurfl, L.A.; Lazo, N.D. Inhibition of the Self-Assembly of Aβ and of Tau by Polyphenols: Mechanistic Studies. *Molecules* 2019, 24, 2316. [CrossRef]
23. Hameed, A.; Galli, M.; Adamska-Patruno, E.; Kretowski, A.; Ciborowski, M. Select Polyphenol-Rich Berry Consumption to Defer or Deter Diabetes and Diabetes-Related Complications. *Nutrients* 2020, 12, 2538. [CrossRef]
24. Pasinetti, G.M.; Wang, J.; Ho, L.; Zhao, W.; Dubner, L. Roles of resveratrol and other grape-derived polyphenols in Alzheimer's disease prevention and treatment. *Biochim. Biophys. Acta* 2015, 1852, 1202–1208. [CrossRef] [PubMed]
25. Krasinski, C.A.; Ivancic, V.A.; Zheng, Q.; Spratt, D.E.; Lazo, N.D. Resveratrol Sustains Insulin-degrading Enzyme Activity toward Aβ42. *ACS Omega* 2018, 3, 13275–13282. [CrossRef] [PubMed]
26. Ivancic, V.A.; Krasinski, C.A.; Zheng, Q.; Meservier, R.J.; Spratt, D.E.; Lazo, N.D. Enzyme kinetics from circular dichroism of insulin reveals mechanistic insights into the regulation of insulin-degrading enzyme. *Biosci. Rep.* 2018, 38, BSR20181416. [CrossRef]
27. Krasinski, C.A.; Zheng, Q.; Ivancic, V.A.; Spratt, D.E.; Lazo, N.D. The Longest Amyloid-β Precursor Protein Intracellular Domain Produced with Aβ42 Forms β-Sheet-Containing Monomers That Self-Assemble and Are Proteolyzed by Insulin-Degrading Enzyme. *ACS Chem. Neurosci.* 2018, 9, 2892–2897. [CrossRef]
28. Sharma, S.K.; Chorell, E.; Steneberg, P.; Vernersson-Lindahl, E.; Edlund, H.; Wittung-Stafshede, P. Insulin-degrading enzyme prevents α-synuclein fibril formation in a nonproteolytical manner. *Sci. Rep.* 2015, 5, 12531. [CrossRef]
29. Manno, M.; Craparo, E.F.; Martorana, V.; Bulone, D.; San Biagio, P.L. Kinetics of insulin aggregation: disentanglement of amyloid fibrillation from large-size cluster formation. *Biophys. J.* 2006, 90, 4585–4591. [CrossRef]
30. Windholz, M.; Budavari, S.; Stroumtsos, L.Y.; Fertig, M.N. *The Merck Index: An Encyclopedia of Chemicals and Drugs*; Merck & Co.: New York, NY, USA, 1976.
31. Calderon, A.A.; Zapata, J.M.; Munoz, R.; Pedreno, M.A.; Barcelo, A.R. Resveratrol production as part of the hypersensitive-like response of grapevine cells to an elicitor from *Trichoderma viride*. *New Phytol.* 1993, 124, 455–463. [CrossRef]
32. Holzwarth, G.; Doty, P. The ultraviolet circular dichroism of polypeptides. *J. Am. Chem. Soc.* 1965, 87, 218–228. [CrossRef]
33. Sang, S.; Lee, M.J.; Hou, Z.; Ho, C.T.; Yang, C.S. Stability of tea polyphenol (-)-epigallocatechin-3-gallate and formation of dimers and epimers under common experimental conditions. *J. Agric. Food Chem.* 2005, 53, 9478–9484. [CrossRef]
34. Nelson, D.L.; Cox, M.M. *Lehninger Principles of Biochemistry*; W. H. Freeman and Company: New York, NY, USA, 2013.
35. Bose, M.; Lambert, J.D.; Ju, J.; Reuhl, K.R.; Shapses, S.A.; Yang, C.S. The major green tea polyphenol, (-)-epigallocatechin-3-gallate, inhibits obesity, metabolic syndrome, and fatty liver disease in high-fat-fed mice. *J. Nutr.* 2008, 138, 1677–1683. [CrossRef]
36. Chen, N.; Bezzina, R.; Hinch, E.; Lewandowski, P.A.; Cameron-Smith, D.; Mathai, M.L.; Jois, M.; Sinclair, A.J.; Begg, D.P.; Wark, J.D.; et al. Green tea, black tea, and epigallocatechin modify body composition, improve glucose tolerance, and differentially alter metabolic gene expression in rats fed a high-fat diet. *Nutr. Res.* 2009, 29, 784–793. [CrossRef]

37. Ueda, M.; Nishiumi, S.; Nagayasu, H.; Fukuda, I.; Yoshida, K.; Ashida, H. Epigallocatechin gallate promotes GLUT4 translocation in skeletal muscle. *Biochem. Biophys. Res. Commun.* **2008**, *377*, 286–290. [CrossRef]
38. Yang, C.S.; Zhang, J.; Zhang, L.; Huang, J.; Wang, Y. Mechanisms of body weight reduction and metabolic syndrome alleviation by tea. *Mol. Nutr. Food Res.* **2016**, *60*, 160–174. [CrossRef]
39. Ni, D.; Ai, Z.; Munoz-Sandoval, D.; Suresh, R.; Ellis, P.R.; Yuqiong, C.; Sharp, P.A.; Butterworth, P.J.; Yu, Z.; Corpe, C.P. Inhibition of the facilitative sugar transporters (GLUTs) by tea extracts and catechins. *FASEB J.* **2020**, *34*, 9995–10010. [CrossRef]
40. Nishiumi, S.; Bessyo, H.; Kubo, M.; Aoki, Y.; Tanaka, A.; Yoshida, K.; Ashida, H. Green and black tea suppress hyperglycemia and insulin resistance by retaining the expression of glucose transporter 4 in muscle of high-fat diet-fed C57BL/6J mice. *J. Agric. Food Chem.* **2010**, *58*, 12916–12923. [CrossRef]
41. Keske, M.A.; Ng, H.L.; Premilovac, D.; Rattigan, S.; Kim, J.A.; Munir, K.; Yang, P.; Quon, M.J. Vascular and metabolic actions of the green tea polyphenol epigallocatechin gallate. *Curr. Med. Chem.* **2015**, *22*, 59–69. [CrossRef]
42. Vingtdeux, V.; Giliberto, L.; Zhao, H.; Chandakkar, P.; Wu, Q.; Simon, J.E.; Janle, E.M.; Lobo, J.; Ferruzzi, M.G.; Davies, P.; et al. AMP-activated protein kinase signaling activation by resveratrol modulates amyloid-β peptide metabolism. *J. Biol. Chem.* **2010**, *285*, 9100–9113. [CrossRef]
43. Karuppagounder, S.S.; Pinto, J.T.; Xu, H.; Chen, H.L.; Beal, M.F.; Gibson, G.E. Dietary supplementation with resveratrol reduces plaque pathology in a transgenic model of Alzheimer's disease. *Neurochem. Int.* **2009**, *54*, 111–118. [CrossRef]

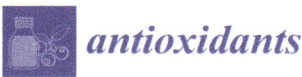

Article

Central Administration of Ampelopsin A Isolated from *Vitis vinifera* Ameliorates Cognitive and Memory Function in a Scopolamine-Induced Dementia Model

Yuni Hong [1,2,†], Yun-Hyeok Choi [3,†], Young-Eun Han [1], Soo-Jin Oh [1,4], Ansoo Lee [1,2], Bonggi Lee [5], Rebecca Magnan [6], Shi Yong Ryu [7], Chun Whan Choi [3,*] and Min Soo Kim [1,2,*]

1. Brain Science Institute, Korea Institute of Science and Technology (KIST), Seoul 02792, Korea; yunihong@kist.re.kr (Y.H.); hye6595@kist.re.kr (Y.-E.H.); osj@kist.re.kr (S.-J.O.); alee@kist.re.kr (A.L.)
2. Division of Bio-Medical Science & Technology, KIST School, University of Science and Technology, Seoul 02792, Korea
3. Natural Product Research Team, Gyeonggi Biocenter, Gyeonggido Business and Science Accelerator, Suwon-si 16229, Korea; choiyh1400@gbsa.or.kr
4. Convergence Research Center for Dementia, KIST, Seoul 02792, Korea
5. Department of Food Science and Nutrition, Pukyong National University, Busan 48513, Korea; bong3257@pknu.ac.kr
6. Department of Neuroscience, Pomona College, Claremont, CA 91711, USA; rmaa2018@mymail.pomona.edu
7. Korea Research Institute of Chemical Technology, Daejeon 34122, Korea; syryu@krict.re.kr
* Correspondence: cwchoi78@gmail.com (C.W.C.); minsoo.kim@kist.re.kr (M.S.K.)
† These authors contributed equally to this work.

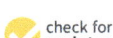

Citation: Hong, Y.; Choi, Y.-H.; Han, Y.-E.; Oh, S.-J.; Lee, A.; Lee, B.; Magnan, R.; Ryu, S.Y.; Choi, C.W.; Kim, M.S. Central Administration of Ampelopsin A Isolated from *Vitis vinifera* Ameliorates Cognitive and Memory Function in a Scopolamine-Induced Dementia Model. *Antioxidants* **2021**, *10*, 835. https://doi.org/10.3390/antiox10060835

Academic Editors: Rui F. M. Silva and Lea Pogačnik

Received: 24 April 2021
Accepted: 19 May 2021
Published: 24 May 2021

Publisher's Note: MDPI stays neutral with regard to jurisdictional claims in published maps and institutional affiliations.

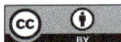

Copyright: © 2021 by the authors. Licensee MDPI, Basel, Switzerland. This article is an open access article distributed under the terms and conditions of the Creative Commons Attribution (CC BY) license (https://creativecommons.org/licenses/by/4.0/).

Abstract: Neurodegenerative diseases are characterized by the progressive degeneration of the function of the central nervous system or peripheral nervous system and the decline of cognition and memory abilities. The dysfunctions of the cognitive and memory battery are closely related to inhibitions of neurotrophic factor (BDNF) and brain-derived cAMP response element-binding protein (CREB) to associate with the cholinergic system and long-term potentiation. *Vitis vinifera*, the common grapevine, is viewed as the important dietary source of stilbenoids, particularly the widely-studied monomeric resveratrol to be used as a natural compound with wide-ranging therapeutic benefits on neurodegenerative diseases. Here we found that ampelopsin A is a major compound in *V. vinifera* and it has neuroprotective effects on experimental animals. Bath application of ampelopsin A (10 ng/µL) restores the long-term potentiation (LTP) impairment induced by scopolamine (100 µM) in hippocampal CA3-CA1 synapses. Based on these results, we administered the ampelopsin A (10 ng/µL, three times a week) into the third ventricle of the brain in C57BL/6 mice for a month. Chronic administration of ampelopsin A into the brain ameliorated cognitive memory-behaviors in mice given scopolamine (0.8 mg/kg, i.p.). Studies of mice's hippocampi showed that the response of ampelopsin A was responsible for the restoration of the cholinergic deficits and molecular signal cascades via BDNF/CREB pathways. In conclusion, the central administration of ampelopsin A contributes to increasing neurocognitive and neuroprotective effects on intrinsic neuronal excitability and behaviors, partly through elevated BDNF/CREB-related signaling.

Keywords: ampelopsin A; *Vitis vinifera*; memory behavioral tests; long-term potentiation; CREB/BDNF signals

1. Introduction

Alzheimer's disease (AD) is the most common neurodegenerative disease with progressive memory loss and cognitive decline in the elderly [1]. The pathological hallmarks of AD include amyloid-β protein accumulation, tau protein aggregation, excessive oxidative stress, and cholinergic dysfunction [2]. Cholinergic circuits have been implicated in cognitive functioning, especially in hippocampus-dependent memory formation, through the modulation of hippocampal synaptic plasticity and transmission [3]. Several studies revealed that deficits in cholinergic signaling, including cholinergic neurons, acetylcholine (ACh), and its receptors were observed in the brain of AD patients [4]. Thus, acetylcholinesterase (AChE) inhibitors, such as donepezil, have become major therapeutic targets for AD treatment, by increasing the availability of ACh at cholinergic synapses within a short period [5]. However, the benefits of current treatments remain controversial due to their lack of efficacy and critical side-effect for long-term use [6].

Scopolamine is a competitive antagonist of ACh at muscarinic receptors which are the main factors underlying the learning process and memory formation by regulating hippocampal synaptic plasticity [7,8]. The scopolamine-induced memory impairment has been widely used as an experimental animal model for the screening of novel therapeutics in AD [9]. Furthermore, the scopolamine appears to be associated with a significant reduction in the expression of brain-derived neurotrophic factor (BDNF) and cAMP-response element-binding protein (CREB) coupled with BDNF activation in the hippocampus [10]. CREB modulates memory formation, consolidation, and long-term memory persistence by positively controlling BDNF expression in the hippocampus [11,12]. Thus, the CREB/BDNF signaling pathways have been suggested as a potential target for the prevention of AD [13].

V. vinifera, the common grapevine, is viewed as the important dietary source of stilbenoids, particularly the widely-studied monomeric resveratrol [14]. Resveratrol has emerged as a natural compound with wide-ranging therapeutic benefits on cancer, cardiovascular, inflammatory, metabolic, and neurodegenerative diseases [15]. Even though resveratrol can be naturally oligomerized to achieve enhanced bioactivity with better potency and selectivity, less attention has been paid to resveratrol oligomers [16,17]. Resveratrol oligomers such as the ampelopsin A have shown promise in the treatment of AD by the interference of neurodegenerative processes, including amyloid cascade, α-synuclein cascade, oxidative damage, and cytotoxicity [18–20]. Furthermore, some stilbenoids were assessed for their anti-AChE activity and appeared to be potent AChE inhibitors from natural sources [21–23]. Among stilbenoids from extracts of *V. vinifera*, resveratrol and ampelopsin A exhibited more potent anti-amyloidogenic activity than the others [24]. Despite these findings, there is limited evidence evaluating the in vivo neuropharmacological activities of ampelopsin A. Thus, we primarily focused on the anti-amnesic potential of ampelopsin A in the scopolamine-injected mice with memory impairment. The actions of ampelopsin A were further examined at the molecular level by assessing the activity of the cholinergic system as well as the expression of CREB/BDNF signals in the hippocampus.

2. Materials and Methods
2.1. General Procedures and Plant Material

Proton nuclear magnetic resonance (^{1}H-NMR), and carbon nuclear magnetic resonance (^{13}C-NMR) spectra were performed on a Bruker (Rheinstetten, Germany) AM 300 NMR spectrometer using TMS as an internal standard. Column chromatography was conducted using a Silica gel 60 (70~230 mesh, Merck KGaA, Darmstadt, Germany), ODS-A (12 nm S-7 μm, YMC GEL, Kyoto, Japan), and Preparative HPLC was performed on LC-8A (Shimadzu, Kyoto, Japan). Thin-layer chromatography analysis was performed on Silica gel 60 F_{254} (Merck KGaA, Darmstadt, Germany) and spots were detected under a UV lamp followed by a 10% H_2SO_4 reagent. The stem bark of *V. vinifera* was harvested in October 2020 from the vineyard, Hwaseong-si, Gyeonggido, Korea. A voucher specimen (G095) was deposited at the Bio-center, Gyeonggi Institute of Science and Technology Promotion, Suwon, South Korea.

2.2. Spectroscopy of Isolated Ampelopsin A from the Stem Bark of V. vinifera

Brown amorphous powder; ^{1}H NMR (300 MHz, acetone-d_6) δ: 7.09 (2H, d, *J* = 8.8, H-2′, 6′), 6.88 (2H, d, *J* = 8.3 Hz, H-2, -6), 6.75 (2H, d, *J* = 8.8 Hz, H-3′, 5′), 6.64 (1H, d, *J* = 1.9 Hz, H-14), 6.62 (2H, d, *J* = 8.3 Hz, H-3, 5), 6.42 (1H, d, *J* = 2.5 Hz, H-12′), 6.21 (1H, br s, H-14′), 6.14 (1H, br d, *J* = 1.9 Hz, H-12), 5.45 (1H, d, *J* = 4.9 Hz, H-7), 5.42 (1H, br d,

J = 4.9 Hz, H-8), 5.42 (1H, d, J = 11.3 Hz, H-7′), 4.15 (1H, br d, J = 11.3 Hz, H-8′); ^{13}C NMR (75 MHz, acetone-d_6) δ: 159.5 (C-9), 158.3 (C-11), 158.3 (C-13′), 157.9 (C-2′, 6′), 156.7 (C-11′), 155.5 (C-9′), 142.5 (C-9′), 139.8 (C-7), 132.0 (C-13), 130.3 (C-1), 129.3 (C-14), 129.3 (C-3, 5), 128.1 (C-2), 118.3 (C-8), 117.7 (C-10′), 115.4 (C-1′), 115.4 (C-4′), 114.9 (C-3), 109.9 (C-12), 104.9 (C-14′), 100.9 (C-12′), 96.5 (C-10), 87.8 (C-7′), 70.6 (C-6), 48.9 (C-8′), 43.3 (C-5). ESI-MS (positive ion mode): m/z 471 [M + H]$^+$.

2.3. Slice Preparation and Electrophysiology

Young adult mice (C57BL/6J, age 5–6 weeks) were anesthetized with isoflurane. The brain was quickly removed and immersed in an ice-cold oxygenated high-magnesium artificial cerebral spinal fluid (aCSF) composed of (mM): 130 NaCl, 24 NaHCO$_3$, 3.5 KCl, 1.25 NaH$_2$PO$_4$, 1 CaCl$_2$, 3 MgCl$_2$, and 10 glucose saturated with 95% O$_2$ and 5% CO$_2$, at pH 7.4. The brain was attached to the stage of a vibratome (DSK Linear Slicer PRO 7, Dosaka EM, Kyoto, Japan) and 300 μm thickness of transverse slices were cut and recovered in an incubation chamber at room temperature for one hour before recording, in standard oxygenated aCSF composed of (mM): 130 NaCl, 24 NaHCO$_3$, 3.5 KCl, 1.25 NaH$_2$PO$_4$, 1.5 CaCl$_2$, 1.5 MgCl$_2$, and 10 glucose saturated with 95% O$_2$ and 5% CO$_2$, at pH 7.4. Slices were placed on the microscope stage and superfused with oxygenated aCSF at room temperature. Whole-cell patch recordings were obtained from CA1 pyramidal neurons in voltage-clamp configuration using a Multiclamp700b (Molecular Devices, Sunnyvale, CA, USA) and a borosilicate patch pipette of 5–7 MΩ resistance. The internal pipette solution for voltage-clamp recordings consisted of (mM): 140 Cs-MeSO$_4$, 10 HEPES, 7 NaCl, 4 Mg-ATP, and 0.3 Na$_3$-GTP with 1 mM QX314. All neurons included in this study have a resting membrane potential below −55 mV, had an access resistance in 10–20 MΩ, and showed only minimal variation during the recordings. Records were filtered at 2 kHz and digitized at 10 kHz using a Digidata1322A (Molecular Devices, CA, USA). The evoked excitatory postsynaptic current (eEPSCs) was recorded by applying 100 μs current injection (1–200 μA) to a bipolar stimulating electrode placed in the CA1 stratum radiatum of schaffer collateral pathway and analyzed using pCLAMP10 software (Axon Instruments, Burlingame, CA, USA). For LTP recordings, electrical stimulations were given as theta-burst stimulation, consisting of 3 trains containing 4 pulses 15 bursts (each with 4 pulses at 100 Hz) of stimuli delivered every 200 ms.

2.4. Animals

Male C57BL/6J mice (8 weeks old; 25–30 g) were purchased from Orient Bio Inc. (Seungnam, Korea). The animals were housed in a room with constant temperature (23 ± 1 °C) and humidity (50 ± 10%) under a 12 h light/dark cycle, and were fed with food and water ad libitum. The experimental procedure was approved by the Institutional Animal Care and Use Committee (IACUC Approval No. KIST-2020-014) and the Institutional Biosafety Committee (IBC), and was conducted in accordance with relevant guidelines and regulation of the IACUC and the IBC in the Korea Institute of Science and Technology (KIST).

2.5. Surgical Procedure and Treatments

After one week of acclimatization, mice underwent stereotaxic surgery for implantation of a cannula in the brain as previously described [25]. Using a stereotaxic frame (Kopf Instruments, Tujunga, CA, USA), a 26-gauge guide cannula (Plastics One, Roanoke, VA, USA) was inserted into the third-ventricle (3 V, coordinates: 2.0 mm posterior to the bregma, 5.3 mm below the surface of skull). Following a week recovery period, mice were randomly divided into three groups (n = 5 per group): control (Con, PBS as a vehicle), scopolamine + vehicle (Scop + Veh, PBS as a vehicle), and scopolamine+ampelopsin A (Scop + AmpA) pretreatment group. All groups were administrated three times a week with either 0.5 μL of phosphate-buffered saline (PBS, as a vehicle) or 0.5 μL ampelopsin A (10 ng/μL, dissolved in PBS) for one month. One month later, scopolamine + vehicle (Scop + Veh) and scopolamine + ampelopsin A (Scop + AmpA) pretreatment groups received 0.8 mg/kg scopolamine ((-)-scopolamine hydrobromide trihydrate, dissolved in 0.9% saline, i.p.) and the control group was injected with 0.9% saline (i.p.) before each behavioral test. The experimental schedule of chemical administration and behavioral tests is shown in Figure 3a.

2.6. Behavioral Tests

All behavioral tests were performed in the behavior testing room. An Anymaze video-tracking system (Stoelting) equipped with a digital camera connected to a computer was used. Following behavioral tests, open field (locomotion), novel object recognition, and passive avoidance were conducted. The study was carried out in compliance with the ARRIVE guidelines. During the behavioral tests, mice were centrally administered PBS or ampelopsin A before every behavioral test, including habituation and test session (60 min before). Subsequently, mice were treated (i.p.) with saline or scopolamine before every behavioral test (30 min before).

2.6.1. Open Field Test

The open-field test (locomotion) was performed as previously described with slight modifications [26]. Specifically, the mouse was located in the center of an open field chamber (40 cm length × 40 cm width × 50 cm height) and was habituated for 20 min. Each mouse was replaced in the same chamber 24 h later. The movements of the mouse were recorded for 10 min and then analyzed via a digital camera connected to the Any-Maze animal tracking system software (Stoelting, Wood Dale, IL, USA). The total distance moved (meters) and the time (seconds) spent in the center/outer of the open field were measured.

2.6.2. Novel Object Recognition Test

The novel object recognition test was performed as described in the previous study [27]. Specifically, the mouse was located in a square arena (40 cm length × 40 cm width × 50 cm height) equipped with a digital camera and was allowed to familiarize with the environment for 10 min before the test. During the first session (familiarization session), two identical objects were put against the center of the opposite wall and the mouse was allowed to explore the objects for 20 min. During the second session (test session), one of the identical objects was replaced by a novel object, and the mouse was allowed to explore the objects for 10 min. In the familiarization session, the mouse contacted with two yellow square-based pyramids(8 cm × 8 cm × 6.5 cm) while in the test session it was with a yellow cube (7 cm × 7 cm × 7 cm) and a yellow square-based pyramid. The amount of time that the mouse spent exploring each object was monitored and analyzed using an ANY-maze video-tracking system (Stoelting, USA). A discrimination index was calculated as (novel − familiar object exploration time)/(novel + familiar object exploration time).

2.6.3. Passive Avoidance Test

The passive avoidance test was performed as previously described [28] using an Avoidance System (B.S Technolab INC., Seoul, Korea). The apparatus (48 cm length × 23 cm width × 28 cm height) consisted of light and dark chambers separated by a gate. On the first day, the mouse was allowed to explore both compartments freely for 10 min. On the following day (training), the mouse was placed in the light compartment and 60 s later the gate was opened. Once the mouse entered the dark compartment, the door was closed and an electrical foot shock (0.3 mA, 3 s) was delivered through the floor. After 24 h (probe trial), the mouse was placed again in the light compartment and then the gate was lifted 60 s later. The step-through latency, or time taken for the mouse to enter the dark compartment, was scored 300 s as the upper limit.

2.7. ChAT Activity

The Choline Acetyltransferase (ChAT) activity in the hippocampus was determined using ChAT Activity Assay Kit (Elabscience, Huston, TX, USA) according to the manufacturer's protocol. Absorbance at 324 nm was measured using a Tecan Infinite 200 microplate reader (Tecan, Männedorf, Switzerland). Enzyme activity was calculated using the following formula: Enzyme activity: (unit/mg protein) = [(ΔA324)/ $\times$ 16.6]/(1.98 $\times$ 10^{-5} nM^{-1} cm^{-1} $\times$ 24)/[protein concentration (mg/mL)]. Protein concentrations were assayed using a Quick Start Bradford Protein Assay kit (Bio-Rad, Hercules, CA, USA).

2.8. Ach Level and AChE Activity

The part of the hippocampus was homogenized on ice using RIPA buffer (Merck KGaA, Darmstadt, Germany) and the homogenates were centrifuged at 16,000$\times$ g for 20 min, then the supernatant was collected to analyze acetylcholine (Ach) level and acetylcholinesterase (AChE) activity using an Amplex Red Ach/AChE Assay Kit (Invitrogen, Waltham, MA, USA) in accordance with the manufacturer's protocol. Absorbance at 563 nm was measured using a Tecan Infinite 200 microplate reader (Tecan, Männedorf, Switzerland). Hippocampal Ach level and AChE activity were calculated from a standard curve.

2.9. Quantitative Real-Time PCR Analysis

The total RNA from the hippocampus tissue was extracted using Trizol reagent (Invitrogen Life Technologies, Waltham, MA, USA) and cDNA synthesized using a SuperScript III First-Strand Synthesis System for RT-PCR (Invitrogen, Waltham, MA, USA) according to the manufacturer's instructions. Complementary DNA amplification was performed using Power SYBR Green PCR Master Mix kit (Applied Biosystems, Waltham, MA, USA) and primers with the following sequences: *Bdnf* (NM_007540), 5'-TCATACTTCGGTTGCATGA AGG-3' and 5'-AGACCTCTCGAACCTGCCC-3'; *TrkB* (NM_001025074), 5'-CTGGGGCTTA TGCCTGCTG-3' and 5'- AGGCTCAGTACACCAAATCCTA-3'; *Akt1* (NM_001165894), 5'-ATGAACGACGTAGCCATTGTG-3' and 5'-TTGTAGCCAATAAAGGTGCCAT-3'; *Creb1* (NM_009952), 5'-AGCAGCTCATGCAACATCATC-3' and 5'-AGTCCTTACAGGAAGACTG AACT-3'; *iNOS* (NM_010927), 5'-GGCAGCCTGTGAGACCTTTG-3' and 5'-TGCATTG GAAGTGAAGCGTTT-3'; *Chrm1* (NM_001112697), 5'-AGTGGCATTCATCGGGATCA-3' and 5'-CTTGAGCTCTGTGTTGACCTTGA-3'; *Ache* (NM_009599), 5'-AGAAAATATTGCAG CCTTTG-3' and 5'-CTGCAGGTCTTGAAAATCTC-3'; *CaMK2* (NM_177407), 5'-GAATCTGC CGTCTCTTGAA-3' and 5'-TCTCTTGCCACTATGTCTTC-3'; *Bcl2* (NM_177410), 5'-AGCTGC ACCTGACGCCCTT-3' and 5'-GTTCAGGTACTCAGTCATCCAC-3'; *Bax* (NM_007527),5'-CGGCGAATTGGAGATGAACTG-3' and 5'-GCAAAGTAGAAGAGGGCAACC-3'; *Actb* (NM_007393), 5'-GGCTGTATTCCCCTCCATCG-3' and 5'-CCAGTTGGTAACAATGCCATG T-3'. The StepOne Real-Time PCR System (Applied Biosystems, Waltham, MA, USA) for quantitative PCR (qPCR) was used for quantitative real-time PCR. PCR results were normalized to those of the control genes encoding β-actin (*Actb*).

2.10. Western Blot Analysis

The part of the hippocampus was homogenized on ice using RIPA buffer (Sigma, Germany) and the homogenates were centrifuged at 16,000$\times$ g for 20 min, then the supernatant was collected. The protein concentration was determined as mentioned above. 30 µg of proteins were separated by 10% polyacrylamide gel electrophoresis and transferred to PVDF membranes (Millipore, Burlington, MA, USA). After blocking in 5% skim milk, the membrane was incubated with rabbit anti-BDNF (1:800, Abcam, Cambridge, UK), rabbit anti-phospho CREB (pCREB; 1:2000, Abcam, Cambridge, UK), mouse anti-CREB (1:1000, Invitrogen, Waltham, MA, USA), and mouse anti- β-actin (1:1000, Cell Signaling Technology, Danvers, MA, USA) overnight at 4 °C. The membranes were washed and incubated for 1 h with HRP conjugated anti-rabbit (Abcam, Cambridge, UK) or anti-mouse IgG antibody (Enzo Life Sciences, Farmingdale, NY, USA). The bands were visualized using Image Quant LAS 4000 (GE Healthcare, Chicago, IL, USA) with ECL reagent (Amersham, Little Chalfont, UK), and the intensity was quantified using Image J software (National Institutes of Health, Bethesda, MD, USA).

2.11. Statistical Analysis

Experimental values were shown as mean ± standard error of the mean (S.E.M.) and evaluated with one-way ANOVA followed by Dunnett's test. The statistical analysis was performed using the GraphPad PRISM software (GraphPad Prism Software Inc., version 8, San Diego, CA, USA). *p*-values of <0.05 were deemed significant.

3. Results

3.1. Isolation and Determination of Compound from the Stem Bark of V. vinifera

The stem bark of *V. vinifera* (3.0 kg) was extracted twice with 15 L of 70% ethanol (EtOH) by two times at room temperature (each time for 2 days). After filtration with a cotton ball, the filtrate was combined and evaporated to dryness to give 221.4 g of dark syrupy extract. The extracts were suspended in distilled water and then partitioned CH_2Cl_2 (5.0 L × 3), EtOAc (5.0 L × 3), and n-butanol (5.0 L × 3) to give CH_2Cl_2 (69.1 g), EtOAc (140.3 g), n-butanol (1.5 g), and water-soluble fractions (2.1 g), (Figure 1a). The EtOAc soluble fraction was subjected to silica gel (2.0 kg) column (10 × 60 cm) chromatography, eluted with MeOH in CH_2Cl_2 in a step-gradient manner from 1% to 50% to give six fractions (F1: 11.0 g, F2: 13.3 g, F3: 9.4 g, F4: 65.3 g, F5: 13.1 g, and F6: 36.7 g). Fraction F3 (9.4 g) was separated by MPLC chromatography that used gradient mixtures as eluents (F31–F38). F34 was also purified in a similar manner with RP-18 preparative HPLC eluted with MeOH in H_2O (1% to 100%) in a stepwise gradient, which finally gave 8.2 mg of compound (Purity 97% in HPLC). The molecular formula of the compound was confirmed by Mass spectrum as $C_{28}H_{20}O_7$, consisting of 19 degrees of unsaturation (Figure 1c). The ^{1}H-NMR spectrum of the compound indicated five pairs of peaks. Two pairs appeared at δ 6.88/6.62 and 7.09/6.75, each peak with characteristic *ortho* and *meta* couplings; Each peak has an integral value of two. They were assigned to the protons of two *para*-disubstituted aromatic rings, A and A'. Two other pairs resonating at δ 6.64/6.14 and 6.42/6.21 were assigned as meta protons on two tetra substituted aromatic rings, B and B' (Figure 1b). With the above data and comparison with literature [29], the compound was identified as ampelopsin A.

3.2. Bath Application of Ampelopsin A Increases the Neuronal Excitability of Hippocampal Neurons

Long-term potentiation (LTP) is a long-lasting increase of postsynaptic responses following electrical stimulation such as theta-burst stimulation (TBS) or a brief, high-frequency stimulation (HFS), leading to an enhancement in the strength of excitatory synaptic transmission and it is considered the generally studied form for examining the synaptic mechanism of learning and memory in the brain [30,31]. We examined whether the bath application of ampelopsin A to the brain rescues the scopolamine-induced deficit in hippocampal LTP. For the measurement of hippocampal LTP, a single dose of ampelopsin A (10 ng/μL) was applied to the hippocampal slices which were perfused with artificial cerebrospinal fluid (aCSF) containing either DMSO vehicle or scopolamine (100 μM) during the baseline recording and for an additional 20 min after LTP induction. In control mice, TBS (consisting of 3 trains containing 4 pulses 15 bursts) induces a robust increase in the percentage of normalized excitatory postsynaptic current (EPSC) (Figure 2a). Scopolamine treatment markedly decreased the mean of normalized EPSC relative to the control group (Figure 2b, $p < 0.05$). In the scopolamine and ampelopsin A combined treatment group, the mean of normalized EPSC significantly increased relative to the scopolamine only treatment group ($p < 0.05$).

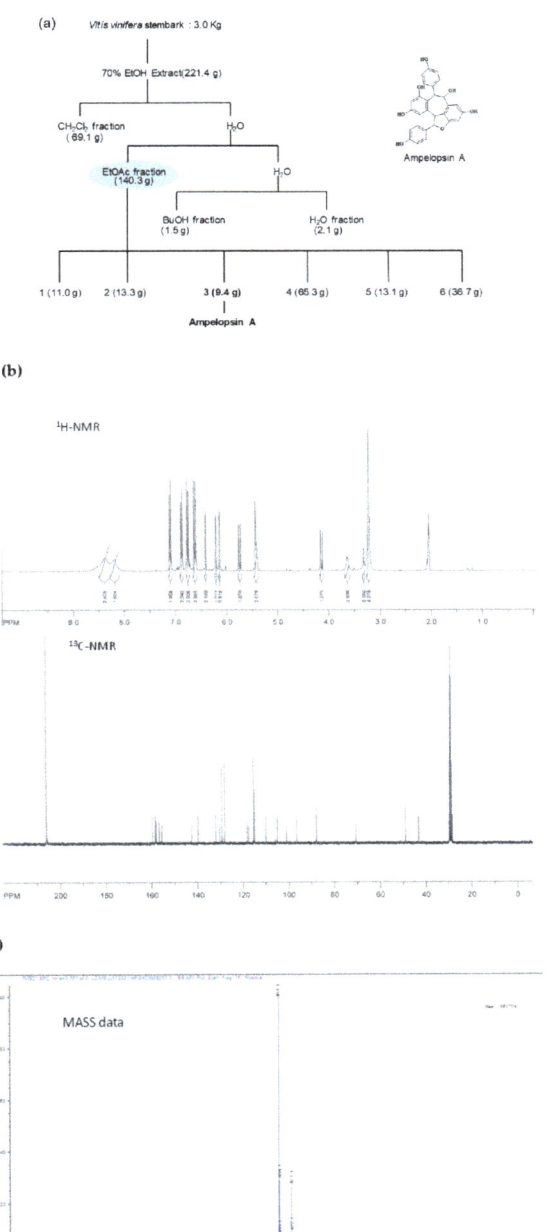

Figure 1. Isolation and structural analysis of ampelopsin A isolated from *V. vinifera*. (**a**) Extraction and purification procedures of ampelopsin A from stembark of *V. vinifera* and its molecular structure. (**b**) ^{1}H-NMR and ^{13}C-NMR (300 MHz, acetone-d_6) spectrums of ampelopsin A from stembark of *V. vinifera*, (**c**) Mass spectrum of ampelopsin A from stembark of *V. vinifera*.

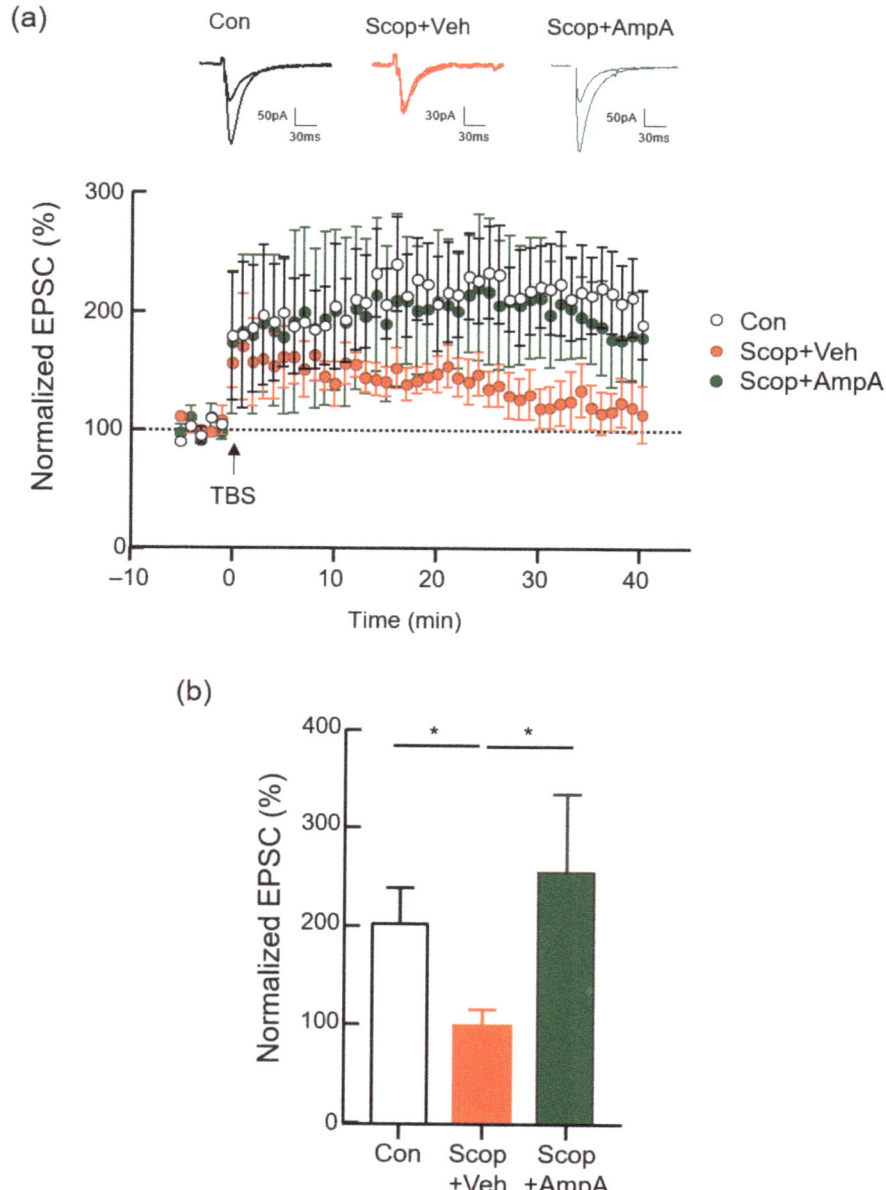

Figure 2. Protective effect of ampelopsin A in hippocampal LTP. A change in the EPSC slope was monitored following LTP induction by theta-burst stimulation (TBS) at SC-CA1 synapses in the hippocampus. The magnitude of LTP was quantified as an increase in the EPSC amplitude relative to the baseline. (**a**) Averaged traces of normalized EPSC amplitude in control, scopolamine (100 μM) with DMSO vehicle, and scopolamine with ampelopsin A (10 ng/μL) group (scale bars, 30 pA or 50 pA, 30 ms). Scopolamine with DMSO or ampelopsin A was treated during the baseline recording and for an additional 20 min after LTP induction by bath application. (**b**) Bar graph of the means for the normalized EPSC amplitude recorded last 5 min, calculated from the data in Figure 2a. Values are expressed as means ± SEM ($n = 4$). * $p < 0.05$; one-way ANOVA with Kruskal-Wallis test with Dunnett's multiple comparisons test.

3.3. Administration of Ampelopsin A into the 3 V Increased Cognitive Memory Behaviors

Based on the rescue effects of ampelopin A in EPSC measurements, we tried to figure out whether central administration of ampeopsin A restores cognition and memory function of the animals which are impaired by scopolamine injection. We designed the experimental schedules (Figure 3a) and conducted stereotaxic surgery on animals which were implanted cannulas into the third ventricle of the brain. We applied the same dose of ampeopsin A (10 ng/µL) via a cannula into the third ventricle of the experimental animals for one month while other animals were applied the PBS as a vehicle in the same way. After this pre-treatment of ampelopsin A (AmpA) over one month, we injected scopolamine (Scop, 0.8 mg/kg, i.p.) into Scop + Veh (pre-treatments of a vehicle then injected the scopolamine) and Scop + AmpA (pre-treatment of ampeopsin A then injected the scopolamine) group before each behavioral test (30 min before).

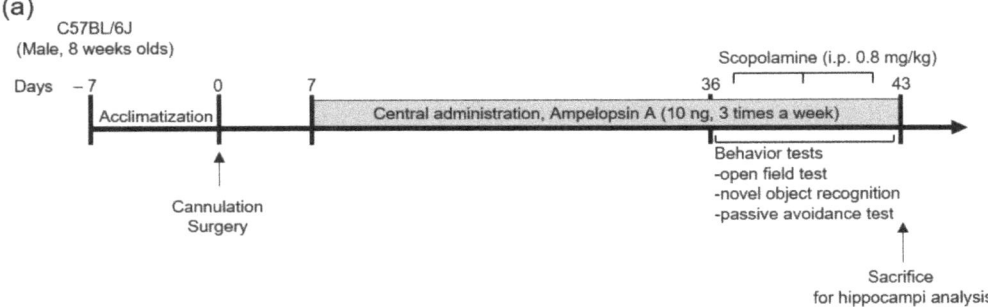

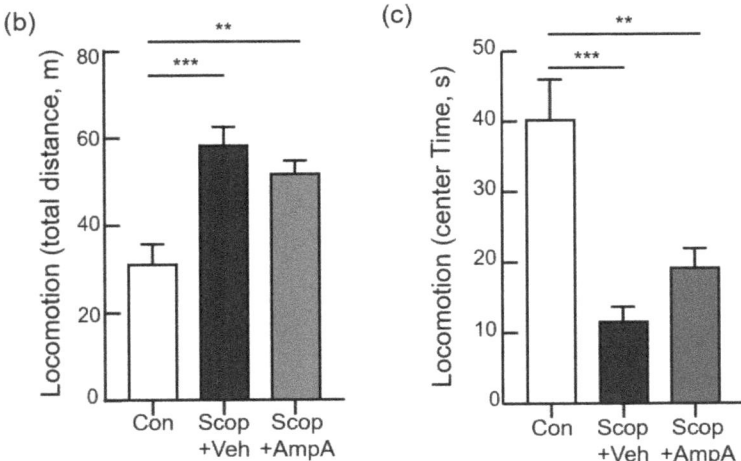

Figure 3. Central administration of ampelopsin A changes the locomotion. Male C57BL/6J mice (10 weeks old) were given 0.5 µL ampelopsin A (10 ng/µL, three times a week) or the same volume of the vehicle (PBS) via the third-ventricle of the brain for one month. 30 min before the behavioral tests, scopolamine (0.8 mg/kg, i.p.) was administered to each group; Scop + Veh (pre-treatment of PBS as a vehicle, scopolamine injection on the experimental day) and Scop + AmpA (pre-treatment of ampelopsin A, scopolamine injection on the experimental day) groups. The control group (Con) was pre-treated with the vehicle into 3 V then was injected PBS (i.p.) instead of scopolamine on the experimental day. (**a**) The schematic timeline of the experiments. (**b**) Total distance and (**c**) time spent exploring the center zone were measured by an open field test (locomotion). Values are expressed as means ± SEM ($n = 5$). ** $p < 0.01$, *** $p < 0.001$; one-way ANOVA with Dunnett's multiple comparisons test.

3.3.1. Open Field Test

An open field test performed before other behavioral analyses ensured that scopolamine worked properly by using its anxiogenic [32] and locomotor stimulant properties [33]. In the open field test, the scopolamine-injected group (Scop + Veh) showed significantly increased total distance traveled by the mice and shortened the time spent in the center zone compared with the control group (Figure 3b, $F_{(2,12)}$ = 12.64 and Figure 3c, $F_{(2,12)}$ = 14.71, $p < 0.001$). In addition, no significant differences were observed between the Scop + Veh group and Scop + AmpA group. It reveals that ampelopsin A was not associated with anxiety and hyper locomotion caused by scopolamine.

3.3.2. Novel Object Recognition Test

We conducted a novel object recognition test and passive avoidance test to confirm the restoration of cognition and memory abilities by the administration of ampelopsin A in memory-impaired models. The time spent with the novel object divided by the total time devoted to exploring both objects, expressed as the discrimination index, was shortened in the Scop + Veh groups than the control group (Figure 4a). However, the Scop + AmpA group markedly increased the discrimination index, indicating that ampelopsin A treatment ameliorated scopolamine-induced recognition memory impairment ($F_{(2,12)}$ = 4.811, $p < 0.05$).

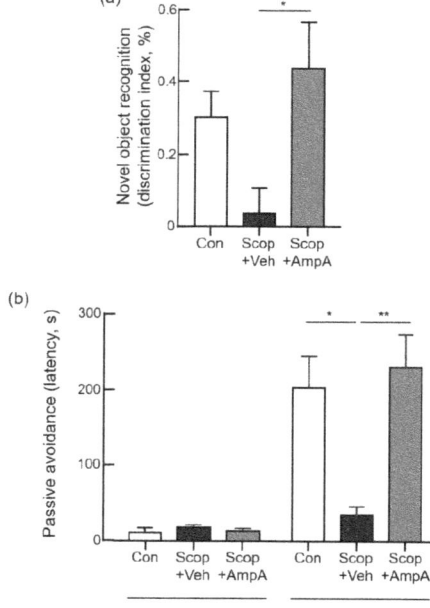

Figure 4. Central administration of ampelopsin A improves cognitive memory behaviors. Male C57BL/6J mice (10 weeks old) were given 0.5 μL ampelopsin A (10 ng/μL, three times a week) or the same volume of the vehicle (PBS) via the third-ventricle of the brain for one month. 30 min before the behavioral tests, scopolamine (0.8 mg/kg, i.p.) was administered to each group; Scop + Veh (pre-treatment of PBS as a vehicle, scopolamine injection on the experimental day) and Scop + AmpA (pre-treatment of ampelopsin A, scopolamine injection on the experimental day) groups. The control group (Con) was pre-treated with the vehicle into 3 V then was injected PBS (i.p.) instead of scopolamine on the experimental day. In the novel object recognition test (**a**), the discrimination index showed the percent time spent with the novel object. In the passive avoidance test (**b**), mice were trained that once the mouse entered the dark compartment, the door was closed, and an electrical foot shock (0.3 mA, 3 s) was delivered through the floor (training session). After 24 h, the moving time to a darkened chamber in a shock-motivated was recorded as a latency time in the test session. Values are expressed as means ± SEM ($n = 5$). * $p < 0.05$, ** $p < 0.01$; one-way ANOVA with Dunnett's multiple comparisons test.

3.3.3. Passive Avoidance Test

In the step-through passive avoidance test, during the training trial, step-through latency was statistically the same amongst all the groups (Figure 4b, $F_{(2,12)} = 0.8304$, $p = 0.459$). The Scop + Veh group showed a significant decrease in step-through latency in comparison with the control group ($F_{(2,12)} = 8.671$, $p < 0.005$). A significant increase of step-through latency was presented in the Scop + AmpA group, suggesting that ampelopsin A recovered scopolamine-induced memory impairment in the experimental animals. Interestingly, the Scop + AmpA group showed similar levels with the control group. It means that scopolamine impairments did not work on memory dysfunction by chronic treatments of ampelopsin A.

3.4. Administration of Ampelopsin A Ameliorates Cholinergic Dysfunction

To elucidate the possible molecular mechanisms of ampelopsin A, the levels of acetylcholine and the activities of choline acetyltransferase and acetylcholinesterase that are involved in the acetylcholine metabolism were measured. The hippocampi of mice given scopolamine significantly decreased acetylcholine (ACh) contents and the levels of choline acetyltransferase (ChAT) were reduced by the scopolamine injection. These levels of the ACh and ChAT were recovered in the Scop+AmpA groups (Figure 5a, $F_{(2,9)} = 4.602$, $p < 0.05$ and Figure 5b, $F_{(2,9)} = 1.308$). In contrast, the levels of acetylcholinesterase (AChE) activities were increased in the Scop + Veh groups but significantly decreased in the Scop + AmpA groups (Figure 5c, $F_{(2,9)} = 4.602$, $p < 0.05$). We also measured gene expressions of muscarinic acetylcholine receptor (*Chrm1*, $F_{(2,9)} = 2.935$) and the acetylcholinesterase (*Ache*, $F_{(2,10)} = 6.650$, $p < 0.05$). These genes were also changed by the central administration of ampelopsin A (Figure 5d).

3.5. Administration of Amplopsin A Elevates BDNF-Related Signaling in the Hippocampus

To further elucidate the underlying molecular mechanisms of ampelopsin A, the mRNA and protein expression of CREB/BDNF-related signaling were determined. The CREB1 ($F_{(2,9)} = 11.30$, $p < 0.001$), BDNF ($F_{(2,9)} = 5.912$, $p < 0.05$), CaMK2 ($F_{(2,9)} = 4.285$, $p < 0.05$), Akt ($F_{(2,9)} = 6.626$, $p < 0.05$), and TrkB ($F_{(2,10)} = 7.323$, $p < 0.05$) mRNA levels were significantly down-regulated by the Scop + Veh group compared with the control group but were up-regulated in the Scop + AmpA group (Figure 6a). Consistently, scopolamine injection decreased protein levels of BDNF and phosphorylation of CREB in the hippocampus, and the administration of ampelopsin A effectively increased BDNF and pCREB protein levels compared with the administration of scopolamine (Figure 6c, $F_{(2,9)} = 8.8$, $p < 0.01$ and Figure 5d, $F_{(2,9)} = 4.772$, $p < 0.05$).

3.6. Antioxidant and Anti-Apoptotic Effects on the Hippocampus by Ampelopsin A

Ampelopsin has been known to have antioxidant and anti-apoptotic activities [34,35]. We examined whether central administration of ampelopsin A is responsible for antioxidant and anti-apoptotic effects. The Scop + Veh group significantly increased the mRNA levels of iNOS compared with the control group. This increase was attenuated when ampelopsin A was administrated (Figure 6b, $F_{(2,12)} = 7.658$, $p < 0.01$). We measured pro-apoptotic and anti-apoptotic effects by the treatments of ampelopsin A. The Scop + Veh group showed a significant increase of Bax ($F_{(2,12)} = 7.658$, $p < 0.01$) as a pro-apoptotic marker, then it was attenuated by the treatment of ampelopsin A. In contrast, anti-apoptotic Bcl-2 expression altered its expression ($F_{(2,10)} = 6.662$, $p < 0.05$) then was restored by the treatments of ampelopsin A. The Administration of ampelopsin A recovered apoptotic gene expression in scopolamine-injected mice. These antioxidant and anti-apoptotic effects also support neuroprotective effects of ampelopsin A administration.

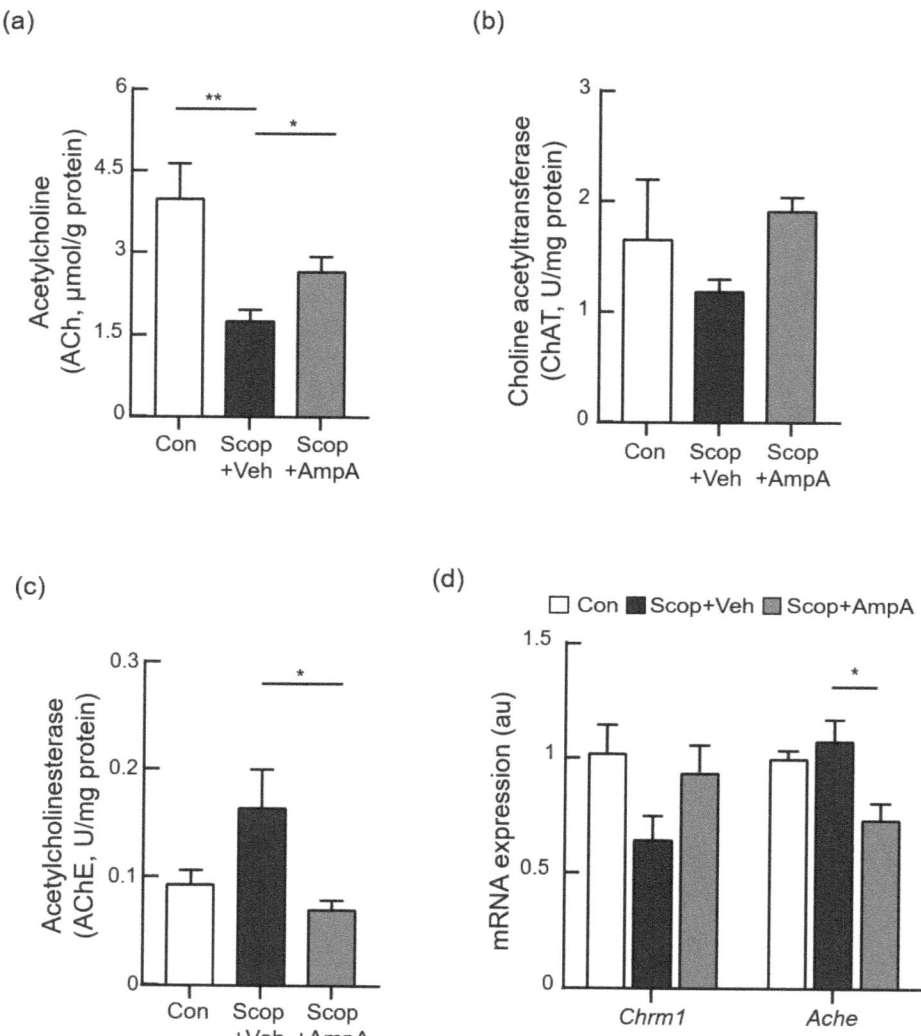

Figure 5. Inhibitory effect of ampelopsin A against scopolamine-induced cholinergic dysfunction. Male C57BL/6J mice (10 weeks old) were given 0.5 μL ampelopsin A (10 ng/μL, three times a week) or the same volume of the vehicle (PBS) via the third-ventricle of the brain for one month. Mice were sacrificed and hippocampi were isolated for measurements of cholinergic parameters and mRNA expression. 30 min before the mice sacrifice, scopolamine (0.8 mg/kg, i.p.) was administered to each group; Scop + Veh (pre-treatment of PBS as a vehicle, scopolamine injection on the experimental day) and Scop + AmpA (pre-treatment of ampelopsin A, scopolamine injection on the experimental day) groups. The control group (Con) was pre-treated with the vehicle into 3 V then was injected PBS (i.p.) instead of scopolamine on the experimental day. (**a**–**c**) Acetylcholine levels and acetylcholinesterase and choline acetyltransferase activities in the hippocampus are shown. (**d**) *Chrm1* and *Ache* mRNA levels determined by real time-PCR. Gene expression was normalized to that of β-actin. Au means the arbitrary units. Values are expressed as means ± SEM ($n = 4$). * $p < 0.05$, ** $p < 0.01$; one-way ANOVA with Dunnett's multiple comparisons test.

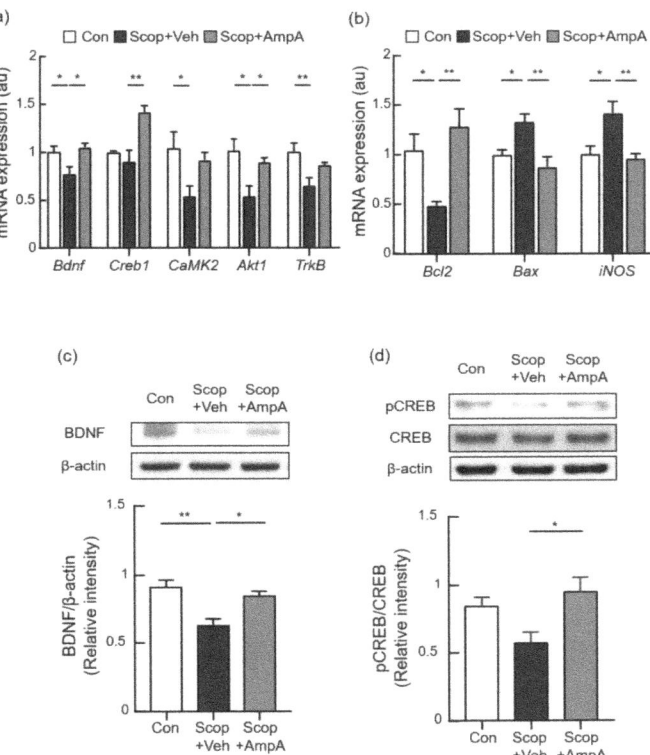

Figure 6. Increase of BDNF-related and anti-apoptotic signaling by central administration of ampelopsin A. Male C57BL/6J mice (10 weeks old) were given 0.5 μL ampelopsin A (10 ng/μL, three times a week) or the same volume of the vehicle (PBS) via the third-ventricle of the brain for one month. Mice were sacrificed and hippocampi were isolated for measurements of mRNA and protein expression. 30 min before the mice sacrifice, scopolamine (0.8 mg/kg, i.p.) was administered to each group; Scop + Veh (pre-treatment of PBS as a vehicle, scopolamine injection on the experimental day) and Scop + AmpA (pre-treatment of ampelopsin A, scopolamine injection on the experimental day) groups. The control group (Con) was pre-treated with the vehicle into 3 V then was injected PBS (i.p.) instead of scopolamine on the experimental day. (**a**) Alterations in the expression of *Bdnf*, *Creb1*, *CaMK2*, *Akt*, and *Trkb* were determined by real time-PCR ($n = 4$). (**b**) *Bcl2*, *Bax*, and *iNOS* mRNA levels determined by real time-PCR ($n = 4$–5). Gene expression was normalized to that of β-actin. Au means the arbitrary units. (**c**) Quantification of BDNF/β-actin and (**d**) phosphorylated CREB/CREB intensity ($n = 4$). Values are expressed as means ± SEM. * $p < 0.05$, ** $p < 0.01$; one-way ANOVA with Dunnett's multiple comparisons test.

4. Discussion

Resveratrol (3,5,4-trihydroxystilbene) is a naturally occurring polyphenol that has attracted the attention of many chemists and pharmacologists due to its diverse biological activities such as chemopreventive, antimicrobial, antioxidant, and anti-inflammatory actions [36–39]. Grapevine is known as an important source of resveratrol and many resveratrol derivatives [40]. The previous other studies showed that extracts, resveratrols, from *V. vinifera* stembark protected the brain cell dysfunction by inhibiting the aggregation of amyloid-β and against α-synuclein cytotoxicity [18–20]. Among these extracts, a dimer of resveratrol from *V. vinifera*, ampelopsin A, exhibited more potent anti-amyloidogenic activity than the others [24]. However, it was questionable whether ampelopsin A works on cognitive function for neuroprotective activities in the animal models. Based on the current study, it is quite clear that the brain administration (3 V) of ampleopsin A significantly improved cognitive behaviors, enhanced synaptic transmission, and the cholinergic system in scopolamine-induced memory dysfunction. The underlying mechanisms include but are not limited to the broad up-regulation of genes associated with CREB-BDNF signaling pathways.

In this study, we administrated the relatively low dose of ampelopsin A (10 ng) into the mice brain compared to other references' uses (μg or mg) [41,42]. The brain responded to this low dose of ampelopsin A to initiate neuroprotective effects in cognition and memory. In addition, we found that chronic administration of ampelopsin A efficiently improved cognition and memory functions whereas acute administration of ampelopsin A did not improve these functions in the experimental animals (data not shown). Usually, chronic treatments were considered as over 10 days to 12 weeks [41,43,44], and similar central treatments for one month showed increases in memory functions [45]. To do so, chronic (a month) and low-dose treatments of ampelopsin A contribute to a change of cognitive and memory abilities.

Cholinesterase (ChE) contributes to the short half-life of released ACh, and it terminates cholinergic neurotransmission by the hydrolysis of ACh in turn. The inhibition of ChEs expression slows down the breakdown of ACh, thereby prolonging ACh presence at synaptic cleft to stimulate their muscarinic receptors. Based on these facts, two major ChEs, AChE and butyrylcholinesterase (BuChE), have been potential targets in AD therapy [46,47]. BuChE is considered to play supportive role in the brain because AChE predominates over BuChE activity [48]. BuChE is also distributed in the hippocampus, but at lower levels than AChE which is mainly located in the synaptic cleft and synaptic membranes in normal status [49,50]. Since our study is the first study suggesting the ampelopsin A as a ChE inhibitor, we focused on the inhibitory activity of AChE as the hippocampal cholinergic mediation. As BuChE has brought much attention compensating for the action of AChE in cognitive impairment, further studies will establish the detailed influence of stilbenoids on BuChE for a beneficial feature in AD treatment [51–53].

Scopolamine, a muscarinic acetylcholine receptor antagonist, is a commonly used chemical that impairs learning and memory in animal models. Scopolamine-induced deficits in a battery of cognitive function are important for comparison of sensitivity and specificity to find therapeutic candidates for neurodegenerative diseases [54,55]. The exact mechanism of scopolamine action to ACh, ChAT, and ChE remains poorly understood. Since scopolamine has been used in the standard cognitive impairment model, there were a lot of literatures to show that the effects of scopolamine treatment can induce cognitive deficit through decreasing ACh contents and ChAT activities while increasing AChE activities in the hippocampus [10,56,57]. The stilbenoids, including ampelopsin A, have been studied as the potent AChE inhibitors for developing AD-targeting drugs [21–23]. Ampelopsin A may be considered as an AD-targeting drug by its anti-AChE activity [24]. In addition, this cholinergic system contributes to neurogenesis in the hippocampus via the CREB/BDNF signaling which is responsible for long-term memory formation [58,59]. Based on our study, administration of ampelopsin A delayed deficit of cholinergic cognitive memory and ameliorated long-term memory by restoring CREB/BDNF signaling. Therefore, ampelopsin A might be considered a strong candidate for treating AD to recover acetylcholine cascades in the hippocampus with reduced symptoms [10,60,61].

The avoidance reaction of an experimental mouse is important for the acquisition of extinction memory. In the passive avoidance test, the animal learns to avoid an unpleasant stimulus by hindering locomotion and investigation [62]. Additionally, treatments with an anti-BDNF antibody or BDNF antisense mRNA produce memory dysfunction in concurrence with a loss of LTP and ERK signaling [62–64]. To do so, the hippocampal BDNF-TrkB signaling is required for the acquisition and consolidation of conditioned fear [65,66]. In addition, hippocampus-specific deletion of BDNF lessens fear extinction, while hippocampal BDNF accelerates the acquisition of extinction memory [67]. BDNF is one of the crucial factors to form fear extinction memory [62,67,68]. Our study showed that ampelopsin A significantly increased the avoidance reaction of experimental mice and up-regulated hippocampal BDNF/CREB cascades, including BDNF, CREB1, CaMK2, Akt, and TrkB. Although cognition and memory functional mechanisms mediated by each gene may be different, these genes are closely associated with avoiding aversive stimulus in the memory regions. We assumed that ampleopsin A may stimulate BDNF-CREB signaling in the hippocampus for increases of memory function although more detailed experiments are necessary. In addition, scopolamine induces an increase in neuro-inflammation (iNOS) and apoptosis (Bax) while it inhibits anti-apoptotic factors (Bcl-2) [69]. Our study showed that ampelopsin A has neuroprotective effects by reversing molecular and cell damages released from neuroinflammation and apoptosis.

Long-term potentiation (LTP) represents a long-lasting increase in the efficacy of excitatory synaptic transmission, and it is widely used to measure a cellular mechanism of learning and memory in the brain [30,31]. Among all neurotransmitters and trophic factors, BDNF and glutamate are mostly related to memory function [62]. BDNF directly works on depolarizing neurons by enhancing glutamatergic transmission for inducing phosphorylation of NMDA receptor through its TrkB receptors [70]. The BDNF utilizes positive regulations on LTP in memory formation at the cellular level. In addition, impairment of LTP in mutant mice lacking BDNF was rescued by recombinant BDNF application [71]. The endogenous BDNF is necessary for LTP formation which comes out from presynaptic neurons and BDNF-dependent LTP formation is responsible for protein synthesis [71,72]. The BDNF mediates the translation of protein synthesis via several intracellular signaling pathways including Akt and PI3K, kinases involved in cell growth, survival, differentiation, and intracellular trafficking. Our study showed that the chronic administration of ampelopsin A into the brain rescues the scopolamine-induced deficit in hippocampal LTP through BDNF activation. The recovered capability of LTP in the brain is important for brain protection in neurodegenerative diseases. Chronic administration of ampelopsin A might be considered a therapy for neurodegenerative disease by recovering functional LTP in the brain.

5. Conclusions

The central administration of ampelopsin A ameliorates scopolamine-induced cognitive impairment in the brain. These effects of ampelopsin A might be related to restored LTP through BDNF activation.

Author Contributions: Y.H. co-designed and performed mice surgery, treatments, qPCR, behavioral tests, cholinergic experiments and prepared all figures; Y.-H.C. did LC/MS and NMR, and A.L. conducted data analysis of LC/MS and NMR; Y.-E.H. and S.-J.O. performed electrophysiology and data analysis; R.M. performed preliminary experiments about AmpA's central treatments; B.L., S.Y.R., C.W.C., and M.S.K. performed all data analysis and wrote the paper; C.W.C. and M.S.K. conceived of the hypothesis and designed the project, and all authors participated in discussions. All authors have read and agreed to the published version of the manuscript.

Funding: This work was supported by the Bio and Medical Technology Development Program of National Research Foundation (NRF) funded by the Ministry of Science and ICT (NRF-2020M3A9D8039920 and NRF-2018M3C7A1056897).

Institutional Review Board Statement: The experimental procedure was approved by the Institutional Animal Care and Use Committee (IACUC Approval No. KIST-2020-014) and the Institutional Biosafety Committee (IBC), and was conducted in accordance with relevant guidelines and regulation of the IACUC and the IBC in the Korea Institute of Science and Technology (KIST).

Informed Consent Statement: Not applicable.

Data Availability Statement: All datasets of this study are generated in the article.

Conflicts of Interest: The authors declare that they have no conflicts of interest with the contents of this article.

References

1. Scheltens, P.; De Strooper, B.; Kivipelto, M.; Holstege, H.; Chetelat, G.; Teunissen, C.E.; Cummings, J.; van der Flier, W.M. Alzheimer's Disease. *Lancet* **2021**, *397*, 1577–1590. [CrossRef]
2. Breijyeh, Z.; Karaman, R. Comprehensive Review on Alzheimer's Disease: Causes and Treatment. *Molecules* **2020**, *25*, 5789. [CrossRef]
3. Drever, B.D.; Riedel, G.; Platt, B. The Cholinergic System and Hippocampal Plasticity. *Behav. Brain Res.* **2011**, *221*, 505–514. [CrossRef]
4. Mufson, E.J.; Counts, S.E.; Perez, S.E.; Ginsberg, S.D. Cholinergic System during the Progression of Alzheimer's Disease: Therapeutic Implications. *Expert Rev. Neurother.* **2008**, *8*, 1703–1718. [CrossRef] [PubMed]
5. Ferreira-Vieira, T.H.; Guimaraes, I.M.; Silva, F.R.; Ribeiro, F.M. Alzheimer's Disease: Targeting the Cholinergic System. *Curr. Neuropharmacol.* **2016**, *14*, 101–115. [CrossRef] [PubMed]
6. Marucci, G.; Buccioni, M.; Ben, D.D.; Lambertucci, C.; Volpini, R.; Amenta, F. Efficacy of Acetylcholinesterase Inhibitors in Alzheimer's Disease. *Neuropharmacology* **2020**, 108352. [CrossRef] [PubMed]
7. Fernandez de Sevilla, D.; Nunez, A.; Buno, W. Muscarinic Receptors, from Synaptic Plasticity to its Role in Network Activity. *Neuroscience* **2021**, *456*, 60–70. [CrossRef] [PubMed]
8. Shinoe, T.; Matsui, M.; Taketo, M.M.; Manabe, T. Modulation of Synaptic Plasticity by Physiological Activation of M1 Muscarinic Acetylcholine Receptors in the Mouse Hippocampus. *J. Neurosci.* **2005**, *25*, 11194–11200. [CrossRef]
9. Klinkenberg, I.; Blokland, A. The Validity of Scopolamine as a Pharmacological Model for Cognitive Impairment: A Review of Animal Behavioral Studies. *Neurosci. Biobehav. Rev.* **2010**, *34*, 1307–1350. [CrossRef]
10. Lee, J.S.; Kim, H.G.; Lee, H.W.; Han, J.M.; Lee, S.K.; Kim, D.W.; Saravanakumar, A.; Son, C.G. Hippocampal Memory Enhancing Activity of Pine Needle Extract against Scopolamine-induced Amnesia in a Mouse Model. *Sci. Rep.* **2015**, *5*, 9651. [CrossRef]
11. Bekinschtein, P.; Cammarota, M.; Igaz, L.M.; Bevilaqua, L.R.; Izquierdo, I.; Medina, J.H. Persistence of Long-term Memory Storage Requires a Late Protein Synthesis- and BDNF- Dependent Phase in the Hippocampus. *Neuron* **2007**, *53*, 261–277. [CrossRef]
12. Ortega-Martinez, S. A New Perspective on the Role of the CREB Family of Transcription Factors in Memory Consolidation via Adult Hippocampal Neurogenesis. *Front. Mol. Neurosci.* **2015**, *8*, 46. [CrossRef] [PubMed]
13. Amidfar, M.; de Oliveira, J.; Kucharska, E.; Budni, J.; Kim, Y.K. The Role of CREB and BDNF in Neurobiology and Treatment of Alzheimer's Disease. *Life Sci.* **2020**, *257*, 118020. [CrossRef] [PubMed]
14. Riviere, C.; Pawlus, A.D.; Merillon, J.M. Natural Stilbenoids: Distribution in the Plant Kingdom and Chemotaxonomic Interest in Vitaceae. *Nat. Prod. Rep.* **2012**, *29*, 1317–1333. [CrossRef] [PubMed]
15. Akinwumi, B.C.; Bordun, K.M.; Anderson, H.D. Biological Activities of Stilbenoids. *Int. J. Mol. Sci.* **2018**, *19*, 792. [CrossRef] [PubMed]
16. Richard, T.; Pawlus, A.D.; Iglesias, M.L.; Pedrot, E.; Waffo-Teguo, P.; Merillon, J.M.; Monti, J.P. Neuroprotective Properties of Resveratrol and Derivatives. *Ann. N. Y. Acad. Sci.* **2011**, *1215*, 103–108. [CrossRef]
17. Lim, K.G.; Gray, A.I.; Anthony, N.G.; Mackay, S.P.; Pyne, S.; Pyne, N.J. Resveratrol and Its Oligomers: Modulation of Sphingolipid Metabolism and Signaling in Disease. *Arch. Toxicol.* **2014**, *88*, 2213–2232. [CrossRef]
18. Biais, B.; Krisa, S.; Cluzet, S.; Da Costa, G.; Waffo-Teguo, P.; Merillon, J.M.; Richard, T. Antioxidant and Cytoprotective Activities of Grapevine Stilbenes. *J. Agric. Food Chem.* **2017**, *65*, 4952–4960. [CrossRef]
19. Temsamani, H.; Krisa, S.; Decossas-Mendoza, M.; Lambert, O.; Merillon, J.M.; Richard, T. Piceatannol and Other Wine Stilbenes: A Pool of Inhibitors against alpha-Synuclein Aggregation and Cytotoxicity. *Nutrients* **2016**, *8*, 367. [CrossRef]
20. Choi, Y.H.; Yoo, M.Y.; Choi, C.W.; Cha, M.R.; Yon, G.H.; Kwon, D.Y.; Kim, Y.S.; Park, W.K.; Ryu, S.Y. A New Specific BACE-1 Inhibitor from the Stembark Extract of V. vinifera. *Planta Med.* **2009**, *75*, 537–540. [CrossRef]
21. Pinho, B.R.; Ferreres, F.; Valentao, P.; Andrade, P.B. Nature as a Source of Metabolites with Cholinesterase-inhibitory Activity: An Approach to Alzheimer's Disease Treatment. *J. Pharm. Pharmacol.* **2013**, *65*, 1681–1700. [CrossRef] [PubMed]
22. Orhan, I.; Tosun, F.; Sener, B. Coumarin, Anthroquinone and Stilbene Derivatives with Anticholinesterase Activity. *Z. Naturforsch. C J. Biosci.* **2008**, *63*, 366–370. [CrossRef] [PubMed]
23. Namdaung, U.; Athipornchai, A.; Khammee, T.; Kuno, M.; Suksamrarn, S. 2-Arylbenzofurans from Artocarpus Lakoocha and Methyl Ether Analogs with Potent Cholinesterase Inhibitory Activity. *Eur. J. Med. Chem.* **2018**, *143*, 1301–1311. [CrossRef]
24. Zga, N.; Papastamoulis, Y.; Toribio, A.; Richard, T.; Delaunay, J.C.; Jeandet, P.; Renault, J.H.; Monti, J.P.; Merillon, J.M.; Waffo-Teguo, P. Preparative Purification of Antiamyloidogenic Stilbenoids from Vitis vinifera (Chardonnay) Stems by Centrifugal Partition Chromatography. *J. Chromatogr. B Analyt. Technol. Biomed. Life Sci.* **2009**, *877*, 1000–1004. [CrossRef]
25. Zhang, G.; Li, J.; Purkayastha, S.; Tang, Y.; Zhang, H.; Yin, Y.; Li, B.; Liu, G.; Cai, D. Hypothalamic Programming of Systemic Ageing Involving IKK-beta, NF-kappaB and GnRH. *Nature* **2013**, *497*, 211–216. [CrossRef] [PubMed]
26. Anchan, D.; Clark, S.; Pollard, K.; Vasudevan, N. GPR30 Activation Decreases Anxiety in the Open Field Test but not in the Elevated Plus Maze Test in Female Mice. *Brain Behav.* **2014**, *4*, 51–59. [CrossRef]
27. Zhang, L.; Seo, J.H.; Li, H.; Nam, G.; Yang, H.O. The Phosphodiesterase 5 Inhibitor, KJH-1002, Reverses a Mouse Model of Amnesia by Activating a cGMP/cAMP Response Element Binding Protein Pathway and Decreasing Oxidative Damage. *Br. J. Pharmacol.* **2018**, *175*, 3347–3360. [CrossRef]
28. Jiang, B.; Song, L.; Huang, C.; Zhang, W. P7C3 Attenuates the Scopolamine-Induced Memory Impairments in C57BL/6J Mice. *Neurochem. Res.* **2016**, *41*, 1010–1019. [CrossRef]

29. Oshima, Y.; Ueno, Y.; Hikino, H.; Yang, L.L.; Yen, K.Y. Ampelopsin-a, Ampelopsin-B and Ampelopsin-C, New Oligostilbenes of Ampelopsis-Brevipedunculata Var Hancei. *Tetrahedron* **1990**, *46*, 5121–5126. [CrossRef]
30. Malenka, R.C.; Nicoll, R.A. Long-term Potentiation–A Decade of Progress? *Science* **1999**, *285*, 1870–1874. [CrossRef]
31. Nicoll, R.A. A Brief History of Long-Term Potentiation. *Neuron* **2017**, *93*, 281–290. [CrossRef] [PubMed]
32. Smythe, J.W.; Murphy, D.; Bhatnagar, S.; Timothy, C.; Costall, B. Muscarinic Antagonists are Anxiogenic in Rats Tested in the Black-white Box. *Pharmacol. Biochem. Behav.* **1996**, *54*, 57–63. [CrossRef]
33. Rosenzweig-Lipson, S.; Thomas, S.; Barrett, J.E. Attenuation of the Locomotor Activating Effects of D-amphetamine, Cocaine, and Scopolamine by Potassium Channel Modulators. *Prog. Neuropsychopharmacol. Biol. Psychiatry* **1997**, *21*, 853–872. [CrossRef]
34. Hou, X.; Zhang, J.; Ahmad, H.; Zhang, H.; Xu, Z.; Wang, T. Evaluation of Antioxidant Activities of Ampelopsin and Its Protective Effect in Lipopolysaccharide-induced Oxidative Stress Piglets. *PLoS ONE* **2014**, *9*, e108314. [CrossRef] [PubMed]
35. Zhou, Y.; Shu, F.; Liang, X.; Chang, H.; Shi, L.; Peng, X.; Zhu, J.; Mi, M. Ampelopsin Induces Cell Growth Inhibition and Apoptosis in Breast Cancer Cells through ROS Generation and Endoplasmic Reticulum Stress Pathway. *PLoS ONE* **2014**, *9*, e89021. [CrossRef] [PubMed]
36. Iliya, I.; Ali, Z.; Tanaka, T.; Iinuma, M.; Furusawa, M.; Nakaya, K.; Murata, J.; Darnaedi, D.; Matsuura, N.; Ubukata, M. Stilbene Derivatives from Gnetum gnemon Linn. *Phytochemistry* **2003**, *62*, 601–606. [CrossRef]
37. Langcake, P.; Pryce, R.J. A New Class of Phytoalexins from Grapevines. *Experientia* **1977**, *33*, 151–152. [CrossRef]
38. Bokel, M.; Diyasena, M.N.C.; Gunatilaka, A.A.L.; Kraus, W.; Sotheeswaran, S. Canaliculatol, an Antifungal Resveratrol Trimer from Stemonoporous-Canaliculatus. *Phytochemistry* **1988**, *27*, 377–380. [CrossRef]
39. Kitanaka, S.; Ikezawa, T.; Yasukawa, K.; Yamanouchi, S.; Takido, M.; Sung, H.K.; Kim, I.H. (+)-Alpha-viniferin, an Anti-inflammatory Compound from Caragana chamlagu Root. *Chem. Pharm. Bull.* **1990**, *38*, 432–435. [CrossRef]
40. Yan, K.X.; Terashima, K.; Takaya, Y.; Niwa, M. A Novel Oligostilbene Named (+)-viniferol A from the Stem of Vitis vinifera 'Kyohou'. *Tetrahedron* **2001**, *57*, 2711–2715. [CrossRef]
41. Valle, A.; Hoggard, N.; Adams, A.C.; Roca, P.; Speakman, J.R. Chronic Central Administration of Apelin-13 over 10 Days Increases Food Intake, Body Weight, Locomotor Activity and Body Temperature in C57BL/6 Mice. *J. Neuroendocrinol.* **2008**, *20*, 79–84. [CrossRef] [PubMed]
42. Treleaven, C.M.; Tamsett, T.; Fidler, J.A.; Taksir, T.V.; Cheng, S.H.; Shihabuddin, L.S.; Dodge, J.C. Comparative Analysis of Acid Sphingomyelinase Distribution in the CNS of Rats and Mice Following Intracerebroventricular Delivery. *PLoS ONE* **2011**, *6*, e16313. [CrossRef]
43. Li, H.Q.; Peng, S.Y.; Li, S.H.; Liu, S.Q.; Lv, Y.F.; Yang, N.; Yu, L.Y.; Deng, Y.H.; Zhang, Z.J.; Fang, M.S.; et al. Chronic Olanzapine Administration Causes Metabolic Syndrome through Inflammatory Cytokines in Rodent Models of Insulin Resistance. *Sci. Rep.* **2019**, *9*. [CrossRef] [PubMed]
44. Zhang, Y.L.; Kim, M.S.; Jia, B.S.; Yan, J.Q.; Zuniga-Hertz, J.P.; Han, C.; Cai, D.S. Hypothalamic Stem Cells Control Ageing Speed Partly through Exosomal miRNAs. *Nature* **2017**, *548*. [CrossRef]
45. Oh, S.Y.; Jang, M.J.; Choi, Y.H.; Hwang, H.; Rhim, H.; Lee, B.; Choi, C.W.; Kim, M.S. Central Administration of Afzelin Extracted from Ribes fasciculatum Improves Cognitive and Memory Function in a Mouse Model of Dementia. *Sci. Rep.* **2021**, *11*, 9182. [CrossRef] [PubMed]
46. Nordberg, A.; Ballard, C.; Bullock, R.; Darreh-Shori, T.; Somogyi, M. A Review of Butyrylcholinesterase as a Therapeutic Target in the Treatment of Alzheimer's Disease. *Prim. Care Companion CNS Disord.* **2013**, *15*. [CrossRef]
47. Grossberg, G.T. Cholinesterase Inhibitors for the Treatment of Alzheimer's Disease: Getting on and Staying on. *Curr. Ther. Res. Clin. Exp.* **2003**, *64*, 216–235. [CrossRef]
48. Giacobini, E. Cholinergic Function and Alzheimer's Disease. *Int. J. Geriatr. Psychiatry* **2003**, *18*, S1–S5. [CrossRef]
49. Schegg, K.M.; Harrington, L.S.; Neilsen, S.; Zweig, R.M.; Peacock, J.H. Soluble and Membrane-bound Forms of Brain Acetylcholinesterase in Alzheimer's Disease. *Neurobiol. Aging* **1992**, *13*, 697–704. [CrossRef]
50. Santarpia, L.; Grandone, I.; Contaldo, F.; Pasanisi, F. Butyrylcholinesterase as a Prognostic Marker: A Review of the Literature. *J. Cachexia Sarcopeni* **2013**, *4*, 31–39. [CrossRef]
51. Li, Q.; Chen, Y.; Xing, S.; Liao, Q.; Xiong, B.; Wang, Y.; Lu, W.; He, S.; Feng, F.; Liu, W.; et al. Highly Potent and Selective Butyrylcholinesterase Inhibitors for Cognitive Improvement and Neuroprotection. *J. Med. Chem.* **2021**. [CrossRef]
52. Kosak, U.; Brus, B.; Knez, D.; Sink, R.; Zakelj, S.; Trontelj, J.; Pislar, A.; Slenc, J.; Gobec, M.; Zivin, M.; et al. Development of an in vivo Active Reversible Butyrylcholinesterase Inhibitor. *Sci. Rep.* **2016**, *6*, 39495. [CrossRef] [PubMed]
53. Li, Q.; Xing, S.; Chen, Y.; Liao, Q.; Xiong, B.; He, S.; Lu, W.; Liu, Y.; Yang, H.; Li, Q.; et al. Discovery and Biological Evaluation of a Novel Highly Potent Selective Butyrylcholinsterase Inhibitor. *J. Med. Chem.* **2020**, *63*, 10030–10044. [CrossRef] [PubMed]
54. Hodges, D.B., Jr.; Lindner, M.D.; Hogan, J.B.; Jones, K.M.; Markus, E.J. Scopolamine Induced Deficits in a Battery of Rat Cognitive Tests: Comparisons of Sensitivity and Specificity. *Behav. Pharmacol.* **2009**, *20*, 237–251. [CrossRef] [PubMed]
55. Nakae, K.; Nishimura, Y.; Ohba, S.; Akamatsu, Y. Migrastatin Acts as a Muscarinic Acetylcholine Receptor Antagonist. *J. Antibiot.* **2006**, *59*, 685–692. [CrossRef]
56. Spignoli, G.; Pepeu, G. Interactions between Oxiracetam, Aniracetam and Scopolamine on Behavior and Brain Acetylcholine. *Pharmacol. Biochem. Behav.* **1987**, *27*, 491–495. [CrossRef]
57. Hu, J.R.; Chun, Y.S.; Kim, J.K.; Cho, I.J.; Ku, S.K. Ginseng Berry Aqueous Extract Prevents Scopolamine-induced Memory Impairment in Mice. *Exp. Ther. Med.* **2019**, *18*, 4388–4396. [CrossRef]

58. Kotani, S.; Yamauchi, T.; Teramoto, T.; Ogura, H. Pharmacological Evidence of Cholinergic Involvement in Adult Hippocampal Neurogenesis in Rats. *Neuroscience* **2006**, *142*, 505–514. [CrossRef] [PubMed]
59. Xu, J.; Rong, S.; Xie, B.; Sun, Z.; Deng, Q.; Wu, H.; Bao, W.; Wang, D.; Yao, P.; Huang, F.; et al. Memory Impairment in Cognitively Impaired Aged Rats Associated with Decreased Hippocampal CREB Phosphorylation: Reversal by Procyanidins Extracted from the Lotus Seedpod. *J. Gerontol. A Biol. Sci. Med. Sci.* **2010**, *65*, 933–940. [CrossRef] [PubMed]
60. Zhang, S.J.; Luo, D.; Li, L.; Tan, R.R.; Xu, Q.Q.; Qin, J.; Zhu, L.; Luo, N.C.; Xu, T.T.; Zhang, R.; et al. Ethyl Acetate Extract Components of Bushen-Yizhi Formula Provides Neuroprotection against Scopolamine-induced Cognitive Impairment. *Sci. Rep.* **2017**, *7*, 9824. [CrossRef] [PubMed]
61. Um, M.Y.; Lim, D.W.; Son, H.J.; Cho, S.; Lee, C. Phlorotannin-rich Fraction from Ishige foliacea Brown Seaweed Prevents the Scopolamine-induced Memory Impairment via Regulation of ERK-CREB-BDNF Pathway. *J. Funct. Foods.* **2018**, *40*, 110–116. [CrossRef]
62. Regue-Guyon, M.; Lanfumey, L.; Mongeau, R. Neuroepigenetics of Neurotrophin Signaling: Neurobiology of Anxiety and Affective Disorders. *Prog. Mol. Biol. Transl. Sci.* **2018**, *158*, 159–193. [CrossRef] [PubMed]
63. Alonso, M.; Vianna, M.R.M.; Depino, A.M.; Souza, T.M.E.; Pereira, P.; Szapiro, G.; Viola, H.; Pitossi, F.; Izquierdo, I.; Medina, J.H. BDNF-triggered Events in the Rat Hippocampus are Required for Both Short- and Long-term Memory Formation. *Hippocampus* **2002**, *12*, 551–560. [CrossRef] [PubMed]
64. Ma, Y.L.; Wang, H.L.; Wu, H.C.; Wei, C.L.; Lee, E.H. Brain-derived Neurotrophic Factor Antisense Oligonucleotide Impairs Memory Retention and Inhibits Long-term Potentiation in Rats. *Neuroscience* **1998**, *82*, 957–967. [CrossRef]
65. Ou, L.C.; Gean, P.W. Transcriptional Regulation of Brain-derived Neurotrophic Factor in the Amygdala during Consolidation of Fear Memory. *Mol. Pharmacol.* **2007**, *72*, 350–358. [CrossRef] [PubMed]
66. Rattiner, L.M.; Davis, M.; French, C.T.; Ressler, K.J. Brain-derived Neurotrophic Factor and Tyrosine Kinase Receptor B Involvement in Amygdala-dependent Fear Conditioning. *J. Neurosci.* **2004**, *24*, 4796–4806. [CrossRef] [PubMed]
67. Rosas-Vidal, L.E.; Do-Monte, F.H.; Sotres-Bayon, F.; Quirk, G.J. Hippocampal-prefrontal BDNF and Memory for Fear Extinction. *Neuropsychopharmacology* **2014**, *39*, 2161–2169. [CrossRef] [PubMed]
68. Peters, J.; Dieppa-Perea, L.M.; Melendez, L.M.; Quirk, G.J. Induction of Fear Extinction with Hippocampal-infralimbic BDNF. *Science* **2010**, *328*, 1288–1290. [CrossRef] [PubMed]
69. Tang, K.S. The Cellular and Molecular Processes Associated with Scopolamine-induced Memory Deficit: A Model of Alzheimer's Biomarkers. *Life Sci.* **2019**, *233*. [CrossRef] [PubMed]
70. Levine, E.S.; Dreyfus, C.F.; Black, I.B.; Plummer, M.R. Brain-derived Neurotrophic Factor Rapidly Enhances Synaptic Transmission in Hippocampal Neurons via Postsynaptic Tyrosine Kinase Receptors. *Proc. Natl. Acad. Sci. USA* **1995**, *92*, 8074–8077. [CrossRef]
71. Zakharenko, S.S.; Patterson, S.L.; Dragatsis, I.; Zeitlin, S.O.; Siegelbaum, S.A.; Kandel, E.R.; Morozov, A. Presynaptic BDNF Required for a Presynaptic but not Postsynaptic Component of LTP at Hippocampal CA1-CA3 Synapses. *Neuron* **2003**, *39*, 975–990. [CrossRef]
72. Kang, H.; Schuman, E.M. A Requirement for Local Protein Synthesis in Neurotrophin-induced Hippocampal Synaptic Plasticity. *Science* **1996**, *273*, 1402–1406. [CrossRef] [PubMed]

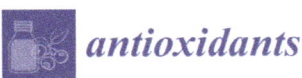

Article

Neurophysiological Effects of Whole Coffee Cherry Extract in Older Adults with Subjective Cognitive Impairment: A Randomized, Double-Blind, Placebo-Controlled, Cross-Over Pilot Study

Jennifer L. Robinson [1,2,3,4,5,*], Julio A. Yanes [1,2,3,4], Meredith A. Reid [2,3,4,5], Jerry E. Murphy [1], Jessica N. Busler [1,2,3,4], Petey W. Mumford [6], Kaelin C. Young [6,7], Zbigniew J. Pietrzkowski [8], Boris V. Nemzer [9], John M. Hunter [9] and Darren T. Beck [4,7]

1. Department of Psychology, Auburn University, Auburn, AL 36849, USA; jay0005@auburn.edu (J.A.Y.); jem0058@auburn.edu (J.E.M.); jzb0046@auburn.edu (J.N.B.)
2. Auburn University MRI Research Center, Auburn University, Auburn, AL 36849, USA; mareid@auburn.edu
3. Alabama Advanced Imaging Consortium, Auburn University, Auburn, AL 36849, USA
4. Initiative for the Center for Neuroscience, Auburn University, Auburn, AL 36849, USA; dbeck@auburn.vcom.edu
5. Department of Electrical and Computer Engineering, Auburn University, Auburn, AL 36849, USA
6. School of Kinesiology, Auburn University, Auburn, AL 36849, USA; pwm0009@auburn.edu (P.W.M.); kyoung@auburn.vcom.edu (K.C.Y.)
7. Edward Via College of Osteopathic Medicine, Auburn, AL 36830, USA
8. VDF FutureCeuticals, Inc., 23 Peters Canyon Road, Irvine, CA 92606, USA; zb@futureceuticals.com
9. VDF FutureCeuticals, Inc., 2692 N. State Route 1-17, Momence, IL 60954, USA; bnemzer@futureceuticals.com (B.V.N.); jhunter@futureceuticals.com (J.M.H.)
* Correspondence: jrobinson@auburn.edu

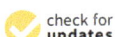

Citation: Robinson, J.L.; Yanes, J.A.; Reid, M.A.; Murphy, J.E.; Busler, J.N.; Mumford, P.W.; Young, K.C.; Pietrzkowski, Z.J.; Nemzer, B.V.; Hunter, J.M.; et al. Neurophysiological Effects of Whole Coffee Cherry Extract in Older Adults with Subjective Cognitive Impairment: A Randomized, Double-Blind, Placebo-Controlled, Cross-Over Pilot Study. *Antioxidants* **2021**, *10*, 144. https://doi.org/10.3390/antiox10020144

Academic Editor: Rui F. M. Silva

Received: 1 December 2020
Accepted: 13 January 2021
Published: 20 January 2021

Publisher's Note: MDPI stays neutral with regard to jurisdictional claims in published maps and institutional affiliations.

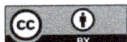

Copyright: © 2021 by the authors. Licensee MDPI, Basel, Switzerland. This article is an open access article distributed under the terms and conditions of the Creative Commons Attribution (CC BY) license (https://creativecommons.org/licenses/by/4.0/).

Abstract: Bioactive plant-based compounds have shown promise as protective agents across multiple domains including improvements in neurological and psychological measures. Methodological challenges have limited our understanding of the neurophysiological changes associated with polyphenol-rich supplements such as whole coffee cherry extract (WCCE). In the current study, we (1) compared 100 mg of WCCE to a placebo using an acute, randomized, double-blind, within-subject, cross-over design, and we (2) conducted a phytochemical analysis of WCCE. The primary objective of the study was to determine the neurophysiological and behavioral changes that resulted from the acute administration of WCCE. We hypothesized that WCCE would increase brain-derived neurotrophic factor (BDNF) and glutamate levels while also increasing neurofunctional measures in cognitive brain regions. Furthermore, we expected there to be increased behavioral performance associated with WCCE, as measured by reaction time and accuracy. Participants underwent four neuroimaging scans (pre- and post-WCCE and placebo) to assess neurofunctional/metabolic outcomes using functional magnetic resonance imaging and magnetic resonance spectroscopy. The results suggest that polyphenol-rich WCCE is associated with decreased reaction time and may protect against cognitive errors on tasks of working memory and response inhibition. Behavioral findings were concomitant with neurofunctional changes in structures involved in decision-making and attention. Specifically, we found increased functional connectivity between the anterior cingulate and regions involved in sensory and decision-making networks. Additionally, we observed increased BDNF and an increased glutamate/gamma-aminobutyric acid (GABA) ratio following WCCE administration. These results suggest that WCCE is associated with acute neurophysiological changes supportive of faster reaction times and increased, sustained attention.

Keywords: functional magnetic resonance imaging; spectroscopy; 7T; polyphenols; nutraceuticals

1. Introduction

Recent studies have demonstrated the promising effects of bioactive phytochemicals (e.g., polyphenols) on cardiovascular and endocrine health outcomes [1–4]. As such, an increasingly intriguing line of inquiry is whether materials with high contents of these compounds may also have effects on neurophysiological and psychological measures. Preliminary evidence suggests that polyphenols may have effects in these domains, particularly in aging populations [4–7]. Whole coffee cherry extract (WCCE), is a proprietary, safe [8], powdered extract of whole coffee cherries from *Coffea arabica* with high levels of polyphenols and substantially low (<2%) levels of caffeine (for a detailed composition profile, please see Table 1 of the study by Reyes-Izquierdo et al. (2013b) [9]). WCCE has been previously associated with increased serum concentrations of both circulating and exosomal brain-derived neurotrophic factor (BDNF), in addition to increased alertness and decreased fatigue [4,9–12]. BDNF is a protein synthesized in neurons and other types of cells, and it is associated with a range of neural (e.g., plasticity) [13–16] and psychological processes [17–20]. As such, BDNF may represent an important target for identifying the pathophysiological mechanisms underlying observed behavioral or cognitive effects associated with WCCE (and possibly other polyphenol-rich materials). However, there is a need for comprehensive studies that simultaneously assess cognition and neurophysiological measures in order to better understand such mechanisms [4,5].

Because of the observed beneficial effects of WCCE in the extant literature that are commensurate with evidence from other polyphenol-rich materials [7,21,22] and in light of the mounting evidence suggesting that polyphenols have neurotrophic effects [23–26], it is important to consider the chemical properties of WCCE that may drive the mechanisms involved in such effects. Recently, the phytochemical profile of WCCE was determined by a high-resolution non-targeted mass spectrometry approach (Figure 1) [27]. Importantly, one of the most abundant and widely distributed polyphenols in plants are chlorogenic acids, which are well-known for their antioxidant, anti-inflammatory, anti-hypertensive, and therapeutic properties [28–30]. Coffee is remarkably rich with chlorogenic acids and other polyphenols. These naturally occurring phytonutrients are concentrated during the WCCE extraction process (please see Table 1). In this study, we extended the chemical profiling of WCCE to include the antioxidant potential, as determined by five separate assays.

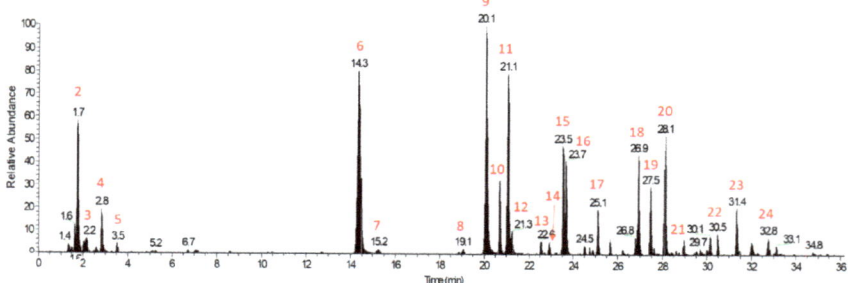

Figure 1. LC–MS base peak chromatogram (BPC) profile of whole coffee cherry extract (WCCE), adapted from the work of Nemzer and colleagues (under review) [27]. The major detected peaks were labelled with peak numbers ranging from 1 to 24, and the compounds corresponding to each peak are identified here: 1. gluconic acid; 2. quinic acid; 3. malic acid; 4. citric acid; 5. 2-hydroxyglutaric acid; 6. 3-O-caffeoylquinic acid (3-CQA); 7. protocatechualdehyde; 8. 3- coumaroylquinic acid (3-CoQA); 9. 5-CQA; 10. 3-feruloylquinic acid (3-FQA); 11. 4-CQA; 12. caffeic acid; 13. 5-CoQA; 14. 4-CoQA; 15. 5-FQA; 16. 4-FQA; 17. quinic acid-glucoside-R*; 18. 3-dicaffeoylquinic acid (3-DiCQA); 19. 5-DiCQA; 20. 4-DiCQA; 21. 3-Caffeoyl-5-FQA; 22. valeroylquinic acid (VQA) diglucoside-R*; 23. caffeoyl tryptophan; and 24. dimethylcaffeic acid. Other compounds identified in WCCE in the positive ion mode include pantothenic acid, trigonelline, choline, and glycerophosphocholine derivatives. Figure adapted from the work of Nemzer et al. (under review) [27]. A listing of the typical polyphenols found in WCCE can be found in Table 1.

Table 1. List of polyphenol compounds in WCCE, expressed in mg/g ± SD. Table adapted from the work of Nemzer et al. (under review) [27].

Polyphenol	mg/g
3-O-Caffeoylquinic acid	41.3 ± 8.4
5-p-coumaroylquinic acid	0.4 ± 0.1
5-O-Caffeoylquinic acid	134.6 ± 16.7
3-Feruloylquinic acid	7 ± 1.2
4-O-Caffeoylquinic acid	74.9 ± 11.1
p-coumaroylquinic acid	0.6 ± 0.1
p-coumaroylquinic acid	2.5 ± 0.5
4-Feruloylquinic acid	8.4 ± 1.7
5-Feruloylquinic acid	38.1 ± 6.3
3-O-Caffeoylquinic lactone	7.8 ± 1.2
4-O-Caffeoylquinic lactone	3.8 ± 0.6
3,4-O-Dicaffeoylquinic acid	37.6 ± 7.3
3,5-O-Dicaffeoylquinic acid	12.1 ± 2.2
4,5-O-Dicaffeoylquinic acid	47.2 ± 7.8
3-O-Feruloyl-4-Caffeoylquinic acid	0.9 ± 0.2
3-O-Caffeoy-4-Feruloylquinic acid	3.3 ± 0.6
3-O-Feruloyl-5-Caffeoylquinic acid	0.2 ± 0
3-O-Caffeoy-5-Feruloylquinic acid	1.1 ± 0.3
4-O-Feruloyl-5-Caffeoylquinic acid	0.7 ± 0.2
4-O-Caffeoy-5-Feruloylquinic acid	3.4 ± 0.7
Total CGA	425.8 ± 63.9
Trigonelline	33.78 ± 5.2
Caffeine	18.2 ± 3.3

Interestingly, mild cognitive impairment (MCI) is associated with a reduced BDNF level [18,31]. MCI represents an intermediate stage between the expected cognitive decline of normal aging and the more serious decline of dementia. MCI is marked by problems with memory, language, thinking, and judgment that are greater than normal age-related changes. Given that earlier studies reported that WCCE may stimulate increases in BDNF [9,11], one remaining question was whether WCCE, potentially through increases in BDNF, could acutely improve cognitive function or provide protective effects in older adults who may be on the verge of or have MCI. To this end, BDNF has been associated with such changes via its effects on N-methyl-D-aspartate-type (NMDA) receptors [32–34]. Furthermore, recent evidence suggests that the long-term administration of WCCE has cognitive effects in such a population in as little as seven days and persisting for 28 days [35]. Thus, understanding the acute neurophysiological effects may provide critical mechanistic information.

Though acute, observable changes may be associated with BDNF, it is also plausible that underlying pathophysiological mechanisms may be related to some other, as-yet unidentified, neural process(es). Unfortunately, even when solely considering BDNF, methodological limitations have led to a dearth of evidence to suggest, define, support, or explain the complex and dynamic mechanistic possibilities. For example, hippocampal BDNF messenger ribonucleic acid (mRNA) expression largely depends on the neuronal excitation/inhibition balance [36], rendering it difficult to elucidate underlying mechanisms. To our knowledge, no previous study has examined neurotransmitters (e.g., glutamate and/or gamma-aminobutyric acid (GABA) concentrations) or neurometabolics concurrent with changes in BDNF levels. Therefore, the purpose of this study was to implement a comprehensive, multi-modal investigation to assess (1) the quantitative profiles of various phenolics inherent in WCCE, (2) the antioxidant properties of WCCE, and (3) the effects of WCCE in older adults on neurofunctional and neurometabolic processes while concurrently measuring associated acute cognitive and behavioral effects.

In this pilot study, representing the first of its kind, we leveraged a randomized, double-blind, placebo-controlled, within-subjects crossover design to assess the neurophysiological, neurofunctional, and cognitive effects of acute WCCE administration. Contributing to the novelty of this study, we employed advanced ultra-high field, high-resolution (i.e., submillimeter) functional magnetic resonance imaging (fMRI) and magnetic resonance spectroscopy (MRS) techniques to identify the neurofunctional and neurometabolic changes, respectively, of the acute administration of WCCE. Performing fMRI and MRS at high field strengths (e.g., 7 Tesla (7T)) offers significant advantages such as an increased signal-to-noise that allows for more sensitive assessments [37–39]. Likewise, using high field strengths also affords better spectral resolution, providing more robust and accurate measurements of glutamate and glutamine [40,41]. Furthermore, the utilization of a within-subjects design allows for the control of individual variability, which has recently been considered an important and necessary step toward understanding brain dynamics, favoring smaller samples with greater density of measurement [42–48]. We also report a complementary analysis outlining the antioxidant potential of WCCE across five separate assays. We hypothesized that WCCE would be associated with increased BDNF, improved cognitive function as measured by accuracy and reaction time during behavioral challenges, and changes in glutamate (increases) and GABA (decreases) compared to the placebo. Given the latter hypothesis, we also anticipated increased glutamate and glutamine ratios with GABA.

2. Materials and Methods

2.1. Ethics and Reproducibility

This protocol was developed at Auburn University and approved by the Auburn University Institutional Review Board (#16-391 MR 1610) in accordance with the ethical standards set forth by the Helsinki Declaration of 1975 (as revised in 1983). The study was retrospectively registered on http://clinicaltrials.gov, identifier NCT03812744 (https://clinicaltrials.gov/ct2/show/NCT03812744), and reporting guidelines for randomized, controlled trials of herbal interventions were followed where applicable [49]. For transparency purposes, we have also included figures demonstrating all data points where applicable. Future studies will be prospectively registered.

2.2. Participants and Recruitment

Participants were recruited from the community using fliers and through information sessions conducted in small senior groups throughout the community. Interested participants were initially screened via phone for contraindications. All potential participants were then invited to the study site for consenting and additional screening. Specifically, participants were screened for contraindications to the imaging environment, as well as memory decline using the Logical Memory (Adult Battery for Ages 16–69) section of the Wechsler Memory Scale IV (WMS) [50], the Mini-Mental State Examination (MMSE) [51,52], and the Clinical Dementia Rating (CDR) [53,54] scale. Inclusion criteria were: (1) memory complaints and memory difficulties, as verified by an informant; (2) no diagnosis of Alzheimer's disease (and no suspected diagnosis on site by research staff); and (3) no significant cerebrovascular disease, as determined by self-reported patient history and confirmed by the informant and neurocognitive measures. Exclusion criteria were: (1) contraindications for magnetic resonance imaging (MRI) scanning, including implanted cardioverter defibrillators, any ferrous implanted metal in the body (e.g., aneurysm clips), certain types of dental work, or claustrophobia; (2) history of cardiovascular disease; and (3) those with a current or recently prescribed medication known to interfere with peripheral and/or cerebral blood flow or vascular function. Written, informed consent was obtained for all participants. Twelve participants were recruited, but 4 dropped out because of discomfort in the scanner or because of the time commitment ($n = 8$, determined by *a priori* power analyses assuming a large effect size ($f = 0.60$), 80% power, and a paired t-test design). Eight participants completed the study (4 men/4 women; 60.75 ± 2.76 (M $\pm$ SD) years of age; CDR = 0.13 ± 0.23; MMSE = 27.25 ± 0.71; and WMS = 15.88 ± 1.64), with recruitment occurring from October 2016 through 2018. Though the sample size may be considered small in the context of traditional fMRI studies, it should be noted that recent research has suggested that within-subjects designs may substantially improve power, given that larger group-based designs may not detect important differences in individual variability [42–45].

2.3. Procedures

This study was conducted as an acute, single-dose, double-blind, placebo-controlled, within-subjects crossover design (for an overview of the study design, please see Figure 2). Recruited participants were offered an opportunity to visit the Auburn University MRI Research Center (AUMRIC) prior to enrolling in the study to acclimate to the neuroimaging environment. Following initial screening and informed consent, basic demographic information was collected and neurocognitive assessments were administered (i.e., MMSE, CDR, and WMS). All participants fasted prior to the MRI study session, which occurred on a different day than the consenting and neurocognitive assessments.

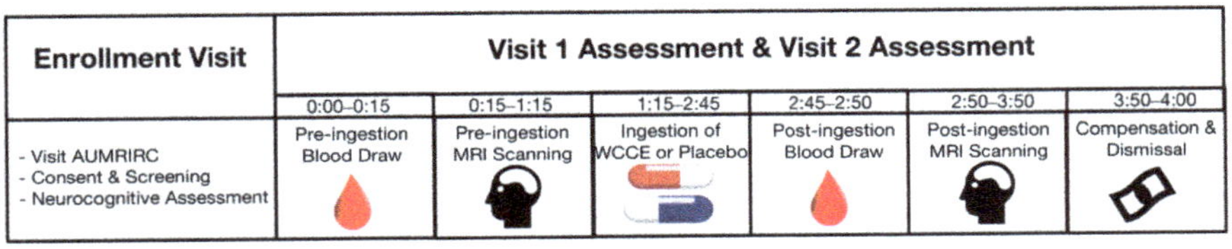

Figure 2. Study design overview. For the Visit 1 and Visit 2 Assessment, 0:00 indicates the participants arrival at the imaging center. Subsequent times indicate hours and minutes since arrival. AUMRIRC: Auburn University MRI Research Center.

2.3.1. Interventions

The nutraceutical intervention used in this study was 100 mg of WCCE, commercially marketed as NeuroFactor™, manufactured by VDF FutureCeuticals, Inc. For a detailed composition profile, please see Table 1 and Figure 1. Dosage, as well as post-administration scan timing, was chosen based on previous research demonstrating significant effects on BDNF [9,11], as well as reductions in mental fatigue and higher levels of alertness [10]. Furthermore, a dosage of 100 mg of WCCE was later corroborated in a longitudinal, double-blind, placebo-controlled study in which cognitive effects were noted in as little as 7 days and persisted throughout a 28-day study period [35]. Silica oxide capsules, identical in appearance to WCCE, served as the placebo. Each capsule contained 100 mg of material. The capsules were provided by VDF FutureCeuticals, Inc., who maintained all blinding information.

2.3.2. MRI Sessions

All MRI sessions were conducted in the morning, beginning between 8 a.m. and 9 a.m. Due to the length of the study session, participants were allowed to eat a small breakfast item between scans. This was held consistent for both sessions for all participants. Additionally, participants were asked to refrain from alcohol, caffeine, heavy exercise, and tobacco for at least 18 h prior to their scanning sessions. Blood samples were acquired upon arriving (to assess baseline BDNF levels) and 90 min following the ingestion of the study material (just prior to the post-ingestion MRI scan). Blood samples (~10 mL per draw) were collected from the antecubital veins using a butterfly catheter and captured in serum and plasma blood collection tubes containing ethylenediaminetetraacetic acid (EDTA). Samples were immediately centrifuged at 3000 rpm for approximately 15 min at 4 °C, and then they were stored at −80 °C. Participants were prepped for the scanning environment and were familiarized to the tasks that they would be performing in the scanner. Each participant had to achieve a level of mastery on the behavioral tasks outside of the scanning environment (>80% accuracy) prior to entering the MRI suite. After achieving mastery, participants underwent the scanning session. The scanning protocol consisted of the following: a localizer, gre-field mapping (36 slices; TR/TE: 400/4.92 ms; 3.1 × 3.1 × 3.0 mm voxels; 60°

flip angle; and base/phase resolution: 64/100), a whole brain functional scan for registration purposes (60 slices; TR/TE: 6000/28 ms; 0.9 × 0.9 × 1.5 mm voxels; 70° flip angle; base/phase resolution 234/100; and GRAPPA acceleration factor of 3), a MPRAGE 3D high resolution structural scan (256 slices; TR/TE: 2200/2.89 ms; 0.7 mm^3 isotropic voxels; 7° flip angle; and base/phase resolution: 256/100), MRS focused on the dorsal anterior cingulate cortex (dACC; Figure 3) (STEAM; TR/TE/TM: 10,000/5/45 ms; 25 × 20 × 12 mm voxel size; 32 averages with water suppression; 2 averages without water suppression; 4 kHz spectral bandwidth; and 2048 points), a resting state fMRI scan (37 slices; TR/TE: 3000/28 ms; 70° flip angle; base/phase resolution: 234/100; GRAPPA acceleration factor of 3; interleaved sequence; 100 volumes; and total acquisition time 5:00), and fMRI n-back and go/no-go tasks (same sequence parameters as the resting state fMRI, but the number of volumes were 151 and 142, respectively). Participants completed all scanning tasks and were escorted out of the scanning environment to the lounge area, where they immediately ingested either WCCE or the placebo. Following a designated 90-min wait time, another blood draw was conducted, and the scanning procedure was repeated. Participants were then dismissed and returned after 72 h to repeat the entire protocol with the alternate test substance. We chose a 72-h interval based on our assessment of the literature that suggested that polyphenols should be fully metabolized within this timeframe [55–57]. Order was randomly assigned (via a random number generator by author D.T.B.), with six individuals assigned to WCCE followed by the placebo and two assigned to the placebo followed by WCCE. Participants and investigators were blind to test substance assignment, and the sponsor was blind to participant assignment until the end of the study. Participants were compensated for their time ($75 for completing the first session and $125 for completing the second session).

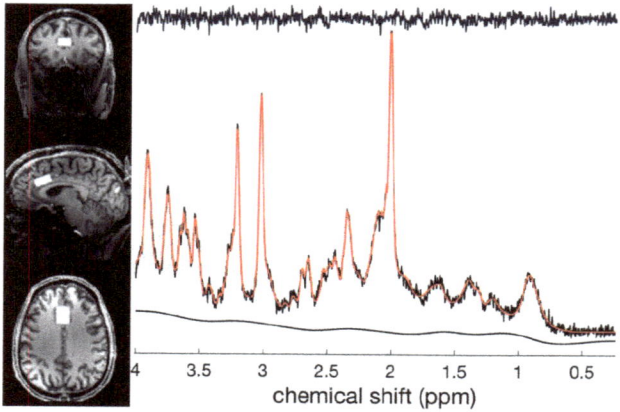

Figure 3. Magnetic resonance spectroscopy (MRS) voxel placement in the dorsal anterior cingulate cortex (dACC) and representative spectra. The 7 Tesla (7T) spectroscopy offers significant advantages, including more accurate assessments of glutamate and glutamine.

2.3.3. Exosomal BDNF

Exosomal BDNF was measured using a commercially available ELISA according to manufacturer's instructions (Sigma Aldrich, St. Louis, MO, USA). Exosomes were isolated from serum aliquots and separated by precipitation using an ExoQuick™ Exosome Precipitation Kit (System Biosciences, Mountain View, CA, USA). Briefly, the supernatant was collected in a clean tube while the pellet was centrifuged for 5 min at 1500× g and any remaining supernatant was removed. The pellet was resuspended in 250 µL of an exosome-binding buffer (System Biosciences, Mountain View, CA, USA) and incubated in an ice bath for 5 min to complete the lytic process. BDNF contained in the exosomal lysate was measured using the previously described BDNF ELISA (Sigma Aldrich, St. Louis, MO, USA). The intra- and inter-assay coefficients of variance were 3.2% and 5.0%, respectively.

2.3.4. Behavioral Tasks

Go/no-go task: The go/no-go task is designed to assess inhibitory responses. Stimuli were presented in a continuous stream, and participants were asked to perform a binary decision on each stimulus (e.g., is the stimulus in an alternating pattern with the previous stimulus?). Participants pressed a button if the stimulus met the criteria (go trial) or withheld their response if it did not (no-go trial/lures). The task was designed to have more 'go' than 'no-go' trials, enticing the participant into a pattern of responses, thus making the 'no-go' trials more difficult in populations with poor impulse control [58–62]. Accuracy and reaction time, two of our primary outcome measures, were recorded by the E-Prime (https://pstnet.com/products/e-prime/) stimulus presentation software. Stimuli were presented once every 1000 ms with an additional 500 ms intertrial interval to allow for responses. Following an instructional slide and a 4-s countdown slide, the task was presented in a block design such that 60 trials were presented followed by a 15 s rest period, which repeated a total of 3 times. A final block of 71 trials was also administered (total time = 7:05, total trials = 251 (247 requiring a response, since the first trial after any rest period did not require a response), total lures = 25, or ~10%). This task reliably activates regions of the prefrontal cortex (PFC), including the middle frontal gyrus, the inferior frontal gyrus, and the anterior cingulate [63,64]. These regions are implicated in cognitive control and response inhibition, making this an ideal task for examining the effects of WCCE on cognitive function.

N-back: The n-back task is widely used in working memory literature. It requires participants to determine if the current stimulus repeats relative to the item that occurred 'n' times before its onset. As such, a 1-back task would require participants to determine if the current stimulus is the same as the one previous to it, whereas a 2-back task would require participants to determine if the present stimulus is the same as 2 stimuli ago. The task becomes increasingly harder with higher numbers of stimuli that need to be recalled. We used the 1-back task as a cognitive challenge. Stimuli were presented for 1500 ms with a 500 ms intertrial interval in blocks of 50 trials for a total of 200 trials. Each block was separated by a 15 s rest period (total time = 7:25). The neural network actively involved in the n-back includes an extensive frontoparietal network, encompassing regions involved in attention and decision making [65,66]. For both cognitive tasks, accuracy, defined as the number of correct responses, and reaction time, measured in ms, were recorded by the E-Prime (https://pstnet.com/products/e-prime/) stimulus presentation software.

2.4. Chemical Analysis

The commercially available WCCE, marketed under the trade name of "Neurofactor™," was standardized to 40% minimum chlorogenic acids. Neurofactor™ was manufactured and supplied by VDF FutureCeuticals, Inc. Chemical analyses were conducted by VDF FutureCeuticals, Inc. (B.V.N.). Below, we report methods for high HPLC analyses.

2.4.1. Chlorogenic Acid

Samples were extracted in 50% methanol, separated by reversed-phase HPLC and detected at 325 nm. Chlorogenic acid and related compounds present in the sample were quantified using a commercially available standard as the external standard. Response factors were used to quantify the related chlorogenic acid compounds against chlorogenic acid.

2.4.2. Trigonelline by HPLC

Trigonelline is naturally found in coffee plants. Trigonelline was extracted from the samples using an ammonium formate buffer, which was separated by reversed-phase HPLC with detection at 265 nm by photodiode-array detection (PDA/DAD), and quantification was calculated using a commercially available standard.

2.4.3. Caffeine

Caffeine was extracted using 70% methanol, separated by reversed-phase HPLC, measured at 272 nm using PDA/DAD, and quantified using a commercially available standard. The caffeine and trigonelline contents were characterized by HPLC Agilent 1100 (Agilent Technologies) equipped with a diode array detector and quantified by UV absorbance.

2.4.4. Sample Preparation for Antioxidant Measurements

Approximately 20 mg of each sample were weighed and extracted with 20 mL of ethanol/water (70:30 v/v) for 1 h at room temperature on an orbital shaker. The extracts were centrifuged at 5900 rpm, and the supernatant was used for the total antioxidant capacity assay. The total antioxidant capacity was determined by calculating the sum of the individual result against five free radicals, namely peroxyl radicals, hydroxyl radicals, peroxynitrite, superoxide anions, and singlet oxygen. All results were expressed as µM Trolox equivalent per gram (µM TE/g). Ethanol (HPLC grade) and 6-hydroxy-2,5,7,8 tetramethyl-2-carboxylic acid (Trolox) were obtained from Sigma-Aldrich (St. Louis, MO, USA).

Peroxyl Radicals Scavenging Capacity (ORAC Assay)

The oxygen radical absorbance capacity (ORAC) assay was conducted on the basis of a report by Huang, Ou, and colleagues [67,68], modified for the FL600 microplate fluorescence reader (Bio-Tek Instruments, Inc., Winooski, VT, USA). The FL600 microplate fluorescence reader was used with fluorescence filters for an excitation wavelength of 485 ± 20 nm and an emission wavelength of 530 ± 25 nm. The plate reader was controlled by the KC4 3.0 software, and 2,2'-Azobis (2-amidinopropane) dihydrochloride (AAPH) was used as the source for the peroxyl radical, which was generated as a result of the spontaneous decomposition of AAPH at 37 °C. AAPH was obtained from Wako Chemicals USA, Inc. (Richmond, VA, USA). Fluorescein was the chosen target protein, with a loss of fluorescence an indicator of the extent of damage from its reaction with the peroxyl radical. The protective effect of the antioxidants was measured by comparing the fluorescence time/intensity area under the curve of the sample compared with a control assay with no antioxidant compounds present. Trolox, a water-soluble analogue of vitamin E, was used as the calibration standard. Fluorescence readings were taken every minute for up to 35 min following the addition of AAPH.

Hydroxyl Radical Scavenging Capacity (HORAC Assay)

The HORAC assay was based on a report by Ou and colleagues (2002) [67] and modified for the FL600. Fluorescein (FL) was used as the probe. The fluorescence decay curve of FL was monitored in the absence or presence of antioxidants. The area under the fluorescence decay curve (AUC) was then integrated, and the net AUC was calculated by subtracting the AUC of the blank from that of the sample antioxidant.

Peroxynitrite Scavenging Capacity (NORAC Assay)

Peroxynitrite (ONOO-) scavenging was measured by monitoring the oxidation of dihydrorhodamine-123 (DHR-123) according to a modification of the method of Chung and colleagues (2001) [69]. Briefly, a stock solution of DHR-123 (5 mM) in dimethylformamide was purged with nitrogen and stored at −80 °C. A working solution with DHR-123 (final concentration (fc) of 5 µM) diluted from the stock solution was placed on ice in the dark immediately prior to study. The buffer of 90 mM sodium chloride, 50 mM sodium phosphate (pH 7.4), and 5 mM potassium chloride with 100 µM (fc) diethylenetriaminepentaacetic acid (DTPA) was purged with nitrogen and placed on ice before use. ONOO- scavenging by the oxidation of DHR-123 was measured with an FL600 microplate fluorescence reader with excitation and emission wavelengths of 485 and 530 nm, respectively, at room temperature. The background and final fluorescent intensities were measured 5 min after treatment with or without SIN-1 (fc 10 µM) or authentic ONOO- (fc 10 µM) in 0.3 N sodium hydroxide. The oxidation of DHR-123 by the decomposition of SIN-1 gradually increased, whereas authentic ONOO- rapidly oxidized DHR-123, with its final fluorescent intensity being stable over time.

Superoxide Anion Scavenging Assay (SORAC Assay)

The SORAC assay was based on the previously described method by Zhang and colleagues (2009) [70]. Simply, hydroethidine was used as a probe in measuring $O_2^{\bullet -}$ scavenging capacity. Nonfluorescent hydroethidine was oxidized by $O_2^{\bullet -}$ generated by the mixture of xanthine and xanthine oxidase to form a species of unknown structure that exhibited a strong fluorescence signal at 586 nm. The addition of SOD inhibited the hydroethidine oxidation.

Singlet Oxygen Scavenging Assay (SOAC Assay)

The SOAC assay was based on the previously described method by Zhang and colleagues (2009) [70]. Singlet oxygen was generated from the mixture of H_2O_2 and MoO_4^{2-}. Hydroethidine (HE) was used as a probe to singlet oxygen. Hydroethidine was prepared in N,N-dimethylacetamide (DMA) in order to make 40 µM solution. Additionally, 2.635 mM Na_2MoO_4 and 13.125 mM H_2O_2 working solutions were prepared in DMA. An HE solution (125 µL) was added to a well, followed by the addition of 25 µL of 2.635 mM $Na_2MoO_4^{2-}$ and 25 µL of 13.125 mM H_2O_2, respectively. The plate was then transferred to an FL600 microplate fluorescence reader with excitation and emission wavelengths of 530 and 620 nm, respectively, to record the change of fluorescence intensity at 37 °C for 35 min. The addition of the samples inhibited the oxidation of hydroethidine induced by singlet oxygen.

2.5. Statistical Analysis Plan

2.5.1. Functional Magnetic Resonance Imaging (fMRI)

FMRI data processing was carried out using FEAT (FMRI Expert Analysis Tool) Version 6.00, part of FSL (FMRIB's Software Library, www.fmrib.ox.ac.uk/fsl) [71,72]. Prior to statistical modeling, non-brain material was removed from the data, slice timing correction was applied using Fourier-space time-series phase-shifting, motion correction was applied using MCFLIRT [73], and a high-pass temporal filter (Gaussian-weighted least-squares straight line fitting, with sigma = 50.0 s) was applied. Data from these analyses were smoothed with a Gaussian kernel of FWHM 5.0 mm. The grand-mean intensity normalization of the entire 4D dataset by single multiplicative factor was also applied. Functional images were registered to a high-resolution T1 anatomical volume and standardized to Montreal Neurological Institute (MNI) space [73,74]. Timeseries statistical analysis was carried out using FILM with local autocorrelation correction [75]. Higher-level analyses were performed with a mixed effects model where subjects were treated as random factors, and images contrasting the 'on' and 'off' conditions were generated for each task (i.e., n-back and go/no-go). For our analyses, we also used motion artifact detection (fsl_motion_outliers, a script in the FSL software suite) to create confound matrices that were subsequently used in the general linear model (GLM) analyses to completely remove the effects of severe motion volumes from the analyses without any adverse effects on the statistics. The format of the confound matrix is a separate column for each time point that is deemed to be an outlier. Within each column, the values are all zeroes except for a value of '1' at the time point that is considered to be the outlier. The effect of adding this to the GLM is that it fully models all the influence of that time point with a separate parameter estimate which means that the intensities at that time point (in any voxel) have no influence on any of the other parameter estimates, effectively removing the effect of this time point from the estimation of all the effects of interest. Group z-statistic images were thresholded on magnitude ($z \geq 2.3$), as well as cluster-extent determined by $z > 2.3$ and a corrected cluster significance threshold of $p < 0.05$ [76] using a within-subjects, repeated measures design (controlling for each individual's average brain activation over their four imaging sessions to account for individual differences in global brain activity). For the go/no-go task, one participant's pre-WCCE task data were excluded due to a scanner reconstruction error. Statistical images were generated for task, rest, and contrasts between task and rest for both go/no-go and n-back tasks. Additionally, for the go/no-go task, we examined differences between go trials and no-go trials, modelled separately.

Connectivity modeling was executed using the 'conn' toolbox [77] (https://www.nitrc.org/projects/conn/) for MATLAB and SPM12 [63–65,70,72,78] (Statistical Parametric Mapping (http://www.fil.ion.ucl.ac.uk/spm)) using standard fMRI pre-processing steps (i.e., brain extraction, slice timing correction, Gaussian smoothing (5 mm FWHM), band-pass filtering (0.008–0.09), regression of motion and physiological artifacts, registration to anatomical space, and normalization to MNI standard space). Voxel-to-voxel and seed-to-voxel connectivity maps were generated.

2.5.2. Magnetic Resonance Spectroscopy (MRS)

For MRS data, spectra were analyzed using the LCModel software (version 6.3-1J) [79]. LCModel performs automatic quantification of in vivo proton MR spectra by analyzing spectra as a linear combination of model spectra from sequence-specific simulations. The water-suppressed spectra were eddy current-corrected and quantified using the unsuppressed water signal. Spectra were analyzed using the default fitting range of 0.2–4.0 ppm. One participant's spectra had a large lipid peak, so a different fit window (1.6–4.0 ppm) was applied. Cramer–Rao lower bounds (CRLBs) were used as a measure of fit, and metabolites with CRLB > 50% were rejected from further analysis [80]. Metabolite concentrations were then calculated. All values were cerebrospinal fluid (CSF)-corrected using methods outlined in Gasparovic, Song [81]. Of note, GABA was not detected by the LCModel in two spectra (one post-WCCE and one post-placebo). Glutamate/GABA and glutamine/GABA ratios were calculated from the spectral fittings of each respective neurometabolite. We conducted paired t-tests in lieu of repeated measures ANOVA because of the pilot nature of this study and because the power analyses were based on main effects only, not interactions.

2.5.3. Exosomal BDNF and Behavioral Data

We conducted paired t-tests to determine differences between timepoints (post–pre) and conditions (WCCE–placebo). Paired t-tests were chosen because of the pilot nature of this study and because the power analyses were based on main effects only, not interactions. Effect sizes are reported for significant results for use in planning larger studies in the future.

3. Results

3.1. FMRI: General Linear Modeling

Go/no-go: When collapsing across trial types, WCCE ingestion was associated with a decreased blood-oxygen level dependent (BOLD) activity during go/no-go trials in the left inferior frontal gyrus (Brodmann area (BA) 9/47), the left cingulate gyrus (BA 24), bilateral superior temporal gyri (BA 22), and portions of the right middle temporal gyrus (BA 39) (Figure 3; for a listing of all coordinates associated with differences in activation patterns, please see the supplemental tables hosted at https://osf.io/qypr8/). Additionally, deactivations were noted in the left precentral and middle frontal gyri (BA 6), as well as the insula during no-go trials, while an extensive fronto-limbic network deactivated during go-trials. Post-placebo ingestion was associated with increased activity throughout key decision-making regions, namely bilateral cingulate/posterior cingulate (BA 23/24/31) during the no-go trials compared to the go trials (please see the supplemental tables hosted at https://osf.io/qypr8/). Furthermore, no-go trials elicited greater activity in bilateral anterior cingulate following the ingestion of the placebo (Figure 4).

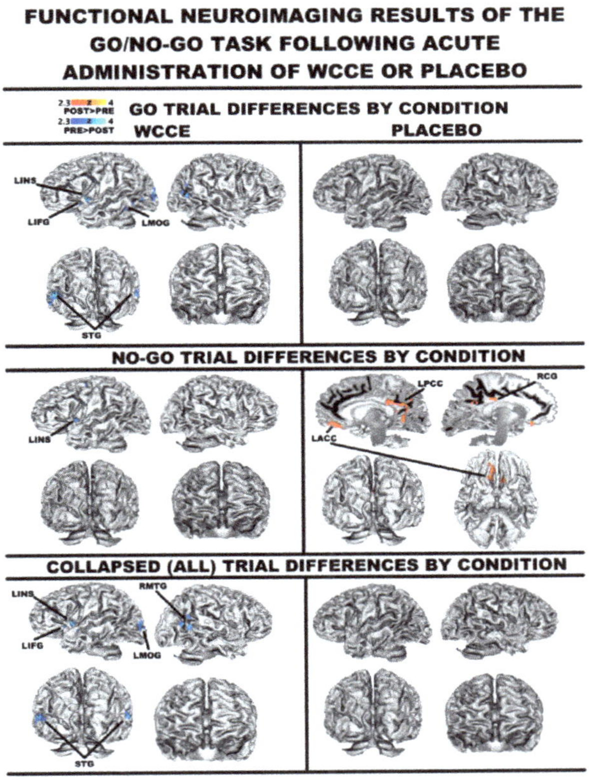

Figure 4. Differences in the pre–post consumption of WCCE or placebo for go trials (uppermost panel), no-go trials (middle panel), and all trials collapsed (bottom panel). In all panels, WCCE is presented on the left side, and the placebo is presented on the right. Statistic images were thresholded on magnitude ($z \geq 2.3$), as well as cluster extent-determined by $z > 2.3$ and a corrected cluster significance threshold of $p < 0.05$. Local maxima tables for each contrast are available at https://osf.io/qypr8/. Abbreviations: LACC = left anterior cingulate cortex; LIFG = left inferior frontal gyrus; LINS = left insula; LMOG = left middle occipital gyrus; LPCC = left posterior cingulate cortex; RCG = right cingulate gyrus; and STG = superior temporal gyrus.

N-back: Post-WCCE ingestion was associated with greater right posterior cingulate (BA 29/30), parahippocampal (BA 30), and culmen activity during rest periods compared to pre-ingestion (please see https://osf.io/qypr8/ for a listing of coordinates). No differences were observed for the placebo.

3.2. FMRI: Connectivity

Functional connectivity differences were observed in the ACC during the go/no-go task such that following WCCE ingestion, the ACC had greater connectivity with the left superior frontal gyrus (height threshold $p_{uncorrected} < 0.01$; cluster threshold $p_{FDR-corrected} < 0.05$). Furthermore, during the n-back task, we found significant differences in post-WCCE > pre-WCCE between the ACC and the precuneus, paracingulate, bilateral superior frontal gyri, and bilateral frontal poles (one-sided t-test, $p_{uncorrected} < 0.01$ height threshold; $p_{FDR-corrected} < 0.05$ cluster threshold). Placebo post > pre ACC connectivity was greater with the precuneus and left inferior and middle frontal gyri (Figure 5).

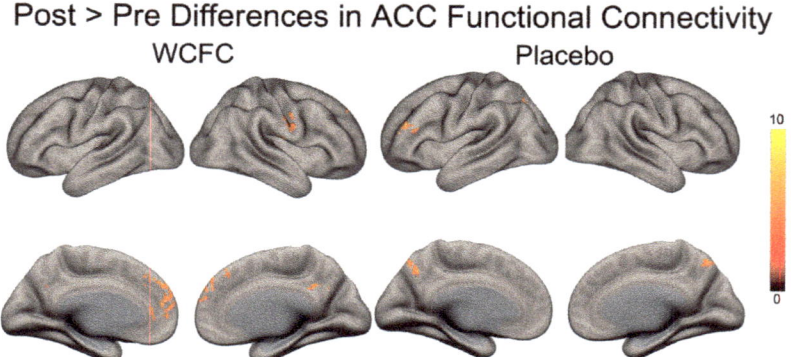

Figure 5. Anterior cingulate functional connectivity differences (post > pre) during the n-back task. WCCE showed greater connectivity post-consumption between the ACC and the paracingulate, the precuneus, and portions of the superior frontal gyrus and frontal poles. The placebo demonstrated a greater connectivity between the ACC and portions of the left dorsolateral prefrontal cortex, as well as the precuneus. Data were thresholded with $p_{uncorrected} < 0.01$ height threshold, $p_{FDR-corrected} < 0.05$ cluster threshold, one-tailed.

3.3. MRS

Treatment differences were not observed for GABA or glutamate independently. Notably, WCCE showed a qualitative decrease in GABA that approached significance. However, both the glutamate/GABA ratio (WCCE: $t(6) = 2.192$; $p = 0.036$; estimated Cohen's $d = 0.83$, one-tailed; placebo: $t(6) = -0.978$; $p > 0.05$) and the glutamine/GABA ratio (WCCE: $t(6) = 2.155$; $p = 0.038$, estimated Cohen's $d = 0.82$, one-tailed; placebo: $t(6) = -1.323$; $p > 0.05$) were significantly different post-consumption of WCCE but not the placebo. Specifically, WCCE demonstrated a significant increase in glutamate/GABA (pre-WCCE (M ± SEM): 6.81 ± 0.54; post-WCCE: 10.35 ± 1.26) and glutamine/GABA ratios (pre-WCCE: 2.26 ± 0.27; post-WCCE: 3.37 ± 0.41), while the placebo demonstrated no change (glutamate/GABA pre-placebo: 10.16 ± 1.20; post-placebo: 9.00 ± 0.97; glutamine/GABA pre-placebo: 3.44 ± 0.63; post-placebo: 2.81 ± 0.71) and qualitatively decreased post-consumption (Figure 6). All descriptive data are presented in the supplemental tables hosted at https://osf.io/qypr8/.

CHANGES IN NEUROTRANSMITTER LEVELS WITHIN THE ANTERIOR CINGULATE FOLLOWING ACUTE ADMINISTRATION OF WCCE OR PLACEBO

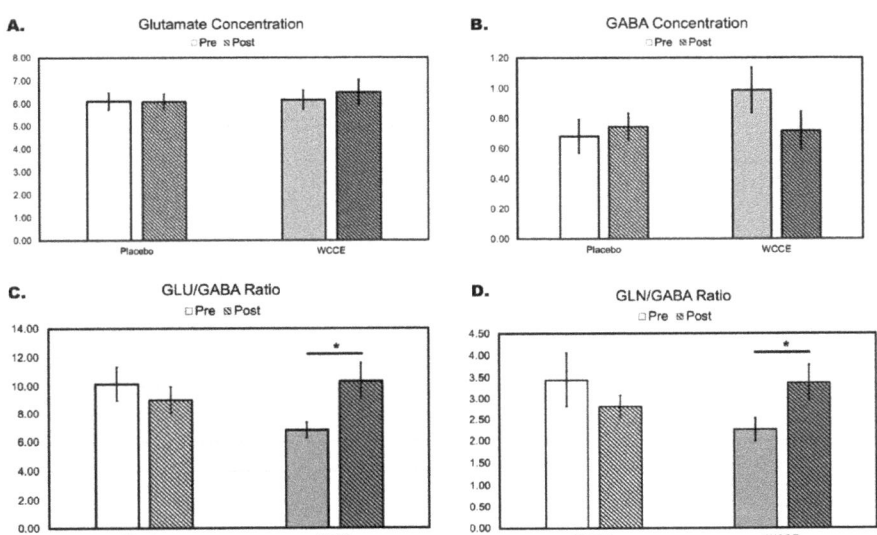

Figure 6. Bar graph with M ± SEM demonstrating the changes in glutamate, gamma-aminobutyric acid (GABA), and the ratios of glutamate/GABA (GLU/GABA) and glutamine/GABA (GLN/GABA) within the anterior cingulate cortex following the administration of either the placebo or WCCE. Y-axis units of measurement are institutional units. A * indicates significance at the $p < 0.05$ level for one-tailed t-tests. For descriptive data, please see the supplemental table hosted at https://osf.io/qypr8/. Clear bars represent the placebo, while gray bars represent WCCE. Striped bars indicate post-measurements.

3.4. BDNF

Despite no differences in exosomal BDNF at baseline between treatment days, there was a significant increase in exosomal BDNF after the ingestion of WCCE when compared to pre-WCCE ingestion ($t(7) = 2.00$; $p = 0.04$, one-tailed; estimated Cohen's $d = 0.71$ (Figure 7, Table 2). No differences in exosomal BDNF were observed post-placebo ingestion when compared to pre-placebo baseline levels ($t(7) = 1.855$; $p > 0.05$, one-tailed).

3.5. Behavioral Results

For both the go/no-go and n-back tasks, we examined reaction time and accuracy. For reaction time, we found significant reductions on correct trials during the n-back task post-consumption for WCCE ($t(7) = -3.649$; $p = 0.004$; estimated Cohen's $d = -1.29$, one-tailed) but not for the placebo ($t(7) = -0.406$; $p > 0.05$). No significant differences were identified for reaction time for the go/no-go task. For accuracy, we found that accuracy during the go/no-go task declined post-consumption of the placebo ($t(7) = -2.758$; $p = 0.014$; estimated Cohen's $d = 0.98$, one-tailed) but not post-consumption of WCCE ($t(7) = -0.406$; $p > 0.05$) (Table 3), thus suggesting a possible protective effect of WCCE. No significant differences were noted during the n-back task with regard to accuracy.

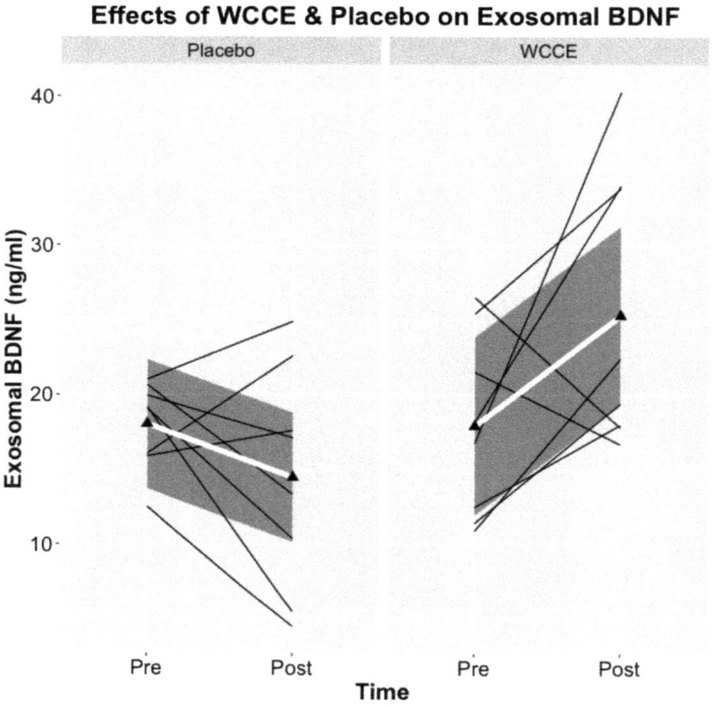

Figure 7. Pre- and post-consumption data for exosomal brain-derived neurotrophic factor (BDNF). Thin black lines indicate individual participant data, while the thicker white line depicts the group average. The dark gray shading surrounding the white line uses locally weighted regression (loess) for a visualization of group variability. Line graphs were created with open-source software ggplot2 in R.

Table 2. Descriptive statistics of exosomal BDNF. Results indicated a significant increase in the exosomal BDNF level after the ingestion of WCCE when compared to pre-WCCE ingestion. No differences in exosomal BDNF were observed post-placebo ingestion when compared to pre-placebo baseline levels. M = mean, SD = standard deviation, SEM = standard error of the mean.

	Exosomal BDNF Results												
	Descriptives							t-Statistics					
	Pre			Post						95% Confidence Interval of the Difference			
	M	SD	SEM	M	SD	SEM	M	SD	SEM	Lower	Upper	t	df	Sig. (1-Tailed)
Post WCCE > Pre WCCE	17.92	6.17	2.18	25.31	9.26	3.27	7.40	10.45	3.69	−1.34	16.13	2.00	7	0.04
Post Placebo > Pre Placebo	18.03	2.95	1.04	14.47	7.50	2.65	−3.56	7.08	2.50	−9.48	2.36	−1.42	7	0.10

Table 3. Descriptive statistics of the behavioral tasks (i.e., n-back and go/no-go) performed in the scanner. Notably, for reaction time, we found significant reductions during the n-back task post-consumption for WCCE but not for the placebo. For accuracy, we found that accuracy during the go/no-go task declined post-consumption of the placebo but not post-consumption of WCCE.

N-back Behavioral Results

		Descriptives							t-Statistics				
		Pre			Post				95% Confidence Interval of the Difference				
		M	SD	SEM	M	SD	SEM	M	SD	SEM	Lower	Upper	t	df	Sig. (1-Tailed)
Post WCCE > Pre WCCE	Number of Errors	2.125	2.532	0.895	2.625	2.774	0.981	0.500	2.070	0.732	−1.231	2.231	0.683	7	0.258
	Reaction Time for Correct Trials	574.670	84.335	29.817	536.527	82.185	29.057	−38.144	29.567	10.454	−62.863	−13.425	−3.649	7	0.004
Post Placebo > Pre Placebo	Number of Errors	3.250	3.770	1.333	3.000	2.828	1.000	−0.250	1.389	0.491	−1.411	0.911	−0.509	7	0.313
	Reaction Time for Correct Trials	568.838	111.814	39.532	559.269	86.193	30.474	−9.569	66.678	23.574	−65.314	46.175	−0.406	7	0.349

Go/No-Go Behavioral Results

		Descriptives							t-Statistics				
		Pre			Post				95% Confidence Interval of the Difference				
		M	SD	SEM	M	SD	SEM	M	SD	SEM	Lower	Upper	t	df	Sig. (1-Tailed)
Post WCCE > Pre WCCE	Reaction Time for Successful Trials	387.953	38.729	15.811	381.654	44.676	18.239	−6.299	23.166	9.457	−30.610	18.011	−0.666	5	0.2675
	Accuracy	242.000	5.967	2.436	242.333	4.082	1.667	0.333	2.805	1.145	−2.610	3.277	0.291	5	0.3915
Post Placebo > Pre Placebo	Reaction Time for Successful Trials	397.013	26.611	9.408	395.563	41.291	14.599	−1.450	25.287	8.940	−22.591	19.691	−0.162	7	0.438
	Accuracy	242.125	5.463	1.931	239.625	7.170	2.535	−2.500	2.563	0.906	−4.643	−0.357	−2.758	7	0.014

3.6. HPLC Analyses

An analysis of the antioxidant capacity of the 5 assays (ORAC, HORAC, NORAC, SORAC, and SOAC), as well as the total value, is presented in Table 4.

Table 4. Antioxidant analysis of WCCE. Results are expressed as μmol Trolox equivalent/g ± SD. ORAC: oxygen radical absorbance capacity.

Antioxidant Assay	μmol Trolox Equivalent/g
ORAC	6097 ± 225
HORAC	18,709 ± 426
NORAC	527 ± 52
SORAC	860 ± 24
SOAC	2042 ± 185
Total ORAC	28,237 ± 782

4. Discussion

Here, we used advanced neuroimaging techniques to identify neurophysiological changes associated with a polyphenol-rich and unique material, WCCE. Following the ingestion of a single dose, our data demonstrated neurophysiological changes concomitant with behavioral improvements. To our knowledge, this represents the first comprehensive study of its kind assessing multi-level outcomes employing a rigorous double-blind, randomized, within-subjects crossover design.

Before discussing the outcome of our acute administration clinical trial, it is important to note the chemical composition of WCCE and its associated antioxidant properties. For this, we report the outcome of a series of five antioxidant assays to characterize the antioxidant properties of WCCE. Using LC–MS, a recent study demonstrated that WCCE is rich in chlorogenic acid compounds and other polyphenols [27], which was in line with previous research by Mullen and colleagues (2011) [30], who had identified 24 such compounds including hydroxycinnamate, flavan-3-ols, and flavonol conjugates in samples of arabica and robusta coffee extracts. Here, we demonstrate that the robust polyphenol profile of WCCE is concomitant with notable antioxidant properties that are consistent with hypothesized mechanisms underlying the neurotrophic and potentially therapeutic effects of polyphenols [21,25,26]. This is particularly important because of the causal links between oxidative stress and inflammation in neurodegeneration and brain aging [5,26,82].

Our primary objective was to examine changes in neurophysiological markers as a result of acute WCCE administration. As a major neurotrophic factor that serves several important regulatory roles in the nervous system, including neuronal development, synaptic plasticity, and neuronal survival, BDNF was postulated to increase following the administration of WCCE. Several studies have shown that exosomes carry neuronal proteins which are able to cross the blood–brain barrier. However, other than one previous report, little is known concerning the presence of BDNF in exosomes in response to nutritional supplementation. Here, we found that exosomal levels of BDNF were increased by roughly 41% in exosomes obtained from the serum of study participants after single-dose WCCE ingestion, whereas the placebo resulted in no significant change. Importantly, polyphenols have had a consistent, robust effect on BDNF in both human and animal models [9,23,25,26].

One mechanism through which BDNF appears to maintain elevated levels of neuronal excitation is through the prevention of GABAergic signaling activities [83]. While glutamate is the brain's major excitatory neurotransmitter and phosphorylation normally activates receptors, GABA is the brain's primary inhibitory neurotransmitter. The phosphorylation of $GABA_A$ receptors tends to reduce their activity. Therefore, increases in exosomal BDNF after the ingestion of WCCE may suggest a relationship with the trends observed in the present study for a decrease in GABA and an increase in glutamate (Figure 5). This may also reflect the glutamate/GABA balance, which has been shown in previous studies to be associated with BDNF [36]. Indeed, we did find significant differences in the glutamate/GABA ratio and the glutamine/GABA ratio. Specifically, WCCE led to greater increases in the ratio post-consumption, suggesting that either glutamine increased, GABA decreased, or a combination of the two occurred. In contrast, the placebo caused no significant change, with qualitative decreases noted. This is an intriguing result, especially given that glutamine has been shown to be a useful predictor of prognosis in psychiatric conditions and has been associated with a number of roles including as a precursor for neurotransmitter and protein synthesis [84–88]. Together with our other observations, these data suggest the bioavailability and bioactivity of the (as yet not fully identified) active principals within WCCE. Additional studies will need to be conducted to further explore these relationships.

While glutamate and GABA have been implicated in BDNF levels, we failed to find significant effects when testing the individual neurotransmitter changes. We did observe trends wherein WCCE increased glutamate and decreased GABA, and we found a significant change in the ratios between these two neurotransmitters. This latter result suggests that WCCE likely has an effect on the glutamine–glutamate cycling. Given that aging has been associated with aberrations in glutamate, GABA, and glutamate/GABA ratios, these results are clinically intriguing [89,90] and should be corroborated by larger studies. It is of note, however, that placebo pre-baseline values were similar to post-administration WCCE values. As such, it is possible that post-WCCE administration was a function of regression to the mean baseline. While we do not suspect this to be the case given the within-subject nature of the design, it is still worthy of consideration and notable for future studies. Furthermore, in exploratory analyses with other neurometabolites/neurotransmitters (data not shown here), we noted differences in taurine that approached significance as a result of WCCE ingestion (M ± SEM: 1.26 ± 0.05 pre-ingestion versus 1.43 ± 0.09 post-ingestion; $t(7) = 1.881; p = 0.10$, two-tailed). Taurine affects neuronal signaling through its interactions on ion channels, particularly calcium, and has been demonstrated to protect against inflammation, apoptosis, and oxidative stress in animals [91,92], all of which have been associated with polyphenols. Additionally, taurine has known effects on GABA receptors, potentially providing a mechanistic explanation for the effects on BDNF. While these inferences should be interpreted with caution, future studies should examine the effects of WCCE and other polyphenol-rich materials on taurine and other neurometabolites.

We also used submillimeter fMRI to identify neurofunctional changes associated with WCCE ingestion. During most clinical investigations, there is an expectation that any tested substance will increase the activity of some physiological or psychological parameter and that the placebo will do little or nothing. Consequently, we found it to be interesting to observe that, under these experimental conditions, our data suggested that WCCE actually reduced BOLD activation throughout fronto-limbic regions, while, in contrast, the placebo increased activity in key structures involved in decision making, suggesting that WCCE may increase the efficiency of pivotal regions contributing to cognition. Specifically, across conditions of the go/no-go task, post-WCCE administration led to less activation in the left inferior frontal gyrus and left insula. In contrast, post-placebo administration was associated with an increased activity in the cingulate and posterior cingulate cortex. These stark post-consumption differences represent an initial finding that WCCE may have distinct neurophysiological effects that should be corroborated with larger studies. Additionally, it should be noted that we did observe increases in activation following the consumption of WCCE within the right posterior cingulate and right parahippocampal gyrus during the rest periods of the n-back task, while we did not find any differences during the task. Furthermore, during the n-back task, we observed connectivity differences such that WCCE was associated with increased connectivity between the ACC and regions involved in working memory, error monitoring, and sensory processing. The latter is particularly interesting given recent results demonstrating changes in measures of concentration and fatigue [10], as well as cognitive improvements in an n-back paradigm noted in a longitudinal study [35]. During the same task, the placebo was associated with greater functional connectivity between the ACC and the precuneus, a region linked to very discrete sensory processing. Coupled with our behavioral results, WCCE appears to affect cognitive processing, including working memory and response inhibition, through specific neurofunctional changes within fronto-limbic and fronto-parietal networks and the altered recruitment of these networks through connectivity changes with neural hubs associated with these networks. Further studies with larger samples will be needed to confirm these findings.

Finally, we examined behavioral performance on two well-known tasks of cognition—the n-back and the go/no-go task. Behaviorally, WCCE resulted in an approximately four times greater reduction in reaction time during the n-back task compared to the placebo. Furthermore, the placebo was associated with a decreased accuracy during the go/no-go task, with participants committing over 50% more errors compared to post-WCCE ingestion. This manifestation within the placebo group may have been due to mental fatigue, decreased alertness, or increased frustration in individuals who, by definition, were untreated and were not availed of the support of the WCCE. These results suggest that WCCE has acute behavioral effects and further corroborates findings demonstrating long-term effects of WCCE administration [35]. Moreover, these acute results may imply longer-term significant effects on cognitive processing, pointing toward an increased efficiency (i.e., reduced reaction time) and potentially protecting against errors through increased sustained attention or other mechanisms. This has been behaviorally supported in recent research [35], also conducted in older adults.

Taken together, our results contribute additional evidence linking polyphenols with significant antioxidant properties to positive neurophysiological and behavioral outcomes in an aging population with subjective cognitive decline. Our data represent the first of their kind examining a nutraceutical using a multimodal approach. Additional studies will be necessary to further characterize the effects of polyphenol-rich compounds on the brain.

Limitations

The current study had several notable limitations. First, the sample size was small ($n = 8$), and both men and women participated. While we leveraged a within-subjects design, future studies should seek larger samples and should explore sex differences. However, it should also be noted that recent studies have highlighted the utility of smaller samples with more robust measurement designs. Specifically, Laumann and colleagues (2015) [45] pointed out that large, group-based functional neuroimaging analyses may hide significant individual variability that could be particularly meaningful. Similar results have been noted in a variety of studies [42–45], suggesting that controlling for individual variability by way of within-subjects designs may substantially improve power, especially in consideration of robust, multi-modal functional neuroimaging studies. Second, because we used a truly random assignment procedure, we had an unbalanced ordering (six received WCCE first and only two received the placebo first). However, one would expect that decreases in reaction time and improvements in accuracy would occur with practice; thus it could be argued that placebo conditions would be at an advantage given that participants would have been overly familiar with the tasks at the time of their fourth administration (i.e., post-placebo ingestion). Thus, we feel confident that the observed behavioral effects were robust, especially since they corroborated with previous evidence [10,35]. Nonetheless, it will be important to conduct larger samples with balanced ordering so that more strict statistical models can be employed (e.g., multivariate analysis of covariance (MANCOVA)). Third, this study was limited to the assessment of observed activities within 90 min following a single dose of WCCE/placebo. Longer term studies may yield a deeper understanding of potential functional benefits and the underlying mechanisms involved. Fourth, we did not control the participants' diets, nor did we evaluate their habits. However, we have no reason to believe that their diets or habits changed between sessions. Regardless, additional studies should employ diaries or other accounts to examine these important lifestyle factors. Finally, it should be noted that numerous bioactive compounds within WCCE could be causing the results demonstrated in this study. Investigations to determine the active principles within WCCE could provide further insight into mechanisms of action and could lead to a greater specificity and amplitude of responses. This could include animal studies that would allow for the more precise identification of potential mechanisms of action. Future studies should employ parametric designs to more specifically assess the effects of unique polyphenol-rich materials on cognition and neurophysiology.

5. Conclusions

To the best of our knowledge, this is the first time that, aside from traditional psychological assessments such as n-back or go/no-go, any well-characterized and quantified dietary supplement material has been reported to induce measurable, acute physiological changes in brain connectivity, as well as potential changes in certain neurometabolites. Here, we demonstrated significant improvements in cognition, with concomitant observed changes in neurofunctional brain networks after a single 100 mg dose of WCCE, a polyphenol-rich plant-based extract that appears to increase exosomal BDNF, an essential neuroprotein. Finally, using a multi-modal approach, we present a robust and potentially useful methodology for the bigger-picture evaluation of candidate materials with possible application for the modulation of neuropsychophysiological activity. Additional well-powered studies should be conducted for a full assessment of WCCE's effects and mechanisms of action.

Supplementary Materials: The following are available online at https://osf.io/qypr8/, Table S1: Differences in the Go/No-Go Task (All Trials Combined), Table S2: Differences in Go Trials During the Go/No-Go Task, Table S3: Differences in No-Go Trials During the Go/No-Go Task, Table S4: Differences in No-Go Trials During the Go/No-Go Task, Table S5: No-Go > Go Trial Differences, Table S6: Differences in Rest During the N-back Task, Table S7: Neurometabolite (MRS) Results.

Author Contributions: Conceptualization, J.L.R., D.T.B., and J.M.H.; methodology, J.L.R., D.T.B., J.M.H., and Z.J.P.; formal analysis, J.L.R., D.T.B., J.A.Y., M.A.R., J.E.M., J.N.B., P.W.M., K.C.Y., and B.V.N.; investigation, J.L.R., D.T.B., J.A.Y., J.E.M., J.N.B., and M.A.R.; resources, J.L.R. and D.T.B.; data curation, J.A.Y., J.N.B., J.E.M., M.A.R., J.L.R., D.T.B., and B.V.N.; writing—original draft preparation, J.L.R.; writing—reviewing and editing, J.L.R., J.M.H., D.T.B., J.A.Y., J.E.M., J.N.B., M.A.R., and B.V.N.; visualization, J.L.R.; supervision, J.L.R. and D.T.B.; project administration, J.L.R. and D.T.B.; funding acquisition, J.L.R. and D.T.B. All authors have read and agreed to the published version of the manuscript.

Funding: This work was supported by VDF FutureCeuticals, Inc. (grant #G00010324, awarded to J.L.R. and D.T.B.).

Institutional Review Board Statement: The study was conducted according to the guidelines of the Declaration of Helsinki (as revised in 1983), and approved by the Institutional Review Board of Auburn University (protocol code 16-391 MR 1610, approved 10/19/16).

Informed Consent Statement: Written informed consent was obtained from all participants involved in the study.

Data Availability Statement: The data presented in this study are openly available at https://osf.io/qypr8/.

Conflicts of Interest: This work was supported by VDF FutureCeuticals, Inc. (grant #G00010324, awarded to J.L.R. and D.T.B.). Study capsules were provided by VDF FutureCeuticals, Inc. Z.J.P., B.V.N., and J.M.H. are employees and receive compensation from VDF FutureCeuticals, Inc. Following completion of the study, data analysis, and manuscript write-up, J.L.R. has since engaged in a paid consultant role with VDF FutureCeuticals, Inc., however all analyses and manuscript development/editing occurred prior to the establishment of this relationship. All other authors report no conflicts of interest. VDF FutureCeuticals, Inc. maintained the blind drug assignment, but otherwise played no part in the data collection or analysis. The sponsor provided minor proofreading comments on the final draft of the manuscript prior to submission, with ultimate approval of any changes to the manuscript contents by all authors unaffiliated with the sponsor.

References

1. Cao, H.; Ou, J.; Chen, L.; Zhang, Y.; Szkudelski, T.; Delmas, D.; Daglia, M.; Xiao, J. Dietary polyphenols and type 2 diabetes: Human Study and Clinical Trial. *Crit. Rev. Food Sci. Nutr.* **2019**, *59*, 3371–3379. [CrossRef]
2. Hurtado-Barroso, S.; Quifer-Rada, P.; Rinaldi de Alvarenga, J.; Pérez-Fernández, S.; Tresserra-Rimbau, A.; Lamuela-Raventos, R. Changing to a Low-Polyphenol Diet Alters Vascular Biomarkers in Healthy Men after Only Two Weeks. *Nutrients* **2018**, *10*, 1766. [CrossRef] [PubMed]
3. Mendonça, R.D.; Carvalho, N.C.; Martin-Moreno, J.M.; Pimenta, A.M.; Lopes, A.C.S.; Gea, A.; Martinez-Gonzalez, M.A.; Bes-Rastrollo, M. Total polyphenol intake, polyphenol subtypes and incidence of cardiovascular disease: The SUN cohort study. *Nutr. Metab. Cardiovasc. Dis.* **2018**, *29*, 69–79. [CrossRef] [PubMed]
4. Schuster, J.; Mitchell, E.S. More than just caffeine: Psychopharmacology of methylxanthine interactions with plant-derived phytochemicals. *Prog. Neuro-Psychopharmacol. Biol. Psychiatry* **2019**, *89*, 263–274. [CrossRef] [PubMed]
5. Sarubbo, F.; Moranta, D.; Pani, G. Dietary polyphenols and neurogenesis: Molecular interactions and implication for brain ageing and cognition. *Neurosci. Biobehav. Rev.* **2018**, *90*, 456–470. [CrossRef] [PubMed]
6. Shukitt-Hale, B.; Miller, M.G.; Chu, Y.-F.; Lyle, B.J.; Joseph, J.A. Coffee, but not caffeine, has positive effects on cognition and psychomotor behavior in aging. *AGE* **2013**, *35*, 2183–2192. [CrossRef]
7. Whyte, R.A.; Cheng, N.; Fromentin, E.; Williams, M.C. A Randomized, Double-Blinded, Placebo-Controlled Study to Compare the Safety and Efficacy of Low Dose Enhanced Wild Blueberry Powder and Wild Blueberry Extract (ThinkBlue™) in Maintenance of Episodic and Working Memory in Older Adults. *Nutrients* **2018**, *10*, 660. [CrossRef]
8. Heimbach, J.T.; Marone, P.A.; Hunter, J.M.; Nemzer, B.V.; Stanley, S.M.; Kennepohl, E. Safety studies on products from whole coffee fruit. *Food Chem. Toxicol.* **2010**, *48*, 2517–2525. [CrossRef]
9. Reyes-Izquierdo, T.; Nemzer, B.; Shu, C.; Huynh, L.; Argumedo, R.; Keller, R.; Pietrzkowski, Z. Modulatory effect of coffee fruit extract on plasma levels of brain-derived neurotrophic factor in healthy subjects. *Br. J. Nutr.* **2013**, *110*, 420–425. [CrossRef]
10. Reed, R.A.; Mitchell, E.S.; Saunders, C.; O'Connor, P.J. Acute Low and Moderate Doses of a Caffeine-Free Polyphenol-Rich Coffeeberry Extract Improve Feelings of Alertness and Fatigue Resulting from the Performance of Fatiguing Cognitive Tasks. *J. Cogn. Enhanc.* **2019**, *3*, 193–206. [CrossRef]
11. Reyes-Izquierdo, T.; Argumedo, R.; Shu, C.; Nemzer, B.; Pietrzkowski, Z. Stimulatory effect of whole coffee fruit concentrate powder on plasma levels of total and exosomal brain-derived neurotrophic factor in healthy subjects: An acute within-subject clinical study. *Food Nutr. Sci.* **2013**, *4*, 984–990. [CrossRef]
12. Abdel-Aziz, K.; Larner, A.J. Six-item cognitive impairment test (6CIT): Pragmatic diagnostic accuracy study for dementia and MCI. *Int. Psychogeriatr.* **2015**, *27*, 991–997. [CrossRef] [PubMed]
13. Glorioso, C.; Sabatini, M.; Unger, T.; Hashimoto, T.; Monteggia, L.M.; Lewis, D.A.; Mirnics, K. Specificity and timing of neocortical transcriptome changes in response to BDNF gene ablation during embryogenesis or adulthood. *Mol. Psychiatry* **2006**, *11*, 633. Available online: https://www.nature.com/articles/4001835#supplementary-information (accessed on 3 January 2019). [CrossRef] [PubMed]
14. Kohara, K.; Yasuda, H.; Huang, Y.; Adachi, N.; Sohya, K.; Tsumoto, T. A Local Reduction in Cortical GABAergic Synapses after a Loss of Endogenous Brain-Derived Neurotrophic Factor, as Revealed by Single-Cell Gene Knock-Out Method. *J. Neurosci.* **2007**, *27*, 7234. [CrossRef]
15. Palizvan, M.R.; Sohya, K.; Kohara, K.; Maruyama, A.; Yasuda, H.; Kimura, F.; Tsumoto, T. Brain-derived neurotrophic factor increases inhibitory synapses, revealed in solitary neurons cultured from rat visual cortex. *Neuroscience* **2004**, *126*, 955–966. [CrossRef]
16. Wang, L.; Chang, X.; She, L.; Xu, D.; Huang, W.; Poo, M.M. Autocrine Action of BDNF on Dendrite Development of Adult-Born Hippocampal Neurons. *J. Neurosci.* **2015**, *35*, 8384. [CrossRef]
17. Oh, H.; Piantadosi, S.C.; Rocco, B.R.; Lewis, D.A.; Watkins, S.C.; Sibille, E. The Role of Dendritic Brain-Derived Neurotrophic Factor Transcripts on Altered Inhibitory Circuitry in Depression. *Biol. Psychiatry* **2019**, *85*, 517–526. [CrossRef]
18. Sun, Z.; Yu, J.; Liu, Y.L.; Hong, Z.; Ling, L.; Li, G.; Zhuo, Y.; Wang, W.; Zhang, Y. Reduced Serum Levels of Brain-Derived Neurotrophic Factor Are Related to Mild Cognitive Impairment in Chinese Patients with Type 2 Diabetes Mellitus. *Ann. Nutr. Metab.* **2018**, *73*, 271–281. [CrossRef]
19. Barha, C.K.; Liu-Ambrose, T.; Best, J.R.; Yaffe, K.; Rosano, C. Sex-dependent effect of the BDNF Val66Met polymorphism on executive functioning and processing speed in older adults: Evidence from the health ABC study. *Neurobiol. Aging* **2019**, *74*, 161–170. [CrossRef]
20. Kumar, A.; Dogra, S.; Sona, C.; Umrao, D.; Rashid, M.; Singh, S.K.; Wahajuddin, M.; Yadav, P.N. Chronic histamine 3 receptor antagonism alleviates depression like conditions in mice via modulation of brain-derived neurotrophic factor and hypothalamus-pituitary adrenal axis. *Psychoneuroendocrinology* **2019**, *101*, 128–137. [CrossRef]
21. Poulose, S.M.; Miller, M.G.; Scott, T.; Shukitt-Hale, B. Nutritional Factors Affecting Adult Neurogenesis and Cognitive Function. *Adv. Nutr.* **2017**, *8*, 804–811. [CrossRef] [PubMed]
22. Barfoot, K.L.; May, G.; Lamport, D.J.; Ricketts, J.; Riddell, P.M.; Williams, C.M. The effects of acute wild blueberry supplementation on the cognition of 7–10-year-old schoolchildren. *Eur. J. Nutr.* **2019**, *58*, 2911–2920. [CrossRef] [PubMed]
23. Jiang, C.; Sakakibara, E.; Lin, W.-J.; Wang, J.; Pasinetti, G.M.; Salton, S.R. Grape-derived polyphenols produce antidepressant effects via VGF- and BDNF-dependent mechanisms. *Ann. N. Y. Acad. Sci.* **2019**, *1455*, 196–205. [CrossRef] [PubMed]

24. Caracci, F.; Harary, J.; Simkovic, S.; Pasinetti, G.M. Grape-Derived Polyphenols Ameliorate Stress-Induced Depression by Regulating Synaptic Plasticity. *J. Agric. Food Chem.* **2020**, *68*, 1808–1815. [CrossRef] [PubMed]
25. Qi, G.; Mi, Y.; Wang, Y.; Li, R.; Huang, S.; Li, X.; Liu, X. Neuroprotective action of tea polyphenols on oxidative stress-induced apoptosis through the activation of the TrkB/CREB/BDNF pathway and Keap1/Nrf2 signaling pathway in SH-SY5Y cells and mice brain. *Food Funct.* **2017**, *8*, 4421–4432. [CrossRef] [PubMed]
26. Moosavi, F.; Hosseini, R.; Saso, L.; Firuzi, O. Modulation of neurotrophic signaling pathways by polyphenols. *Drug Des. Dev. Ther.* **2015**, *10*, 23–42. [CrossRef]
27. Nemzer, B.; Abshiru, N.; Al-Taher, F. Identification of phytochemical compounds in coffea arabica whole coffee cherries and their extracts by LC-MS/MS. *J. Agric. Food Chem.*. under review.
28. Mullen, W.; Nemzer, B.; Stalmach, A.; Ali, S.; Combet, E. Polyphenolic and Hydroxycinnamate Contents of Whole Coffee Fruits from China, India, and Mexico. *J. Agric. Food Chem.* **2013**, *61*, 5298–5309. [CrossRef]
29. Li, L.; Su, C.; Chen, X.; Wang, Q.; Jiao, W.; Luo, H.; Tang, J.; Wang, W.; Li, S.; Guo, S. Chlorogenic Acids in Cardiovascular Disease: A Review of Dietary Consumption, Pharmacology, and Pharmacokinetics. *J. Agric. Food Chem.* **2020**, *68*, 6464–6484. [CrossRef]
30. Mullen, W.; Nemzer, B.; Ou, B.; Stalmach, A.; Hunter, J.; Clifford, M.N.; Combet, E. The Antioxidant and Chlorogenic Acid Profiles of Whole Coffee Fruits Are Influenced by the Extraction Procedures. *J. Agric. Food Chem.* **2011**, *59*, 3754–3762. [CrossRef]
31. Zheng, T.; Liu, H.; Qin, L.; Chen, B.; Zhang, X.; Hu, X.; Xiao, L.; Qin, S. Oxidative stress-mediated influence of plasma DPP4 activity to BDNF ratio on mild cognitive impairment in elderly type 2 diabetic patients: Results from the GDMD study in China. *Metab. Clin. Exp.* **2018**, *87*, 105–112. [CrossRef] [PubMed]
32. Miranda, M.; Kent, B.A.; Morici, J.F.; Gallo, F.; Saksida, L.M.; Bussey, T.J.; Weisstaub, N.; Bekinschtein, P. NMDA receptors and BDNF are necessary for discrimination of overlapping spatial and non-spatial memories in perirhinal cortex and hippocampus. *Neurobiol. Learn. Mem.* **2018**, *155*, 337–343. [CrossRef] [PubMed]
33. Niculescu, D.; Michaelsen-Preusse, K.; Güner, Ü.; van Dorland, R.; Wierenga, C.J.; Lohmann, C. A BDNF-Mediated Push-Pull Plasticity Mechanism for Synaptic Clustering. *Cell Rep.* **2018**, *24*, 2063–2074. [CrossRef]
34. Zhen, L.; Shao, T.; Luria, V.; Li, G.; Li, Z.; Xu, Y.; Zhao, X. EphB2 Deficiency Induces Depression-Like Behaviors and Memory Impairment: Involvement of NMDA 2B Receptor Dependent Signaling. *Front. Pharmacol.* **2018**, *9*. [CrossRef] [PubMed]
35. Robinson, J.L.; Hunter, J.M.; Reyes-Izquierdo, T.; Argumedo, R.; Brizuela-Bastien, J.; Keller, R.; Pietrzkowski, Z. Cognitive short- and long-term effects of coffee cherry extract in older adults with mild cognitive decline. *Aging Neuropsychol. Cogn.* **2019**, *12*, 1–17. [CrossRef] [PubMed]
36. Zafra, F.; Castrén, E.; Thoenen, H.; Lindholm, D. Interplay between glutamate and gamma-aminobutyric acid transmitter systems in the physiological regulation of brain-derived neurotrophic factor and nerve growth factor synthesis in hippocampal neurons. *Proc. Natl. Acad. Sci. USA* **1991**, *88*, 10037. [CrossRef] [PubMed]
37. Yang, X.; Holmes, M.J.; Newton, A.T.; Morgan, V.L.; Landman, B.A. A Comparison of Distributional Considerations with Statistical Analysis of Resting State fMRI at 3T and 7T. *Proc. SPIE-Intern. Soc. Opt. Eng.* **2012**, *8314*, 831416. [CrossRef]
38. Trattnig, S.; Springer, E.; Bogner, W.; Hangel, G.; Strasser, B.; Dymerska, B.; Cardoso, P.L.; Robinson, S.D. Key clinical benefits of neuroimaging at 7T. *NeuroImage* **2018**, *168*, 477–489. [CrossRef]
39. Pohmann, R.; Speck, O.; Scheffler, K. Signal-to-noise ratio and MR tissue parameters in human brain imaging at 3, 7, and 9.4 tesla using current receive coil arrays. *Magn. Reson. Med.* **2016**, *75*, 801–809. [CrossRef]
40. Reid, M.A.; Salibi, N.; White, D.M.; Gawne, T.J.; Denney, T.S.; Lahti, A.C. 7T Proton Magnetic Resonance Spectroscopy of the Anterior Cingulate Cortex in First-Episode Schizophrenia. *Schizophr. Bull.* **2018**, *45*, 180–189. [CrossRef]
41. Strasser, A.; Xin, L.; Gruetter, R.; Sandi, C. Nucleus accumbens neurochemistry in human anxiety: A 7 T 1H-MRS study. *Eur. Neuropsychopharmacol.* **2019**, *29*, 365–375. [CrossRef] [PubMed]
42. Gordon, E.M.; Laumann, T.O.; Adeyemo, B.; Gilmore, A.W.; Nelson, S.M.; Dosenbach, N.U.F.; Petersen, S.E. Individual-specific features of brain systems identified with resting state functional correlations. *NeuroImage* **2017**, *146*, 918–939. [CrossRef] [PubMed]
43. Gordon, E.M.; Laumann, T.O.; Adeyemo, B.; Petersen, S.E. Individual Variability of the System-Level Organization of the Human Brain. *Cereb. Cortex* **2015**, *27*, 386–399. [CrossRef] [PubMed]
44. Gordon, E.M.; Laumann, T.O.; Gilmore, A.W.; Newbold, D.J.; Greene, D.J.; Berg, J.J.; Ortega, M.; Hoyt-Drazen, C.; Gratton, C.; Sun, H.; et al. Precision Functional Mapping of Individual Human Brains. *Neuron* **2017**, *95*, 791–807.e797. [CrossRef] [PubMed]
45. Laumann, T.O.; Gordon, E.M.; Adeyemo, B.; Snyder, A.Z.; Joo, S.J.; Chen, M.-Y.; Gilmore, A.W.; McDermott, K.B.; Nelson, S.M.; Dosenbach, N.U.F.; et al. Functional System and Areal Organization of a Highly Sampled Individual Human Brain. *Neuron* **2015**, *87*, 657–670. [CrossRef]
46. Poldrack, R.A. Precision Neuroscience: Dense Sampling of Individual Brains. *Neuron* **2017**, *95*, 727–729. [CrossRef]
47. Braga, R.M.; Buckner, R.L. Parallel Interdigitated Distributed Networks within the Individual Estimated by Intrinsic Functional Connectivity. *Neuron* **2017**, *95*, 457–471.e455. [CrossRef]
48. Feilong, M.; Nastase, S.A.; Guntupalli, J.S.; Haxby, J.V. Reliable individual differences in fine-grained cortical functional architecture. *NeuroImage* **2018**, *183*, 375–386. [CrossRef]
49. Gagnier, J.J.; Boon, H.; Rochon, P.; Moher, D.; Barnes, J.; Bombardier, C. Reporting Randomized, Controlled Trials of Herbal Interventions: An Elaborated CONSORT Statement. *Ann. Int. Med.* **2006**, *144*, 364–367. [CrossRef]
50. Wechsler, D. *Wechsler Memory Scale*, 4th ed.; Pearson Assessment: San Antonio, TX, USA, 2009.

51. Folstein, M.F.; Folstein, S.E.; McHugh, P.R. "Mini-mental state": A practical method for grading the cognitive state of patients for the clinician. *J. Psychiatr. Res.* **1975**, *12*, 189–198. [CrossRef]
52. Rovner, B.W.; Folstein, M.F. Mini-mental state exam in clinical practice. *Hosp. Pract.* **1987**, *22*, 140–141.
53. Hughes, C.P.; Berg, L.; Danziger, W.L.; Coben, L.A.; Martin, R.L. A new clinical scale for the staging of dementia. *Br. J. Psychiatry* **1982**, *140*, 566–572. [CrossRef] [PubMed]
54. Lynch, C.A.; Walsh, C.; Blanco, A.; Moran, M.; Coen, R.F.; Walsh, J.B.; Lawlor, B.A. The clinical dementia rating sum of box score in mild dementia. *Dement. Geriatr. Cogn. Disord.* **2006**, *21*, 40–43. [CrossRef] [PubMed]
55. Santos-Buelga, C.; González-Paramás, A.M.; Oludemi, T.; Ayuda-Durán, B.; González-Manzano, S. Plant phenolics as functional food ingredients. *Adv. Food Nutr. Res.* **2019**, *90*, 183–257. [PubMed]
56. Lavefve, L.; Howard, L.R.; Carbonero, F. Berry polyphenols metabolism and impact on human gut microbiota and health. *Food Funct.* **2020**, *11*, 45–65. [CrossRef] [PubMed]
57. Hussain, M.B.; Hassan, S.; Waheed, M.; Javed, A.; Farooq, M.A.; Tahir, A. Bioavailability and Metabolic Pathway of Phenolic Compounds. In *Plant Physiological Aspects of Phenolic Compounds*; Soto-Hernández, M., García-Mateos, R., Palma-Tenango, M., Eds.; InTechOpen: London, UK, 2019. [CrossRef]
58. Rubia, K.; Smith, A.B.; Brammer, M.J.; Taylor, E. Right inferior prefrontal cortex mediates response inhibition while mesial prefrontal cortex is responsible for error detection. *Neuroimage* **2003**, *20*, 351–358. [CrossRef]
59. Braver, T.S.; Barch, D.M.; Gray, J.R.; Molfese, D.L.; Snyder, A. Anterior cingulate cortex and response conflict: Effects of frequency, inhibition and errors. *Cereb Cortex* **2001**, *11*, 825–836. [CrossRef]
60. Rubia, K.; Russell, T.; Bullmore, E.T.; Soni, W.; Brammer, M.J.; Simmons, A.; Taylor, E.; Andrew, C.; Giampietro, V.; Sharma, T. An fMRI study of reduced left prefrontal activation in schizophrenia during normal inhibitory function. *Schizophr. Res.* **2001**, *52*, 47–55. [CrossRef]
61. Shibata, T.; Shimoyama, I.; Ito, T.; Abla, D.; Iwasa, H.; Koseki, K.; Yamanouchi, N.; Sato, T.; Nakajima, Y. The time course of interhemispheric EEG coherence during a GO/NO-GO task in humans. *Neurosci. Lett.* **1997**, *233*, 117–120. [CrossRef]
62. Roberts, L.E.; Rau, H.; Lutzenberger, W.; Birbaumer, N. Mapping P300 waves onto inhibition: Go/No-Go discrimination. *Electroencephalogr. Clin. Neurophysiol. Evoked Potential.* **1994**, *92*, 44–45. [CrossRef]
63. Menon, V.; Adleman, N.E.; White, C.D.; Glover, G.H.; Reiss, A.L. Error-related brain activation during a Go/NoGo response inhibition task. *Hum. Br. Mapp.* **2001**, *12*, 131–143. [CrossRef]
64. Swick, D.; Ashley, V.; Turken, U. Are the neural correlates of stopping and not going identical? Quantitative meta-analysis of two response inhibition tasks. *NeuroImage* **2011**, *56*, 1655–1665. [CrossRef] [PubMed]
65. Mencarelli, L.; Neri, F.; Momi, D.; Menardi, A.; Rossi, S.; Rossi, A.; Santarnecchi, E. Stimuli, presentation modality, and load-specific brain activity patterns during n-back task. *Hum. Br. Mapp.* **2019**, *40*, 3810–3831. [CrossRef] [PubMed]
66. Wang, H.; He, W.; Wu, J.; Zhang, J.; Jin, Z.; Li, L. A coordinate-based meta-analysis of the n-back working memory paradigm using activation likelihood estimation. *Br. Cogn.* **2019**, *132*, 1–12. [CrossRef]
67. Ou, B.; Hampsch-Woodill, M.; Flanagan, J.; Deemer, E.K.; Prior, R.L.; Huang, D. Novel Fluorometric Assay for Hydroxyl Radical Prevention Capacity Using Fluorescein as the Probe. *J. Agric. Food Chem.* **2002**, *50*, 2772–2777. [CrossRef]
68. Huang, D.; Ou, B.; Hampsch-Woodill, M.; Flanagan, J.A.; Prior, R.L. High-Throughput Assay of Oxygen Radical Absorbance Capacity (ORAC) Using a Multichannel Liquid Handling System Coupled with a Microplate Fluorescence Reader in 96-Well Format. *J. Agric. Food Chem.* **2002**, *50*, 4437–4444. [CrossRef]
69. Chung, H.Y.; Choi, H.R.; Park, H.J.; Choi, J.S.; Choi, W.C. Peroxynitrite Scavenging and Cytoprotective Activity of 2,3,6-Tribromo-4,5-dihydroxybenzyl Methyl Ether from the Marine Alga Symphyocladia latiuscula. *J. Agric. Food Chem.* **2001**, *49*, 3614–3621. [CrossRef]
70. Zhang, L.; Huang, D.; Kondo, M.; Fan, E.; Ji, H.; Kou, Y.; Ou, B. Novel High-Throughput Assay for Antioxidant Capacity against Superoxide Anion. *J. Agric. Food Chem.* **2009**, *57*, 2661–2667. [CrossRef]
71. Jenkinson, M.; Beckmann, C.F.; Behrens, T.E.J.; Woolrich, M.W.; Smith, S.M. FSL. *NeuroImage* **2012**, *62*, 782–790. [CrossRef]
72. Smith, S.M.; Jenkinson, M.; Woolrich, M.W.; Beckmann, C.F.; Behrens, T.E.; Johansen-Berg, H.; Bannister, P.R.; De Luca, M.; Drobnjak, I.; Flitney, D.E.; et al. Advances in functional and structural MR image analysis and implementation as FSL. *Neuroimage* **2004**, *23*. [CrossRef]
73. Jenkinson, M.; Bannister, P.R.; Brady, J.M.; Smith, S.M. Improved optimisation for the robust and accurate linear registration and motion correction of brain images. *NeuroImage* **2002**, *17*, 825–841. [CrossRef] [PubMed]
74. Jenkinson, M.; Smith, S.M. A global optimisation method for robust affine registration of brain images. *Med. Image Anal.* **2001**, *5*, 143–156. [CrossRef]
75. Woolrich, M.W.; Ripley, B.D.; Ripley, J.M.; Smith, S.M. Temporal autocorrelation in univariate linear modeling of fMRI data. *NeuroImage* **2001**, *14*, 1370–1386. [CrossRef] [PubMed]
76. Worsley, K.J. Statistical analysis of activation images. In *Functional MRI: An Introduction to Methods*; Jezzard, P., Matthews, P.M., Smith, S.M., Eds.; OUP: Cary, NC, USA, 2001.
77. Whitfield-Gabrieli, S.; Nieto-Castanon, A. Conn: A functional connectivity toolbox for correlated and anticorrelated brain networks. *Br. Connect.* **2012**, *2*, 125–141. [CrossRef]
78. Statistical Parametric Mapping. Available online: http://www.fil.ion.ucl.ac.uk/spm (accessed on 3 January 2019).

79. Provencher, S.W. Estimation of metabolite concentrations from localized in vivo proton NMR spectra. *Magn. Reson. Med.* **1993**, *30*, 672–679. [CrossRef]
80. Kreis, R. The trouble with quality filtering based on relative Cramér-Rao lower bounds. *Magn. Reson. Med.* **2016**, *75*, 15–18. [CrossRef]
81. Gasparovic, C.; Song, T.; Devier, D.; Bockholt, H.J.; Caprihan, A.; Mullins, P.G.; Posse, S.; Jung, R.E.; Morrison, L.A. Use of tissue water as a concentration reference for proton spectroscopic imaging. *Magn. Reson. Med.* **2006**, *55*, 1219–1226. [CrossRef]
82. Han, X.; Shen, T.; Lou, H. Dietary Polyphenols and Their Biological Significance. *Int. J. Mol. Sci.* **2007**, *8*, 950–988. [CrossRef]
83. Henneberger, C.; Jüttner, R.; Rothe, T.; Grantyn, R. Postsynaptic Action of BDNF on GABAergic Synaptic Transmission in the Superficial Layers of the Mouse Superior Colliculus. *J. Neurophysiol.* **2002**, *88*, 595–603. [CrossRef]
84. Newsholme, P.; Procopio, J.; Lima, M.M.; Pithon-Curi, T.C.; Curi, R. Glutamine and glutamate—Their central role in cell metabolism and function. *Cell Biochem. Funct.* **2003**, *21*, 1–9. [CrossRef]
85. Watford, M. Glutamine and glutamate: Nonessential or essential amino acids? *Anim. Nutr.* **2015**, *1*, 119–122. [CrossRef] [PubMed]
86. Shen, J. Modeling the glutamate–glutamine neurotransmitter cycle. *Front. Neuroenerg.* **2013**, *5*. [CrossRef] [PubMed]
87. Strużyńska, L.; Sulkowski, G. Relationships between glutamine, glutamate, and GABA in nerve endings under Pb-toxicity conditions. *J. Inorg. Biochem.* **2004**, *98*, 951–958. [CrossRef] [PubMed]
88. Al-Otaish, H.; Al-Ayadhi, L.; Bjørklund, G.; Chirumbolo, S.; Urbina, M.A.; El-Ansary, A. Relationship between absolute and relative ratios of glutamate, glutamine and GABA and severity of autism spectrum disorder. *Metab. Br. Dis.* **2018**, *33*, 843–854. [CrossRef]
89. Huang, D.; Liu, D.; Yin, J.; Qian, T.; Shrestha, S.; Ni, H. Glutamate-glutamine and GABA in brain of normal aged and patients with cognitive impairment. *Eur. Radiol.* **2017**, *27*, 2698–2705. [CrossRef]
90. Liguz-Lecznar, M.; Lehner, M.; Kaliszewska, A.; Zakrzewska, R.; Sobolewska, A.; Kossut, M. Altered glutamate/GABA equilibrium in aged mice cortex influences cortical plasticity. *Br. Struct. Funct.* **2015**, *220*, 1681–1693. [CrossRef]
91. Niu, X.; Zheng, S.; Liu, H.; Li, S. Protective effects of taurine against inflammation, apoptosis, and oxidative stress in brain injury. *Mol. Med. Rep.* **2018**, *18*, 4516–4522. [CrossRef] [PubMed]
92. Seidel, U.; Huebbe, P.; Rimbach, G. Taurine: A Regulator of Cellular Redox Homeostasis and Skeletal Muscle Function. *Mol. Nutr. Food Res.* **2018**, *63*, 1800569. [CrossRef] [PubMed]

MDPI
St. Alban-Anlage 66
4052 Basel
Switzerland
Tel. +41 61 683 77 34
Fax +41 61 302 89 18
www.mdpi.com

Antioxidants Editorial Office
E-mail: antioxidants@mdpi.com
www.mdpi.com/journal/antioxidants

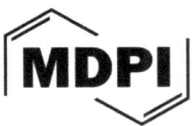

www.ingramcontent.com/pod-product-compliance
Lightning Source LLC
LaVergne TN
LVHW070645100526
838202LV00013B/884